D0984816

Neuroepidemiology

Neuroepidemiology
Theory and Method

Edited by

Craig A. Molgaard

Division of Epidemiology and Biostatistics
Graduate School of Public Health
San Diego State University
San Diego, California

Academic Press, Inc.
Harcourt Brace Jovanovich, Publishers

San Diego   New York   Boston   London   Sydney   Tokyo   Toronto

Copyright © 1993 by ACADEMIC PRESS, INC.

All Rights Reserved.

No part of this publication may be reproduced or transmitted in any form or by any means, electronic or mechanical, including photocopy, recording, or any information storage and retrieval system, without permission in writing from the publisher.

Academic Press, Inc.
1250 Sixth Avenue, San Diego, California 92101-4311

United Kingdom Edition published by
Academic Press Limited
24–28 Oval Road, London NW1 7DX

Library of Congress Cataloging-in-Publication Data

Neuroepidemiology : theory and method / edited by Craig Molgaard.
    p.   cm.
   Includes index.
   ISBN 0-12-504220-5
   1. Nervous system–Diseases–Epidemiology.   I. Molgaard, Craig.
   [DNLM: 1. Epidemiologic methods.   2. Nervous System Diseases–
   epidemiology.   WL 100 N4933]
   RA652.N48   1993
   614.5'98–dc20
   DNLM/DLC
   for Library of Congress   92-49989
                                           CIP

PRINTED IN THE UNITED STATES OF AMERICA
93 94 95 96 97 98   MM   9 8 7 6 5 4 3 2 1

To

Freya

•

Danny

•

Mandy

Contents

Contributors   *xvii*
Preface   *xxi*

An Introduction to Neuroepidemiology

Craig A. Molgaard

POLIOMYELITIS   **3**

KURU   **4**

MINIMATA'S DISEASE   **4**

PARKINSON'S DISEASE   **5**

STROKE   **6**

MULTIPLE SCLEROSIS   **7**

AMYOTROPHIC LATERAL SCLEROSIS   **8**

DEMENTIA OF THE ALZHEIMER'S TYPE   **9**

HUNTINGTON'S DISEASE   **10**

NEURAL TUBE DEFECTS   **10**

PERTUSSIS VACCINES   **11**

CEREBRAL PALSY   **12**

**GUILLAIN–BARRE SYNDROME AND THE SWINE FLU
    VACCINE AFFAIR**   **13**

CREUTZFELDT–JAKOB DISEASE   **14**

HEAD INJURY   **14**

EPILEPSY   **15**

BRAIN TUMORS   **15**

CONCLUSION   **16**

REFERENCES   **16**

I
International Research in Neuroepidemiology

1 Multiple Sclerosis in the Faroe Islands
John F. Kurtzke • Kay Hyllested • Anne Heltberg

EPITOME OF THE EPIDEMIOLOGY OF MULTIPLE
    SCLEROSIS   24

THE FAROE ISLANDS   26

MULTIPLE SCLEROSIS IN THE FAROES   28

MULTIPLE SCLEROSIS: INTRODUCTION AND
    TRANSMISSION   40

THE NATURE OF MULTIPLE SCLEROSIS   49

REFERENCES   50

2 The Epidemiology of Alzheimer's Disease in the People's Republic of China
Elena Yu • Robert Katzman • William T. Liu • Ming-Yuan Zhang • Zheng-Yu Wang • Paul Levy • David Salmon • Guang-Ya Qu

BACKGROUND   54

METHODS   55

RESULTS   59

DISCUSSION   62

APPENDIX   69

REFERENCES   70

3 An Update of the Epidemiology of Western Pacific Amyotrophic Lateral Sclerosis

Leonard T. Kurland • Kurupath Radhakrishnan

EPIDEMIOLOGIC DATA FROM GUAM AND THE MARIANA
   ISLANDS   75
PATTERNS OF DISTRIBUTION AND ETIOLOGIC
   IMPLICATIONS   80
ENVIRONMENTAL CONSIDERATIONS   81
REFERENCES   84

4 The Epidemiology of Stroke-Related Disability

Craig Anderson • Konrad Jamrozik

INTRODUCTION   90
METHODOLOGICAL ISSUES   92
THE EPIDEMIOLOGICAL STUDY OF CEREBROVASCULAR
   DISEASE IN AUSTRALIA   93
THE PERTH COMMUNITY STROKE STUDY   94
CONCLUSION   105
REFERENCES   106

5 The Neuroepidemiology of Human T-Cell Lymphotrophic Virus-I

Stephanie K. Brodine • Richard J. Thomas

TROPICAL MYELONEUROPATHIES   109
HUMAN T-CELL LEUKEMIA VIRUS-I-ASSOCIATED
   MYELOPATHY   111

ISOLATION OF HUMAN T-CELL LYMPHOTROPHIC
VIRUS-I   112

HUMAN T-CELL LYMPHOTROPHIC VIRUS-I   113

EPIDEMIOLOGIC PATTERN OF INFECTION   114

TRANSMISSION OF HUMAN T-CELL LYMPHOTROPHIC
VIRUS-I   115

EPIDEMIOLOGY OF HUMAN T-CELL LYMPHOTROPHIC
VIRUS-I-ASSOCIATED MYELOPATHY–TROPICAL SPASTIC
PARAPARESIS   116

DIAGNOSIS OF HUMAN T-CELL LYMPHOTROPHIC VIRUS-I
INFECTION   118

CLINICAL FEATURES OF HUMAN T-CELL LYMPHOTROPHIC
VIRUS-I-ASSOCIATED MYELOPATHY–TROPICAL SPASTIC
PARAPARESIS   119

OTHER HUMAN T-CELL LYMPHOTROPHIC VIRUSES   121

CONCLUSION   122

REFERENCES   122

II

Social and Behavioral Components
of Neuroepidemiology

6   Patient-Based Assessments of Health Status and Outcome for Some Neurologic Disorders

Ray Fitzpatrick • Ian Robinson • Graham Scambler

EPILEPSY   132

MULTIPLE SCLEROSIS   136

CHRONIC HEADACHE   139

DISCUSSION   142

REFERENCES   145

7 The Epidemiology of Wernicke–Korsakoff Syndrome and Related Neurologic Disorders Due to Alcoholism
Heather Spencer Feigelson • Craig A. Molgaard

REVIEW OF DESCRIPTIVE STUDIES   151
CURRENT RESEARCH TOPICS   157
SUGGESTIONS FOR FUTURE EPIDEMIOLOGIC
  RESEARCH   160
PUBLIC HEALTH INTERVENTION   161
REFERENCES   162

8 Cerebrovascular Disease and Smoking
Deborah M. Parra-Medina • Erin Kenney • John P. Elder

ANALYTICAL STUDIES   166
CAUSATION   175
CONCLUSION   177
REFERENCES   178

9 Alien Hand
Rachelle Smith Doody

PHENOMENOLOGY OF ALIEN HAND   182
ANATOMY AND ETIOLOGY OF ALIEN HAND   186
SOCIOCULTURAL ASPECTS OF ALIEN HAND   187
UNANSWERED QUESTIONS   191
REFERENCES   192

10 Alzheimer's Disease and Related Disorders among African Americans
E. Percil Stanford • Barbara Du Bois

DEMENTIA AND CULTURE   196

DEMENTIA IN THE AFRICAN AMERICAN
    POPULATION   198

CONCERNS FOR CONDUCTING DEMENTIA RESEARCH IN
    THE AFRICAN AMERICAN COMMUNITY   206

CONCLUSION   208

REFERENCES   208

_____ III _____

Population Surveillance in Neuroepidemiology

11 Prevalence at Birth of Neural Tube Defects in California: A Population-Based Study

Margarita E. Villarino • Amanda L. Golbeck • Craig A. Molgaard

FREQUENCY OF NEURAL TUBE DEFECT BIRTHS IN THE
    UNITED STATES   214

EPIDEMIOLOGIC CHARACTERISTICS OF NEURAL TUBE
    DEFECT BIRTHS   214

METHODS   221

RESULTS   223

DISCUSSION   228

REFERENCES   231

12 Lapse of Consciousness: The Impact of Litigation on Surveillance in a Defined Population

Louise S. Gresham • Michelle M. Ginsberg

METHODS   234

RESULTS   235

CONCLUSIONS   238

REFERENCES   240

13 Neuroepidemiology of Intrauterine Radiation Exposure

Lowell E. Sever

EARLY STUDIES OF HEAD CIRCUMFERENCE AND MENTAL RETARDATION AMONG ATOMIC BOMB SURVIVORS, WITH RADIATION EXPOSURE BASED ON DISTANCE FROM THE HYPOCENTER   242

STUDIES OF HEAD CIRUMFERENCE AND MENTAL RETARDATION AMONG ATOMIC BOMB SURVIVORS, WITH RADIATION EXPOSURE BASED ON T65DR DOSIMETRY   245

STUDIES OF MENTAL RETARDATION AND IQ AMONG ATOMIC BOMB SURVIVORS, WITH RADIATION EXPOSURE BASED ON DS86 DOSIMETRY   247

NEUROEPIDEMIOLOGIC ENDPOINTS, IN ADDITION TO HEAD CIRCUMFERENCE, MENTAL RETARDATION, AND IQ, STUDIED IN THE ATOMIC BOMB SURVIVORS   249

PROPOSED MECHANISMS FOR RADIATION EFFECTS ON CENTRAL NERVOUS SYSTEM DEVELOPMENT   251

POSSIBLE CONFOUNDERS AND CONTRIBUTORS TO DIFFERENCES IN MENTAL RETARDATION BETWEEN HIROSHIMA AND NAGASAKI   253

SUMMARY AND CONCLUSIONS   254

REFERENCES   255

14 Childhood Convulsions Associated with Cerebral Malaria in Ghana: An Example of Shoe-Leather Neuroepidemiology

Kathryn Bartmann • Laura K. Wyman • Paul Dagbui

BACKGROUND   257

METHODS   259

RESULTS   259

DISCUSSION   261

REFERENCES   262

15   The Epidemiology of Childhood Lead
     Poisoning
     Omar Shafey

     BACKGROUND   263
     PREDISPOSING FACTORS   271
     PREVALENCE OF LEAD POISONING   272
     EFFECTS OF CHILDHOOD LEAD POISONING   274
     PREVENTION AND TREATMENT OF CHILDHOOD LEAD
          POISONING   278
     CONCLUSION   280
     REFERENCES   281

IV

Methodological Considerations in Neuroepidemiology

16   The Utility of Stroke Data Banks in the
     Epidemiology of Cerebrovascular Disease
     John F. Rothrock • Patrick D. Lyden • Mark L. Brody

     WHY?   287
     WHAT IS SOUGHT AND HOW TO SEEK IT   289
     THE UNIVERSITY OF CALIFORNIA, SAN DIEGO, STROKE
          DATA BANK   297
     APPLICATIONS   302
     SUMMARY   305
     REFERENCES   305

17   Biostatistics and Neuroepidemiology
     Amanda L. Golbeck • Patricia Silva

     NEUROLOGICAL DISEASES AND STOCHASTIC
          PROCESSES   310

NEUROEPIDEMIOLOGY AND SAMPLING
   METHODOLOGY   321
MEDICAL TECHNOLOGY ASSESSMENT AND STOCHASTIC
   MODELS   323
DISCUSSION   325
REFERENCES   326

18   A Case-Control Study of Head Injury to Elementary School Children

Monica Brown • Louise K. Hofherr • Craig A. Molgaard

REVIEW OF THE LITERATURE: RISK FACTORS FOR
   INJURIES TO CHILDREN AT SCHOOL AND MINOR HEAD
   TRAUMA   330
METHODS   336
RESULTS   338
DISCUSSION   342
REFERENCES   346

19   The Epidemiology of Alzheimer's Disease and Dementia among Hispanic Americans

Richard L. Hough • Bohdan Kolody • Barbara Du Bois

COMMUNITY STUDIES OF THE PREVALENCE OF
   COGNITIVE IMPAIRMENT   352
STUDIES OF DIFFERENTIALLY DIAGNOSED
   DEMENTIAS   357
METHODOLOGICAL ISSUES IN THE CROSS-CULTURAL
   ASSESSMENT OF COGNITIVE IMPAIRMENT AND
   DEMENTIA   359
RISK FACTORS   362
SUMMARY   364
REFERENCES   365

Index   369

Contributors

Numbers in parentheses indicate the pages on which the authors' contributions begin.

Craig Anderson[1] (89), Department of Neurology, Royal Perth Hospital, Perth, Western Australia 6009

Kathryn Bartmann (257), Division of Epidemiology and Biostatistics, Graduate School of Public Health, San Diego State University, San Diego, California 92182

Stephanie K. Brodine (109), Department of Epidemiology, Naval Health Research Command, San Diego, California 92134

Mark L. Brody (287), Department of Neurosciences, University of California at San Diego, UCSD Medical Center, San Diego, California 92103

Monica Brown (329), Division of Epidemiology and Biostatistics, Graduate School of Public Health, San Diego State University, San Diego, California 92182

Paul Dagbui[2] (257), St. Anthony's Hospital, Dzodze, Ghana

Rachelle Smith Doody (181), Department of Neurology, Baylor College of Medicine, Houston, Texas 76703

Barbara Du Bois (195, 351), University Center on Aging, College of Health and Human Services, San Diego State University, San Diego, California 92182

John P. Elder (165), Division of Health Promotion, Graduate School of Public Health, San Diego State University, San Diego, California 92182

Heather Spencer Feigelson (149), Department of Epidemiology, School of Public Health, University of California, Los Angeles, Los Angeles, California 90049

---

[1] *Present address:* Department of Medicine (Neurology), Flinders Medical Center, Adelaide, South Australia 5042.

[2] *Present address:* District Health Administration, Aflao, Ghana.

Ray Fitzpatrick (131), Department of Public Health and Primary Care, University of Oxford, Oxford OX1 INF, United Kingdom

Michelle M. Ginsberg (233), Division of AIDS and Community Epidemiology, San Diego County Department of Health Services, San Diego, California 92101

Amanda L. Golbeck (213, 309), Division of Statistics, Department of Mathematical Sciences, San Diego State University, San Diego, California 92182

Louise S. Gresham (233), San Diego County Department of Health Services, and Graduate School of Public Health, San Diego State University, San Diego, California 92182

Anne Heltberg (23), Neurology Service, Roskilde Hospital, 4000 Roskilde, Denmark

Louise K. Hofherr (329), Division of Epidemiology and Biostatistics, Graduate School of Public Health, San Diego State University, San Diego, California 92182

Richard L. Hough (351), Department of Sociology, San Diego State University, San Diego, California 92182

Kay Hyllested (23), Danish Multiple Sclerosis Registry, DS Registret, Rigshospitalet, DK-4000 Roskilde, Copenhagen, Denmark

Konrad Jamrozik (89), Department of Public Health, Queen Elizabeth II Medical Center, University of Western Australia, Nedlands, Perth, Australia 6009

Robert Katzman (53), Alzheimer's Disease Research Center, University of California at San Diego, San Diego, California 92093

Erin Kenney (165), Center for Behavioral and Community Health Studies, Graduate School of Public Health, San Diego State University, San Diego, California 92182

Bohdan Kolody (351), Department of Sociology, San Diego State University, San Diego, California 92182

Leonard T. Kurland (73), Section of Clinical Epidemiology, Department of Health Science Research, Mayo Clinic, Rochester, Minnesota 55905

John F. Kurtzke (23), Veterans Affairs Medical Center, and Georgetown University, Washington, D. C. 20422

Paul Levy (53), Department of Sociology, University of Illinois at Chicago, Chicago, Illinois 60680

William T. Liu (53), Department of Sociology, University of Illinois at Chicago, Chicago, Illinois 60680

Patrick D. Lyden (287), Department of Neurosciences, UCSD Medical Center, University of California at San Diego, San Diego, California 92103

Craig A. Molgaard (1, 149, 213, 329), Division of Epidemiology and Biostatistics, Graduate School of Public Health, San Diego State University, San Diego, California 92182

Deborah M. Parra-Medina (165), Center for Behavioral and Community Health Studies, Graduate School of Public Health, San Diego State University, San Diego, California 92182

Guang-Ya Qu (53), Shanghai Mental Health Center, Shanghai, China

Kurupath Radhakrishnan (73), Section of Clinical Epidemiology, Department of Health Science Research, Mayo Clinic, Rochester, Minnesota 55905

Ian Robinson (131), Department of Human Sciences, Brunel, University of West London, Middlesex UB8 3PH, United Kingdom

John F. Rothrock (287), Department of Neurosciences, UCSD Medical Center, University of California at San Diego, San Diego, California 92103

David Salmon (53), Alzheimer's Disease Research Center, University of California at San Diego, San Diego, California 92093

Graham Scambler (131), Academic Department of Psychiatry, University College and Middlesex School of Medicine, University of London, London WC1E 7HU, United Kingdom

Omar Shafey (263), Medical Anthropology Program, Division of Epidemiology, University of California, San Francisco, San Francisco, California 94143

Lowell E. Sever (241), Epidemiology and Biometry Department, Pacific Northwest Laboratory, Battelle Seattle Research Center, Seattle, Washington 98105

Patricia Silva (310), Children's Hospital, San Diego, California 92123

E. Percil Stanford (195), University Center on Aging, College of Health and Human Services, San Diego State University, San Diego, California 92182

Richard J. Thomas (109), Epidemiology Department, Navy Environmental Health Center, Norfolk, Virginia 23513

Margarita E. Villarino (213), Office of Epidemiology, Centers for Disease Control, Atlanta, Georgia 30309

Zheng-Yu Wang (53), Department of Sociology, University of Illinois at Chicago, Chicago, Illinois 60680

Laura K. Wyman (257), Division of Epidemiology and Biostatistics, Graduate School of Public Health, San Diego State University, San Diego, California 92182

Elena Yu (53), Division of Epidemiology and Biostatistics, Graduate School of Public Health, San Diego State University, San Diego, California 92182

Ming-Yuan Zhang (53), Shanghai Mental Health Center, Shanghai, China

Preface

This book presents a sampling of original neuroepidemiologic papers that hopefully capture the range and excitement of the discipline. It is intended for epidemiologists, neurologists, and social and behavioral scientists with research interests in the area of biomedicine and disease.

The focus of this book is fourfold: international neuroepidemiology, the social and behavioral aspects of neuroepidemiology, issues in population surveillance, and methodological concerns in the field. The organization and selection of contributions is essentially a result of my own research and teaching interests. No doubt others would have done things differently.

This work was initiated while I was on sabbatical at the University of Oxford in 1990 in what was then the Department of Community Medicine and General Practice (now the Department of Public Health and Primary Care). I would like to offer a special thanks for the hospitality and support provided by Martin Vessey and his faculty and staff during my stay in his department. Also to Peter Armitage of the Statistics Department, University of Oxford, for his many acts of kindness before, during, and after my time at Oxford. A special thank you also to Ray Fitzpatrick for the High Dinner at Nuffield College and to Tim Hames for a similar treat at Exeter College.

I also wish to thank F. Douglas Scutchfield of the Graduate School of Public Health, San Diego State University, for the sabbatical per se, and Peter Dual, Dean of the College of Health and Human Services, San Diego State University, for his support in the form of a Research, Service, and Creativity Award (RSCA) from the California State University system. The RSCA was an invaluable assist in the initial support of this book.

Finally, I have had good help from friends during some trying personal times. I have been lucky in many ways to know such fine people as well as having a good and loyal family. To you all, thank you.

Craig A. Molgaard
San Diego, California

An Introduction to Neuroepidemiology

Craig A. Molgaard

The field of neuroepidemiology has reached a period of steady and sure growth following decades of hard work by researchers throughout the world. At present, programs exist in neuroepidemiology at Charing Cross Hospital, London, England, under the direction of Clifford Rose and the Medical College of Philadelphia in the United States under Milton Alter. The first regularly scheduled graduate class in neuroepidemiology in a School of Public Health was initiated in 1985 in the Graduate School of Public Health at San Diego State University. The University of Michigan Summer Epidemiology Program (formerly of the University of Minnesota) offered its first class in neuroepidemiology in 1991, taught by James Mortimer. Several new texts devoted to neuroepidemiology have been published (Anderson, 1991). In addition, the journal *Neuroepidemiology*, currently edited by Alter, reached its 10th anniversary in 1991 (Kurland *et al.*, 1982).

The rise of neuroepidemiology as a specific subdiscipline within the field of modern epidemiology has occurred parallel to the evolution of a number of other subdisciplines (Jaret, 1991). These include cardiovascular epidemiology, reproductive epidemiology, cancer epidemiology, social epidemiology, psychiatric epidemiology, behavioral epidemiology, and genetic epidemiology as well as others.

Yet common sense tells us that, just as the classic distinction between infectious and chronic disease epidemiology is not nearly as clear-cut as we pretend, such subdivisions of epidemiology must surely intersect and overlap at a number of critical points. The same statements can be made about neuroepidemiology. It overlaps with other "kinds" of epidemiology. It has both infectious and chronic disease emphases. Yet neuroepidemiology is distinct as a research field in several ways.

Neuroepidemiology: Theory and Method

First, it is one of the oldest subdisciplines in modern epidemiology, ranking with cardiovascular epidemiology in this regard. By the 1950s, large-scale multiple sclerosis (MS) surveys had been carried out by Kurland and his colleagues. Hyllestad had already founded the Danish Multiple Sclerosis Registry. Most importantly, the basic epidemiology of an obscure neurological disease called kuru among the stone-age Fore tribe of highland New Guinea had been made clear by Carleton Gadjusek, who was on his way to a Nobel Prize for his discovery and delineation of the class of diseases known as slow viruses.

Second, long before international travel was easy and relatively comfortable, neuroepidemiologists were extremely active in the search for geographic foci of disease. Kuru, of course, is one such example of a geographic isolate. Others would include the cluster of neurologic diseases on Guam [amyotrophic lateral sclerosis (ALS) and parkinsonism–dementia], Creutzfeldt–Jakob disease (CJD) in Libya, MS in both the Faeroe Islands of Denmark and the Orkney and Shetland islands of Scotland, human T-cell lymphotrophic virus-I- (HTLV-I) related transient spastic paraparesis in Okinawa and Jamaica, and Minimata's disease in Japan.

Finally, neuroepidemiology was characterized by a unique breed of epidemiologist. Most either were trained in neurology or had interests in it. Many were oriented toward anthropology and cross-cultural research. They also overlapped their careers with those of R. A. Fisher, Jerzy Neyman, Karl Pearson, and Elizabeth Scott, so that they had watched in person the development of modern statistics in this century. The result was that they were not in the least overawed by statistics but, rather, were users of the tools of statistics as they would use any other tool in the armementarium of epidemiology. These neuroepidemiologists were also very good descriptive and analytic epidemiologists. As the eradication of polio in the United States was to show, they were also very good at vaccine development, field trials, and many other things important in the battle against neurologic disease.

A large part of the development of the population–laboratory approach to the study of neurologic disease (as opposed to a purely clinical or surgical approach) was derived from neuropathology. Historically known as geographic pathology, the role of cross-cultural studies in neuropathology in the development of neuroepidemiology was reviewed by Kurland in 1978 (Kurland, 1978). He carefully noted that the study of geographic isolates (defined as a population that may be inbred, remote, isolated, or otherwise distinct) is of interest because a high incidence of a new or rare disease or an unusual prevalence of a well-known disease in such an isolate may reveal genetic or ecological associations that otherwise might be missed.

Neuroepidemiology has been characterized by significant progress against a large number of specific diseases, perhaps more so than any other subfield of epidemiology. Yet no complete "summarization" of these accomplishments has yet appeared in the literature. Listed here are but a few, mentioned in brief.

POLIOMYELITIS

The classic example of an infection of the central nervous system (CNS) in which epidemiology was crucial in controlling the disease was poliomyelitis. Poliomyelitis results from gastrointestinal infection with a virus, followed by viremia and invasion of the CNS in some individuals with resulting paralysis. There are three types of virus. Nonparalytic forms of poliomyelitis are not clinically distinguishable from other enteroviral diseases. Prior to mass immunization, large epidemics of poliomyelitis occurred in the United States and Western Europe. A dramatic upsurge occurred in the United States from 1945 to 1954.

Oddly, the initial flourishing of this disease in the late 1800s seems to be related to public health victories of that century. As improvements in sanitation and sewage disposal spread in industrialized nations, there was no longer widespread distribution of the polio virus. Individuals who formerly were commonly exposed to the virus during the era of poor sanitation, becoming mildly infected with nonparalytic disease, then recovering and moving into an immune state during adolescence and adulthood, no longer were having such an opportunity. The result was that those who encountered the virus later in life as older children or adults had a much greater chance of developing paralytic disease. Many still remember that polio had a "season" (late summer or early fall) when there was a peak of incidence. Small children were often restricted from attending county and state fairs and other social events during the season prior to mass immunization, a form of pseudo-quarantine that served to dramatically increase fear and anxiety in young minds.

Mass vaccination began in the United States in 1955. Initially this was with inactivated polio vaccine (developed by Jonas Salk and his colleagues). This was followed in 1961 with oral polio vaccine (developed by Albert Sabin and his colleagues). The annual incidence of poliomyelitis declined from 13.7 cases per 100,000 in 1952 to 0.003 per 100,000 in 1981 (Polio Network News, 1990).

The stunning success of the polio vaccination campaign is perhaps second only to the eradication of smallpox in its completeness and speed in the history of public health. However, controversy still continues over whether inactivated polio vaccine or oral polio vaccine is preferable.

In addition, in recent years considerable attention has focued on polio survivors who have developed post-polio syndrome. In post-polio syndrome, accumulated strain from overworked muscles that have been chronically overused for many years results from both simple loss of motor nerve cells and recovery of function, when reduction in the number of total motor neuron cells forces remaining cells to drive orphaned muscle fibers in a less efficient manner (Alter *et al.*, 1982).

KURU

In the mid-1950s, Australian researchers identified a degenerative neurological disease known as kuru among the Fore speakers of tribespeople in the New Guinea highlands. Carleton Gadjusek, then working in Australia, began a series of landmark investigations that revolutionized our concepts of viral diseases (Molgaard, 1981). Diverse clinical, pathological, and genetic studies were carried out in a search for the elusive cause of this disease. Moving from a genetic hypothesis in the late 1950s with the critical input of Kurland, Fisher, and others, by the early 1960s Gadjusek and his colleagues had (1) demonstrated transmissibility of the disease in the laboratory following a long incubation period, (2) noted that scrapie, a disease of the CNS of sheep, had very similar lesions when compared to kuru, and (3) theorized that the disease was caused by the ritual endocannabalism of the Fore people. The mechanism was assumed to be inoculation of the agent through breaks in the skin rather than by means of the gastrointestinal tract, explaining the high mortality in women and children involved in food handling and preparation. As cannibalism has decreased in New Guinea during the last four decades, so has the incidence of kuru. For his work on slow viruses, Gadjusek received a Nobel Prize in medicine in 1976.

Work in this area continues in terms of CJD, Gerstmann–Straussler syndrome, transmissible mink encephalopathy, scrapie, wasting disease, and bovine spongiform encephalopathy (Collee, 1990; Marsh *et al.*, 1991; Molgaard and Golbeck, 1990; Wilesmith *et al.*, 1991).

MINIMATA'S DISEASE

In a number of fishing villages adjacent to Minimata, Japan, during the early 1950s, a strange, new disease developed. Characterized by ataxia, sensory disturbances, and tremor, as well as loss of vision, hearing, and intellect, it was progressive and often fatal. Most of the cases were local fisherman and their families. An infectious etiology was presumed.

Because the cases were nonseasonal, and cats and seabirds from the bay also showed evidence of neurological disease, the fish from Minimata Bay and a neurotoxin were suspected. In 1957, fishing in Minimata Bay was banned. There was a cessation of new cases.

The neurotoxin was eventually identified—mercury. A large factory producing vinyl chloride used mercuric chloride in its process and had been discharging it into the bay, where it had apparently been biotransformed into methyl mercury. Once taken up into the aquatic chain, the methyl mercury had reached high concentrations in certain species of fish.

As an aside, it should be noted that there have been a number of instances where populations have been exposed to the neurotoxicity of methyl mercury. This has often been associated with human consumption of fish, but some outbreaks have occurred with grains when methyl mercury compounds as a fungicidal agent have been misused. A noteworthy example of such an occurrence was in Iraq in 1971 and 1972, when 6000 known cases of mercury neurotoxicity occurred. Also, the Mad Hatter character from the delightful children's stories of the Oxford mathematician Dr. Dodgson (also known as Lewis Carroll) reflected a real phenomenon of Victorian neuroepidemiology. This was the use of mercury compounds in the manufacture of hats and the consequent poisoning and erratic behavior of those involved in this occupation.

PARKINSON'S DISEASE

James Parkinson's paper in 1817 on what he called the "shaking palsy" contained the description of the major symptoms of Parkinson's disease (tremor, bradykinesia, and rigidity). In the 1960s, the brain defect that is the driving force of this disease was identified (failure to manufacture dopamine in the substantia nigra as a result of loss of dopamine nerve cells).

During this same time, a successful drug therapy was discovered, which has been called one of the triumphs of modern medical research. Levadopa (or L-dopa), a natural brain chemical that nerve cells can use to make dopamine, was found to restore normal function in terms of reduction of rigidity, tremor, and bradykinesia. As modified by extracerebral decarboxylase inhibitors such as carbidopa and benserazide, which keep levadopa from changing to dopamine before reaching the brain, symptoms are reduced in about three of every four patients.

Although the prevalence of Parkinson's disease increases with age, the risk factor profile for this disease is unclear (Herzman *et al.*, 1990). Some studies have shown a differential by sex, whereas others have not. Even the apparently well-founded racial difference in Parkinson's disease was not in evidence in the Copiah County, Mississippi, study. Several lines of evidence, including the discovery of the meperdine derivative 1-methyl-4-phenyl-1,2,3,6-tetrahydropyridine (MPTP), which is associated with parkinsonism by oxidative biotranformation to MPP+, indicate that environmental chemicals, if the exposure is chronic, may lead to parkinsonian syndromes (Tanner and Langston, 1990). An intriguing aspect of the environmental chemicals hypothesis is that the prevalence of Parkinson's disease is higher in countries that have been industrialized the longest. However, to what extent better case ascertainment in older industrialized countries drives such a pattern is unclear. It should also be noted that the risk of acquiring parkinsonism–dementia complex on Guam has declined since the late 1950s, with hypothesized exposure to an unknown environmental factor appearing to be during adolescence or adulthood (X. Zhang *et al.*, 1990). Other issues in the epidemiology of Parkinson's disease include the prevalence of associated dementia, a north–south geographic gradient in terms of mortality, and an often reported protective effect for tobacco use (Marder *et al.*, 1991; Kurtzke and Goldberg, 1988; Martilla and Rinne, 1976; Rajput *et al.*, 1987).

STROKE

Epidemiologists have identified major risk factors that can lead to stroke as well as ways to maintain good health to prevent stroke, such as anti-platelet therapy (Sivenius *et al.*, 1991). Yet stroke remains the leading neurological disorder in the United States, ranking third among all causes of death and carrying an immense public health burden in terms of disability and cost to patients and families.

One clear risk factor for stroke is a transient ischemic attack (TIA), where a person experiences vague symptoms of stroke such as numbness, loss of muscle strength, difficulty with speech, and difficulty with sight or hearing in some cases. These symptoms, however, quickly fade. A number of TIA registries have been established by the National Institute of Neurological and Communicative Disorders and Stroke (NINCDS) at various cerebrovascular research centers to examine the frequency of TIAs, survivorship, and other epidemiologic aspects of this crucial risk factor (National Institute of Neurological and Communicative Disorders and Stroke, 1990).

Another risk factor for stroke is hypertension, where early detection and medicated control are crucial. Similarly, atherosclerosis affects blood circulation within the brain and is a risk factor in its own right. Other known risk factors for stroke are heart disease (clots may form, break loose, and travel into the brain), diabetes (accompanying destructive changes in blood vessels throughout the body), obesity, lack of exercise, and high levels of stress. Other risk factors such as cigarette smoking and use of birth control pills have been implicated in stroke (Dunbabin and Sandercock, 1990). Evidence also continues to accumulate that recreational drug use is a major risk factor for stroke in young adults (Kaku and Lowenstein, 1990; Rothrock *et al.*, 1988; Levine and Welch, 1988).

Recent research has suggested that small daily doses of aspirin can protect against thrombotic stroke by lessening the severity or number of TIAs. The mechanism appears to be by means of interference with platelet enzyme messenger manufacture. Similarly, recent research has indicated that eicosapentaenic acid in fish oil diets may protect against atherosclerosis.

Other important research on stroke using population-based survey techniques was that carried out by Bruce Schoenberg in 1978 on over 25,000 residents in Copiah County, Mississippi. In this study, Schoenberg determined the first racial differentials in the magnitude and clinical presentation of stroke and other neurological disorders in the United States (Goldstein, 1987). That such research efforts are bearing fruit is clear from the decline in the national stroke death rate, which was approximately 27% during the last decade.

Yet the decline in stroke mortality is not necessarily associated with a decline in stroke incidence; it may be due instead to both heightened public awareness concerning blood pressure and other risk factors for stroke as well as advances in treatment of acute stroke events. The use of carotid endarterectomy for prophylaxis against stroke now appears to be highly beneficial to patients with recent hemispheric and retinal TIAs (North American Symptomatic Carotid Endarterectomy Trial Collaborators, 1991; McCarthy *et al.*, 1991).

MULTIPLE SCLEROSIS

Initially described by the great French neurologist Charcot, MS affects both the sensory and motor (muscle) functions of the body with a great deal of variability and often an initially relapsing course. A demyelinating disease, symptoms, severity, and course are often determined by the extent and location of myelin lesions, as well as myelin repair processes and type of function of the nerve and the specific and general nature of that function. Risk factors are difficult to identify because the disease is so variable (Riise *et al.*, 1991). Optic neuritis is suspected to be a risk factor or, more accurately, a partial form of MS. A slow virus may be implicated in the etiology of this disease. Evidence for this includes the following: MS usually does not occur until early adulthood; the highest prevalence of the disease worldwide is in the temperate regions of the northern United States, Canada, and Europe; and predisposing events related to onset of MS seem to occur before the age of 15 years. However, it has been established that women are almost twice as likely as men to develop MS, and that Whites are more than twice as likely to develop MS as other races. Suspicion continues to focus on an autoimmune malfunction related to the nervous system.

The search for an MS virus has occupied investigators for most of the last two decades. At this point, a viral subgroup of retroviruses (HTLV-I, -II, and -III) have seemingly been excluded as potential etiologic agents, as well as coronaviruses. Given that many viruses have been implicated in the etiology of MS, a number of different viruses, whether acting alone or together, may trigger an autoimmune response. It should also be noted that twin studies have indicated that expression of the disease is partially but not entirely genetically controlled. More than one gene—two for T-cell receptors and at least one for DR2 antigen—may be necessary in determining risk of developing MS (Weinshenker *et al.*, 1990).

Once again, population-based epidemiology has been actively carried out. Study sites have included Olmsted County, Minnesota, the Shetland and Orkney islands of Scotland, and the Faeroe Islands of Denmark (Kurtzke and Hyllested, 1979).

AMYOTROPHIC LATERAL SCLEROSIS

Neuroepidemiologists have thoroughly developed the descriptive epidemiology of ALS (Armon *et al.*, 1991; Kurland and Radhakrishnan, 1992). The geographic distribution is even throughout most of the world, the average age at diagnosis is about 56 years, there is a slight male-to-female preponderance, and approximately 10% of cases appear to be familial with transmission in a dominant pattern of inheritance. However, the agent that actually causes the death of motor neurons has been very difficult to identify. An environmental cause of ALS has been suggested based on studies of the Chamorro population of Guam in the Western Pacific. ALS occurs much more frequently than normal on Guam, the Kii Peninsula of

Japan, and a region of western New Guinea. Because of this, the NINCDS established a research station on Guam in the late 1950s.

The etiology of Guamanian ALS has been hotly disputed. Much attention has focused on the distributions of certain minerals in the soil and water of Guam. Similarly, studies have focused on diet as the island modernized. During the last 30 years, the incidence of ALS on Guam has declined from approximately 1 in 10 people to less than 1 in 100. The incidence of ALS declined even more for those Chamorros who migrated to Hawaii or the mainland United States.

This cohort effect has provided the strongest evidence for the environmental hypothesis (Kurland and Molgaard, 1982). At this point, the cycad nut, used by Guamanians as a starch substitute during times of food shortage during World War II and at other times as an inexpensive food product, has been shown to cause a similar disease when fed to laboratory animals (Spencer *et al.*, 1986; Spencer, 1987).

DEMENTIA OF THE ALZHEIMER'S TYPE

Demographic changes in the world's population have led to an increased emphasis on the epidemiology of age-associated dementia or, rather, senile dementia of the Alzheimer's type. Given a world population that is increasingly aged, and an age-associated disorder, the population at risk for Alzheimer's disease (AD) will continue to grow rapidly into the next century.

With the establishment of a number of Alzheimer's Research Centers in the United States during the 1980s, our knowledge of this disease has increased considerably (Van Duijn and Hofman, 1991). Distinction is now made among idiopathic AD, multiinfarct dementia, and secondary dementias due to specific conditions such as endocrine or infectious disease (Molgaard, 1987). In terms of pathology, the role of amyloid protein continues to be debated (Glenner, 1989; Marx, 1990). The significance of the prion for understanding AD remains unclear (Prusiner, 1987).

The last decade has also witnessed a focusing of methodological attention and work on AD (Rocca and Amaducci, 1991). *Diagnostic and Statistical Manual*, 3rd ed. (DSM-III), criteria for diagnosing dementia and specific dementing disorders were introduced by the American Psychiatric Association in 1980. The Alzheimer's Disease and Related Disorders Association (ADRDA) became increasingly active during the 1980s in terms of both sponsoring primary research and supporting Alzheimer's caregivers. In 1984 a joint NINCDS–ADRDA work group established clinical diagnostic criteria for possible, probable, and definite AD. Histologic criteria for diagnosis were added in 1985, and the DSM-III criteria were revised in 1987. National Institute of Health Consensus Conference criteria for the differential diagnosis of dementing disorders were also added that year. The Eurage Group on Aging of the Brain and Senile Dementia introduced neuropathologic diagnostic criteria for AD in 1988, and the World Health Organization has produced both clinical and research diagnostic criteria in the latest revision of the International Classification of Disease.

The epidemiology per se of AD has begun to emerge as a result of a number of excellent population-based studies and surveys (Yu *et al.*, 1989; Jin *et al.*, 1989). The occurence of AD is generally higher in females, and geographically diverse areas tend to produce similar prevalence estimates (Japan, Europe, North America, China) of this disease (M. Zhang *et al.*, 1990).

Methodological problems in assessing risk factors for AD have been abundant, yet some issues are being resolved (M. Zhang *et al.*, 1989). Familial aggregation in some instances has been accepted as real. A possible familial predisposition of Down's syndrome in association with AD was hypothesized and investigated, but it now seems to carry little weight in the research community. Head trauma and AD has received considerable attention, but a number of case-control studies have produced conflicting results, suggesting the existence of some form of bias (Molgaard *et al.*, 1990). A great deal of clinical trial and pharmalogical research is currently being carried out on AD.

HUNTINGTON'S DISEASE

Huntington's disease (HD) is now, through the techniques of molecular genetics, thought to be ascertainable by means of polymorphic segments of DNA closely linked to the Huntington chorea gene (Pavoni *et al.*, 1990). Also, the descriptive epidemiology (age at onset, chance of inheriting the HD gene, natural history, and survivorship) has been well developed by means of rosters of affected families (Pridmore, 1990). Two important rosters are the Huntingdon's Disease Research Roster maintained at Indiana University ($n = 85,701$) and the Venezuelan Roster for the largest known HD family ($n = 10,000$) found in the Lake Maracaibo district of that country (Young *et al.*, 1986).

HD genetics have proved difficult but illuminating. It is now known that those cases who manifest symptoms at a younger age usually inherit the gene from their father. Also, the younger the onset, the faster the progression of the disease. A great deal of attention has focused on the cause of toxin-induced neuronal degeneration in HD. One suspect has been the neurotoxin quinolinic acid, which occurs naturally in the brains of humans. Research has also been focused on neuropsychological deficits and brain abnormalities in HD.

NEURAL TUBE DEFECTS

Neural tube defects (NTDs), perhaps because of their dramatic nature, have received considerable attention from neuroepidemiologists. To a large extent, both the descriptive and analytic epidemiology have been worked out.

In terms of descriptive epidemiology, the picture is as follows. More female than male babies are afflicted. A woman who has had one child with NTD is at an elevated risk to have a second such birth. Whites are at a higher risk for such a birth than Blacks, Asians, or Ashkenazi Jews. Geographic foci are well known in NTDs. Examples commonly noted in the literature are from Wales, Ireland, the Punjab, West Virginia, and the southeastern United States. Seasonal trends have been noted in Great Britain and the United States. It terms of time of conception, infants conceived February through April have a higher risk of developing a NTD. Time trend analysis clearly shows that the rate of NTD births has been declining in most Western countries since the 1950s from what appears to have been an epidemic of reported cases in the 1930s. A consistent finding has been that women in lower socioeconomic groups, that is, those suffering from either acute or chronic poverty, are at an elevated risk for a NTD birth.

The last has led to a well-developed analytic focus on diet and associated factors as etiologic agents for NTD births. Suspected agents have included tea, blighted potatoes, low calcium intake, and nitrates and nitrites. Although no consistent associations have been noted for these risk factors, current attention has focused on folic acid. This recent work has been well reviewed by Slattery and Janerich (1991) in terms of both study design and biological plausibility issues.

Folic acid is necessary for normal reproduction, growth, lactation, and antibody formulation. A deficiency of folic acid in early pregnancy could lead to faulty cell division and result in NTDs. Several recent case-control studies and one cohort study have examined the issue of chronic maternal malnutrition and the occurrence of NTD births. The focus has been on vitamin/mineral supplementation and dietary counseling as a means of decreasing the risk of an NTD. As usual, the results are conflicting, but there was some evidence for a protective effect associated with multivitamin supplement use or high levels of dietary folate intake. However, it should be noted that a recent report published by the Institute of Medicine (1990) noted a lack of research evidence for multivitamin supplements in the prevention of NTDs. Research in this area continues at present.

PERTUSSIS VACCINES

The true risks and benefits of pertussis vaccination have been the source of much controversy (Cherry *et al.*, 1988). The question of whether pertussis vaccine can cause serious neurological illness or death was often based on anecdotal case reports prior to the National Childhood Encephalopathy Study (Committee on Infectious Diseases, 1991). Carried out in Great Britain from 1976 to 1979, this large case-control study examined whether or not acute neurological illness associated with diphtheria-pertussis-tetanus (DPT) immunization could result in permanent brain damage (Department of Health and Social Security, 1981). An increase in risk was noted (3.3, CI = 1.7–6.5). This result was later criticized by a workshop at the Institute of Medicine sponsored by the Centers for Disease Control (CDC) as being suspect because of limited case ascertainment and study design limitations (Marcuse and Wentz, 1989). A recent updated review of the epidemiologic evidence for a causal relationship between pertussis vaccine and acute neurological illness in children has appeared (Wentz and Marcuse, 1991). There is evidence to support an association between DPT vaccine and serious acute neurological illness, but this is a very rare event (between 1 per 100,000 immunizations and 1 per 1,000,000 immunizations). The evidence for pertussis vaccine causing permanent brain damage is very unclear. If possible, it is even more rare that an acute neurological illness.

A definitive study testing the brain damage hypothesis would have to be very large and will probably never occur for reasons of expense. This is unfortunate, because the public's perception of the risks of pertussis vaccination has shifted radically in recent years as a result of publicity concerning adverse reactions to the vaccine. Such a change in public opinion threatens the efficiency of immunization programs. Current research is examing the safety and efficacy of acellular pertussis vaccines to replace current whole-cell pertussis vaccine (Menkes and Kinsbourne, 1990). Recently, the Immunization Practices Advisory Committee noted that one such acellular pertussis vaccine (ACEL-IMUNE) has been licensed for fourth and fifth doses in the DPT series (CDC 1992). Until now, acellular vaccines have been licensed only in Japan, where they have been routinely administered to children since 1981.

CEREBRAL PALSY

Movement disorders in this group are of varying symptoms and severity. The brain injury often also may be accompanied by mental/emotional impairment, epilepsy, and impairment of the senses. Its developmental base is assumed to be during pregnancy approximately 90% of the time and often perinatal.

A major research effort was mounted by the NINCDS to search for the leading causes of cerebral palsy. Known as the Collaborative Perinatal Project (CPP), this cohort study followed 55,000 women through pregnancy and delivery, with periodic examinations of their children from birth to the age of 7 years. Although sometimes controversial, the results of the CPP have indicated a number of specific environmental events as leading to cerebral palsy. These included convulsive seizures, prematurity and low birth weight, cigarette smoking, excessive use of alcohol, and drug use as well as complications of labor and delivery (Kallen, 1988).

Preventative approaches in this area have included the following: a vaccine for rubella (German measles), increased emphasis on drug- and alcohol-free pregnancies in prenatal counseling, screening and treatment for RH incompatibility, and screening and treatment for newborn hyperbilirubinemia (jaundice). Although major causes of cerebral palsy have been controlled in this fashion, idiopathic cerebral palsy is still common in full-term and full-weight infants (58% of all cases according to results from the CPP). Diseases such as toxoplasmosis and cytomeglovirus continue to be highly dangerous to the fetus.

GUILLAIN–BARRE SYNDROME AND THE SWINE FLU VACCINE AFFAIR

The most notable intersection of neuroepidemiological research and public policy was the series of events surrounding the swine flu vaccine campaign of 1976 in the United States. A national program of immunization against the "swine flu" strain of influenza was stopped when the Public Health Service noted what appeared to be a relatively large number of cases of Guillain–Barre syndrome among the inoculated. Suspicion of an apparent excess of this rare neuromuscular disorder could not be confirmed without knowledge of the baseline incidence of the disease in a population in the absence of any other disturbing factors. Because the Federal government had rushed manufacture and distribution of the vaccine in the face of the perceived "epidemic" of influenza, it had also been forced to assume product liability for adverse reactions to the vaccine, because the manufacturers refused to accept such liability in an increasingly litigious environment. A systematic adverse reaction such as Guillain–Barre, if it truly existed, therefore had great importance.

A study carried out in 1973 by Lesser in Olmsted County using the Mayo Clinic records-linkage system provided the baseline rates for Guillain–Barre syndrome (Kurland and Molgaard, 1981). The ratio of observed to expected cases of this disease among vaccine recipients seemed to indicate that recipients were developing Guillain–Barre syndrome at a rate several times the normal. The program of immunization was not resumed.

Unfortunately, this had the effect of generating large numbers of swine flu injury claims against the Federal government. These suits ran into tens of millions of dollars and often were generated by individuals who developed neurological diseases and syndromes very distant from Guillain–Barre or nonneurological diseases and syndromes altogether.

The issue of whether or not there was truly an excess of cases has continued to be debated in the literature. Research studies examining this matter have been mounted by investigators at the CDC, the Mayo Clinic, and the University of California at San Diego (Kurland *et al.*, 1984a,b; Molgaard and Gresham, 1986).

CREUTZFELDT–JAKOB DISEASE

The etiology of CJD remains most unclear, despite transmissibility in laboratory experiments and some known iatrogenic transmissions through surgical instruments and tissues (Raubertas *et al.*, 1989). Occurring primarily between the ages of 55 and 75 years, CJD is characterized by a rapid progressive dementia and death in approximately 1 year. For the vast majority of cases, the iatrogenic source is not obvious, and case clusters are sporadic. Ethnic and family clusters have been reported among Libyan-born immigrants to Israel. Both the Libyan community and an area with high rates in Czechoslovakia were reproductively isolated prior to World War II. A study from England and Wales examining CJD mortality from 1970 to 1979 noted female excess (Will *et al.*, 1986), but no other suggestive relationships. A detailed review by Brown *et al.* (1987)

concluded that CJD is a minimally contagious disease that may be acquired in early life in several different ways.

More recent research has examined the association of CJD cases with participation in the National Hormone and Pituitary Program (Fradkin *et al.*, 1991). This followed the deaths of three individuals from CJD in 1985, who had been administered human growth hormone (HGH) by means of the national program of acquiring human pituitary glands for extraction of the hormone. Termination of distribution of HGH was then ordered by the National Institutes of Health and a study launched in conjunction with the CDC to examine the entire recipient population. It now appears that those who started HGH therapy prior to 1970 might be at risk and that duration of pituitary HGH therapy might be another iatrogenic risk factor for CJD.

HEAD INJURY

The descriptive epidemiology of head injury has been well developed. Young men are more than twice as likely as women to suffer a head injury. Head injuries occur most often in the 15–24 year-old group. The elderly and infants are also at high risk—the former from falls and the latter from dropping or sometimes abuse. Much of what is known concerning penetrating head injuries has been learned from Veterans Administration and Department of Defense studies on veterans.

Analytic epidemiology has been less well developed in this area, because rehabilitation has tended to receive more attention than in-depth studies of risk factors for injury per se. NINCDS has sponsored four Traumatic Coma Data Banks to examine outcome and survivorship for those with head injuries. It should also be noted that more and more evidence is accruing that head injury is a significant risk factor for dementia of the Alzheimer's type (Molgaard *et al.*, 1990).

EPILEPSY

After stroke, epilepsy is the second-most prevalent neurological disorder in the United States, with approximately 2 million individuals being afflicted. A long tradition of involvement and study from neurologists dating from the 19th century has resulted in clear-cut classifications of seizures and well-honed drug programs that are remarkably effective. At present, 16 antiepileptic drugs are on the market, including Dilantin, Tegretol, and Clouopin.

A variety of etiologies can lead to epilepsy, including complications of infections, head injury, cerebral palsy, mental retardation, and other neurological conditions. Although medication is especially effective in epilepsy, precise knowledge of what causes specific neurons to become epileptic is not available. Prevention focuses on prenatal care and diet, quality medical care during delivery, and avoidance of infant bacterial meningitis and head trauma. Special attention has been devoted to febrile seizures as a risk factor. The epidemiology of this disorder has been considerably elaborated by Allen Hauser of Columbia University and J. Fred Annegars of the University of Texas at Houston (Annegars *et al.*, 1982).

BRAIN TUMORS

Brain tumors are relatively rare, accounting for less than 2% of all cancers diagnosed in the United States each year. In adults, they are most common between the ages of 40 and 60 years, with a slight predilection for males. In children, the peak is between the ages of 6 and 9. Primary tumors of the CNS are the second-most common in children after leukemia.

It is known that brain tumors seldom occur in neurons per se but, rather, in the surrounding and supporting glial cells. Also, the type and location of childhood tumors are different from those of adults, reflecting a nervous system that is still in development.

However, the risk factor picture is very unclear. A possible clustering of brain tumors in workers in petrochemical plants was noted in the late 1970s (Selikoff and Hammond, 1982), but little was learned. Currently, interest focuses on the possible association of brain tumors and leukemia with electromagnetic force fields from high powerlines (Pool, 1990).

CONCLUSION

Similar advances and achievements have been made by epidemiologists in regard to a wide range of other neurological diseases and syndromes [spinal cord injuries, developmental and genetic speech and language disorders (cri du chat syndrome, Tourette's syndrome, aphasia), headache (migraine, cluster), Meniere's disease, chronic pain syndrome, shingles, Korsakoff's syndrome].

For example, an extensive research literature has developed pertaining to the neurologic abnormalities found in association with acquired immunodeficiency syndrome, or AIDS (Koralnik *et al.*, 1990; Nakamura and Molgaard, 1986). Specific attention has focused on the neuropsychiatric dysfunction often associated with human immunodeficiency virus (HIV) infection, with several studies suggesting HIV-associated cognitive abnormalities may be reduced following treatment with Zidovudine, or AZT (Frederick *et al.*, 1988; Portegies *et al.*, 1989). The exact incidence of what is now known as AIDS dementia complex (ADC) is unknown, and to what extent observed cognitive deficits are due to drug use rather that the insidious onset of AIDS dementia complex is unclear (Egan *et al.*, 1990). It may well be that true ADC occurs late in the natural history of the disease. As research continues, these and other medical conundrums will come more within the reasoning system and elucidation of epidemiology.

References

Alter, M., Kurland, L., and Molgaard, C. A. (1982). Progressive muscular atrophy and antecedent poliomyelitis. *In* "Advances in Neurology: Human Motor Neuron Diseases," (L. Rowland, ed.), pp. 303–310. Raven Press, New York.

American Psychiatric Association. (1980). "Diagnostic and Statistical Manual of Mental Disorders," 3rd ed. American Psychiatric Association, Washington, D.C.

Anderson, D. W. (ed.) (1991). "Neuroepidemiology: A Tribute to Bruce Schoenberg." CRC Press, Boca Raton, Florida.

Annegers, J. F., Hanser, W. A., Anderson, V. E., and Kurland, L. T. (1982). The risks of seizure disorders among relatives of patients with childhood onset epilepsy. *Neurology* **32**, 174–180.

Armon, C., Kurland, L. T., Daube, J., and O'Brien, P. C. (1991). Epidemiologic correlates of sporadic amyotrophic lateral sclerosis. *Neurology* **41**, 1077–1084.

Bharucha, N. E., Raven, R. H., and Schoenberg, B. S. (1991). Epidemiology of infections of the central nervous system. *In* (D. W. Anderson ed.). "Neuroepidemiology: A Tribute to Bruce Schoenberg," CRC Press, Boca Raton, Florida.

Brown, P., Cathala, F., Raubertas, R. F., Gadjusek, D. C., and Castaigne, P. (1987). The epidemiology of Creutzfeldt–Jakob disease: Conclusion of a 15-year investigation in France and review of the world literature. *Neurology* **37**, 895–904.

Centers for Disease Control (1992). Pertussis vaccination: acellular pertussis vaccine for reinforcing and booster use—supplementary ACIP statement. Recommendations of the Immunization Practices Advisory Committee (ACIP). *MMWR* **41** (No. RR-1), 1–10.

Cherry, J. B., Brunell, P., Golden, G., and Karzon, D. (1988). Report of the task force on pertussis and pertussis immunization—1988. *Pediatrics* **81**, 939–977.

Collee, J. G. (1990). Bovine spongiform encephalopathy. *Lancet* **336**, 1300–1303.

Committee on Infectious Diseases. (1991). The relationship between pertussis vaccine and brain damage: Reassessment. *Pediatrics* **88**(2), 397–400.

Department of Health and Social Security. (1981). Whooping Cough. Reports from the Committee on Safety of Medicines and the Joint Committee on Vaccination and Immunization, pp. 79–169. Her Majesty's Stationery Office, London.

Dunbabin, D. W., and Sandercock, P. A. G. (1990). Preventing stroke by the modification of risk factors. *Stroke* **21**(Suppl. IV), 12, 36–39.

Egan, V. G., Crawford, J. R., Brettle, R. P., and Goodwin, G. M. (1990). The Edinburgh Cohort of HIV-positive users: Current intellectual function is impaired, but not due to early AIDS dementia complex. *J. AIDS* **7**, 651–655.

Fradkin, J. E., Schonberger, L. B., Mills, J. L., *et al.* (1991). Creutzfeldt–Jakob disease in pituitary growth hormone recipients in the United States. *JAMA* **265**(7), 880–884.

Frederick, A. S., Bigley, J. W., McKinnis, R., Lougue, P. E., Evans, R. W., and Drucker, J. L. (1988). Neuropsychological outcome of zidovudine (AZT) treatment of patients with AIDS and AIDS-related complex. *N. Engl. J. Med.* **319,** 1573–1578.

Glenner, G. G., (1989). The pathobiology of Alzheimer's disease. *Ann. Int. Med.* **40,** 45–51.

Goldstein, M. (1987). A tribute to neuroepidemiologist Dr. Bruce Schoenberg 1942–1987. *Stroke* **18**(6), 985–986.

Herzman, C., Wiens, M., Bowering, D., Snow, B., and Calne, D. (1990). Parkinson's disease: A case-control study of occupational and environmental risk factors. *Am. J. Ind. Med.* **17,** 349–355.

Institute of Medicine. (1990). "Nutrition during Pregnancy," Ch. 21. National Academy Press, Washington, D.C.

Jaret, P. (1991). The disease detectives: Stalking the world's epidemics. *Nat. Geo.* **179,** 114–140.

Jin, H., Zhang, M. Y., Qu, O. Y., Wang, Z. Y., *et al.* (1989). Cross-cultural studies of dementia: Use of a Chinese version of the Blessed–Roth Information–Memory–Concentration Test in a Shanghai dementia survey. *Psychol. Aging* **4**(4) 471–479.

Kaku, D. A., and Lowenstein, D. H. (1990). Emergence of recreational drug abuse as a major risk factor for stroke in young adults. *Ann. Int. Med.* **113,** 821–827.

Kallen, B. (1988). Epidemiology of Human Reproduction. CRC Press, Boca Raton, Florida.

Koralnik, I. J., Beaumanoir, A., Hausler, R., Kohler, A., *et al.* (1990). A controlled study of early neurologic abnormalities in men with asymptomatic human immunodeficiency virus infection. *N. Engl. J. Med.* **323,** 864–870.

Kurland, L. (1978). Geographic isolates: Their role in neuroepidemiology. *Adv. Neurol.* **19,** 69–81.

Kurland, L., and Molgaard, C. (1981). The patient record in epidemiology. *Sci. Am.* **245**(4) 54–63.

Kurland, L. T., and Molgaard, C. A. (1982). Guamanian ALS: Hereditary or acquired? *In* "Advances in Neurology: Human Motor Neuron Disease," Vol. 36 (L. Rowland, ed.), pp. 165–172. Raven Press, New York.

Kurland, L. T., and Radhakrishnan, K. (1992). An update of the epidemiology of Western Pacific amyotrophic lateral sclerosis. *In* "Neuroepidemiology: Theory and Method" (C. Molgaard, ed.). Academic Press, San Diego.

Kurland L., Molgaard, C. A., and Schoenberg, B. (1982). Mayo Clinic Records–Linkage: Contributions to neuroepidemiology. *Neuroepidemiology* **1,** 102–114.

Kurland, L., Molgaard, C. A., Kurland, E., Erdtmann, F., and Stebbing, G. (1984a). Lack of association of swine flu vaccine and rheumatoid arthritis. *Mayo Clin. Proc.* **59,** 816–821.

Kurland, L., Molgaard, C. A., Kurland, E., Wiederholt, W., and Kirkpatrick, J. (1984b). Swine flu vaccine and multiple sclerosis. *J. Am. Med. Assoc.* **251,** 2672–2675.

Kurtzke, J. F., and Goldberg, I. D. (1988). Parkinsonism death rates by race, sex, and geography. *Neurology* **40,** 42–49.

Kurtze, J. F., and Hyllested, K. (1979). Multiple sclerosis in the Faroe Islands. I. Clinical and epidemiologic features. *Ann. Neurol.* **5,** 6–21.

Levine, S. R., and Welch, K. M. (1988). Cocaine and stroke. *Stroke* **19,** 779–783.

Marcuse, E. K., and Wentz, K. R. (1989). The NCES reconsidered: A summary of 1989 workshop. *Vaccine* **7,** 199–210.

Marder, K., Leung, D., Tang, M., Bell, K., Dooneief, G., Cote, L., Stern, Y., and Mayeux, R. (1991). Are demented patients with Parkinson's disease accurately reflected in prevalence surveys? A survival analysis. *Neurology* **41,** 1240–1243.

Marsh, R. F., Bessen, R. A., Lehmann, S., and Hartsough, G. R. (1991). Epidemiological and experimental studies on a new incident of transmissible mink encephalopathy. *J. Gen. Virol.* **72,** 589–594.

Martilla, R. J., and Rinne, U. K. (1976). Dementia in Parkinson's disease. *Acta Neurol. Scand.* **54,** 431–441.

Marx, J. (1990). Alzheimer's pathology explored. *Science* **249,** 984–988.

McCarthy, P. E., McDermott, W. M., and Amorosino, C. S. (1991). Carotid endarterectomy—Specific therapy based on pathophysiology. *N. Engl. J. Med.* **325**(7), 505–507.

Menkes, J. H., and Kinsbourne, M. (1990). Workshop on neurologic complications of pertussis and pertussis vaccination. *Neuropediatrics* **21,** 171–176.

Molgaard, C. A. (1981). Review of Kuru: Early letters and field notes from the collection of D. Carleton Gajdusek. (J. Farquhar and D. Gajdusek, eds.). Raven Press, New York. *Mayo Clin Proc* **56,** 529–530.

Molgaard, C. A. (1987). A multivariate analysis of Hachinski's scale for discrimating senile dementia of the Alzheimer's type from multi-infarct dementia. *Neuroepidemiology* **6,** 153–160.

Molgaard, C. A., and Golbeck, A. L. (1990). Mad cows and Englishmen: Bovine spongiform encephalopathy. *Neuroepidemiology* **9,** 285–286.

Molgaard, C. A., and Gresham, L. (1986). Swine flu vaccine and amyotrophic lateral sclerosis. *J. Am. Med. Assoc.* **255,** 2294 (letter).

Molgaard, C. A., Stanford, E. P., Morton, D. J., Ryden, L. A., Golbeck, A. L., and Schubert, K. R. (1990). The epidemiology of head trauma and neurocognitive impairment in a multiethnic population. *Neuroepidemiology* **9,** 233–242.

Nakamura, C., and Molgaard, C. A. (1986). Neuroepidemiology and acquired immune deficiency syndrome. *Neuroepidemiology* **5,** 181–193.

National Institute of Neurological and Communicative Disorders and Stroke. (1990). "Stroke 1990 Research Program." U.S. Department of Health and Human Services, Washington, D.C.

North American Symptomatic Carotid Endarterectomy Trial Collaborators. (1991). Beneficial effect of carotid endarterectomy in symptomatic patients with high grade carotid stenosis. *N. Engl. J. Med.* **325**(7), 445–453.

Pavoni, M., Granieri, E., Govoni, V., Del Senno, L., and Mapelli, G. (1990). Epidemiologic approach to Huntington's disease in Northern Italy (Ferrara area). *Neuroepidemiology* **9,** 306–314.

Polio Network News. (1990). Polio update. **7,** 1.

Pool, R. (1990). Is there an EMF–cancer connection? *Science* **249,** 1096–1099.

Portegies, P., DeGans, J., Lange, J., *et al.* (1989). Declining incidence of AIDS dementia complex after introduction of zidovudine treatment. *Br. J. Med.* **299,** 819–821.

Pridmore, S. A. (1990). The prevalence of Huntington's disease in Tasmania. *Med. J. Aust.* **153,** 133–134.

Prusiner, S. B. (1987). Prions causing degenerative neurological diseases. *Ann. Rev. Med.* **38,** 381–398.

Rajput, A. H., Offord, K. P., Beard, C. M., and Kurland, L. T. (1987). A case-control study of smoking habits, dementia, and other illnesses in idiopathic Parkinson's disease. *Neurology* **37,** 226–232.

Raubertas, R. F., Brown, P., Cathala, F., and Brown, I. (1989). The question of clustering of Creuzfeldt–Jakob disease. *Am. J. Epidemiol.* **129,** 146–153.

Riise, T., Gronning, M., Klauber, M. R., Barrett-Connor, E., Nyland, H., and Albrektsen, G. (1991). Clustering of residence of multiple sclerosis patients at age 13 to 20 years in Hordaland, Norway. *Am. J. Epidemiol.* **133,** 932–939.

Rocca, W., and Amaducci, L. (1991). Epidemiology of Alzheimer's disease. *In* "Neuroepidemiology: A Tribute to Bruce Schoenberg," (D. W. Anderson, ed.). CRC Press, Boca Raton, Florida.

Rothrock, J. F., Rubenstein, R., and Lyden, P. D. (1988). Ischemic stroke associated with methamphetamine inhalation. *Neurology* **38**, 589–592.

Selikoff, I. J., and Hammond, E. C. (1982). Brain tumors in the chemical industry. *Ann. N.Y. Acad. Sci.*, Vol. 381, New York.

Sivenius, J., Laakso, M., Penttila, I. M., Smets, P., Lowenthal, A., and Riekkinen, P. J. (1991). The European Stroke Prevention Study: Results according to sex. *Neurology* **41**, 1189–1192.

Slattery, M., and Janerich, D. (1991). The epidemiology of neural tube defects: A review of dietary intake and related factors as etiologic agents. *Am. J. Epidemiol.* **133**(6), 526–540.

Spencer, P. S. (1987). Guam ALS/parkinsonism–dementia: A long-latency neurotoxic disorder caused by slow toxin(s) in food? *Can. J. Neurolog. Sci.* **14**, 347–357.

Spencer, P. S., Nunn, P. B., Hugon, J., Ludolph, A., and Roy, D. (1986). Motor neuron disease on Guam: Possibility of a food neurotoxin. *Lancet* **i**, 965.

Tanner, C. M., and Langston, J. W. (1990). Do environmental toxins cause Parkinson's disease? A critical review. *Neurology* **40**(suppl.), 17–30.

Van Duijin, C., and Hofman, A. (1991). Risk factors for Alzheimer's disease: A collaborative re-analysis of case-control studies. *Int. J. Epidemiol.* **20**(suppl. 2).

Weinshenker, B. G., Bulman, D., Carriere, W., Baskerville, J., and Ebers, G. C. (1990). A comparison of sporadic and familial multiple sclerosis. *Neurology* **40**, 1354–1358.

Wentz, K. R., and Marcuse, E. K. (1991). Diptheria–tetanus–petussis vaccine and serious neurologic illness: An updated review of the epidemiologic evidence. *Pediatrics* **87**(3), 287–296.

Wilesmith, J. W., Ryan, J. B. M., and Atkinson, M. J. (1991). Bovine spongiform encephalopathy: Epidemiological studies on the origin. *Vet. Rec.* **128**, 199–203.

Will, R. G., Matthews, W. B., Smith, P. G., and Hudson, C. (1986). A retrospective study of Creutzfeldt–Jakob disease in England and Wales 1970–1979 II: Epidemiology. *J. Neurol. Neurosurg. Psychiatry* **49**, 749–755.

Young, A. B., Shoulson, I., Penney, J. B., Starosta-Rubinstein, S., Gomez, F., Travers, H., Ramos-Arroyo, M. A., Snodgrass, S. R., Bonilla, E., Moreno, H., and Wexler, N. S. (1986). Huntington's disease in Venezuela: Neurologic features and functional decline. *Neurology* **36**, 244–249.

Yu, E. S., Liu, W. T., Levy, P., Zhang, M. Y., Katzman, R., *et al.* (1989). Cognitive impairment among elderly adults in Shanghai, China. *J. Gerentol.* **44**(3), S97–S106.

Zhang, M., Katzman, R., Salmon, D., Jin, H., Cai, G., Wang, Z., *et al.* (1990). The prevalence of dementia and Alzheimer's disease in Shanghai, China: Impact of age, gender, and education. *Am. Neurol. Assoc.* **27**(4), 428–436.

Zhang, X., Anderson, D. W., Lavine, L., and Mantel, N. (1990). Patterns of acquiring parkinsonism–dementia complex on Guam. *Arch. Neurol.* **47**, 1019–1024.

I

International Research in Neuroepidemiology

1

Multiple Sclerosis in the Faroe Islands

John F. Kurtzke • Kay Hyllested • Anne Heltberg

Multiple sclerosis (MS) remains a disease of unknown cause, inadequate treatment, and unpredictable course, despite intense work by all manner of neural scientists for well over a century. Some have thought that an epidemiologic approach might be of benefit in attacking these problems. In essence, epidemiology is the study of the natural history of disease—an attempt to answer the reporter's questions of "who, what, when, and where," with the hope that sufficient data will arise as to "why."

In 1956, John Sutherland published the results of his survey of the prevalence of MS in northern Scotland: The rates in the Shetland–Orkney Islands were then by far the highest in the world (Sutherland, 1956). At that time, MS was considered rare on the Faroe Islands, and this was curious because of their similarity to the Shetland–Orkneys in geography, climate, and origin—both lands having been settled or occupied by Norse Vikings around the ninth century. For these reasons, a comparative study of MS in the Faroes and the Shetland–Orkney Islands was undertaken by Mogens Fog of Denmark and Allison of Northern Ireland. This intensive work was never reported in detail. It was included in Allison's (1963) presidential address, and a summary was presented in 1963 by Fog and Hyllested (1966). Intriguing for the Faroese MS was what appeared to be their young age at prevalence day. However, nothing further was done until the original Faroese case abstracts were reviewed from 1972 to 1974 (J.F.K.). It then became obvious that there were no patients on the list who were calculated to have had clinical onset of MS before 1945. Hyllested concurred; therefore, we both initiated this study, which continues to date, having been joined a few years ago by Anne Heltberg. In our first presentation, we had indeed called the occurrence of MS on the Faroes an epidemic (Kurtzke and Hyllested, 1975). We believe this study is *the* most critical work in the common efforts to define the nature of this disease. If we are correct, the answer to the cause of MS is in the Faroes.

We are well aware of the many claims to etiology that have foundered on the rocks of negative evidence. We also know that the road to fame for workers in MS is to deny whatever is the latest hypothesis. Why then are we out on this limb?

EPITOME OF THE EPIDEMIOLOGY OF MULTIPLE SCLEROSIS

We shall summarize without documentation here an overview of the state of the art as to the epidemiology of MS, based on several recent reviews by one of us (Kurtzke, 1977, 1980a,b, 1983, 1985, 1988, in press).

The best measures of the geographic distribution of MS come from prevalence studies, of which there are now over 300. These works indicate that, geographically, MS is distributed throughout the world within three zones of high, medium, and low frequency. High-frequency areas, with prevalence rates of 30 and above per 100,000 population, and now mostly 50–120 per 100,000 population, comprise northern and central Europe into Italy and the Soviet Union, Canada and the northern United States, and New Zealand and southeastern Australia. These regions are bounded by areas of medium frequency with prevalence rates of 5–29 per 100,000 population, which then comprise much of Australia, the southern United States, southwestern Norway and northernmost Scandinavia, much of the northern Mediterranean basin and possibly its eastern and southern shores as well, and probably the Soviet Union from the Urals into Siberia as well as the Ukraine, together with South African Whites and perhaps central South America. All other known areas of Asia, Africa, and the Caribbean region, including Mexico and possibly northern South America, are all low, with prevalence rates under 5 per 100,000 population. A number of nationwide prevalence studies in Europe provide evidence for geographic clustering of the disease, which is stable over time, but with evidence as well of diffusion over time.

MS death rates have, for the most part, been declining, while in many areas, prevalence rates have been increasing. This is explicable by better case ascertainment and longer survival, the latter providing more deaths in MS unrelated to the disease and, therefore, not listed as underlying-cause deaths from MS.

There is a female preponderance in incidence, prevalence, and mortality rates of about 1.5:1 (female : male). Annual incidence rates in high-risk areas are some 3–5 per 100,000 population, in medium-risk areas about 1 per 100,000, and in low-risk areas about 1 per 1,000,000.

All high- and medium-risk areas are among predominantly white populations: MS is the white man's burden. In America, blacks and Orientals, and possible American Indians, have much lower rates of MS than do Whites, but each group still demonstrates the geographic gradients found for Whites.

Aside from geography, age, sex, and race, risk factors for MS include high socioeconomic status and urbanization of pre-illness residence, at least in one U.S. Army series. No meteorologic correlate of geography is a risk factor for MS when latitude is controlled.

There is an increased familial frequency in MS, with sibs at least 6–8 times and parents 3–4 times more likely than the general population to develop the disease. Twin studies are inconclusive in terms of a genetic component, and I (J.F.K.) believe the familial excess reflects common environment more than common genes.

Migration studies indicate that, on the whole, migrants retain much of the risk of their birthplace. However, this risk is clearly *not* defined at birth: MS death rates for migrants born in one risk area and dying in another are intermediate between those characteristic of their birthplace and their death residence regardless of the direction of the move. Prevalence studies for migrants from high- to low-risk areas indicate the age of adolescence to be critical for risk retention: Those migrating beyond age 15 retain the MS risk of their birthplace; those migrating under age 15 acquire the lower risk of their new residence. Several low-to-high studies show that those migrating in childhood or adolescence do in fact increase their risk of MS, with age 11 apparently the minimum age of susceptibility.

These data may be consolidated into the following conclusions. (1) MS is a place-related disorder, (2) an acquired, exogenous, environmental disease (3) to which whites are especially prone. (4) Migration studies show that the risk of MS can be altered in either direction by moves into regions of appropriately differing MS frequency, and (5) this risk is ordinarily determined by one's location in early adolescence and, thus, (6) well before clinical onset. This is interpreted to mean that (7) the disease itself is acquired long before symptom onset, perhaps near the age of puberty for residents of high-risk areas, with then (8) a prolonged latent or "incubation" period during which one's residence is irrelevant to disease expression; and (9) with the likelihood that at least part of this latent period is one of lesion formation, because (10) on clinical grounds, symptoms occur only when there are "enough" plaques in the appropriate neural pathway. (11) The *simplest* explanation for all these points would be that MS is the result of an infectious agent that has a unique geographic distribution and an age-limited host susceptibility. If this were true, then either (12) MS, like polio, would have to be a much more widespread affection than clinical cases suggest in order to maintain itself in the populace, or (13) there would need to be a nonhuman reservoir (Kurtzke and Hyllested, 1988).

THE FAROE ISLANDS

General Features

The Faroes are a group of 18 major volcanic islands, 17 being inhabited, lying in the North Atlantic Ocean located at 7°W longitude and 62°N latitude. They were first settled by Vikings from western Norway around 825 A.D. The Faroes remained a possession of Norway until the Scandinavian Union of 1387 under Queen Margrethe I of Denmark. This union comprised Denmark, Norway, Sweden, much of Finland, Greenland, Iceland, the Faroes, and, for about a century, the Shetland–Orkneys. The Faroes were ruled as a province of Norway until 1536, when both territories became provinces of Denmark. When Norway became independent and joined with Sweden in 1814, Denmark retained the Faroes, in addition to Greenland and Iceland. The Faroes, or *Færø amt*, were a standard county (*amt*) of Denmark until 1948. The islands then achieved a semiindependent status, though remaining a part of the Kingdom of Denmark. The Faroese people have their own language (a development of Old Norse, and similar to Icelandic), literature, art, currency, stamps, parliament, and laws; however, for international affairs, and for most of their health and welfare services, they still depend on Denmark (Rutherford and Taylor, 1982; Young, 1979).

The islands' principal industries have been fishing and sheep raising (the most accepted translation of *Føroyar* is sheep islands). Only some 3% of the land area is habitable or arable. Trees were unknown until after World War I, when a small grove was planted in the capital, Tórshavn (meaning Thor's Harbor). The terrain is that of steep hills and fjords with only a thin layer of soil. Virtually all villages (*bygdir*) are clustered along the shores of the bays, fjords, and inlets. In 1986, the Faroes consisted of 120 *bygdir* within 50 parishes (*kommunur*) comprising seven districts (*sýslur*)—plus the capital (Fig. 1). However, there has since been some change in *kommunur*. Tórshavn, on the island of Streymoy, now has a population of over 14,000; the next largest town of Klaksvík on the island of Borðoy has some 5000 inhabitants.

In medieval times, the population of the Faroes probably did not exceed 4000 or so, but by 1900 their number had risen to 15,000 and they have continued to grow, reaching some 48,000 in 1990 (Danmarks Statistisk, 1982, 1990).

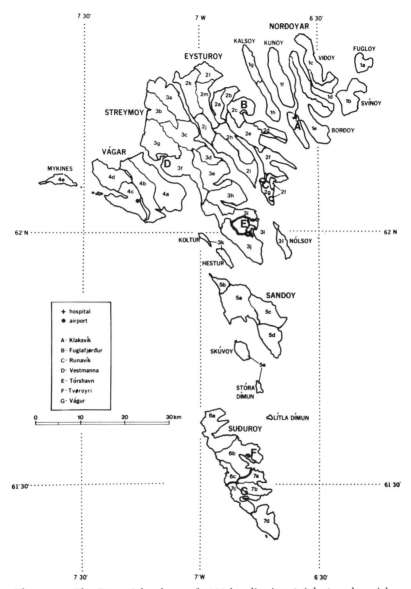

Figure 1 The Faroe Islands as of 1986 by districts (*sýslur*) and parishes (*kommunur*), the latter containing one or more villages (*bygdir*). Parishes are identified in Table III. Tórshavn Uttanb (3i) is now included partly in Tórshavn Bykommuna and partly in Argir. [Reproduced, with permission, from J. F. Kurtzke and K. Hyllested, 1986, Multiple sclerosis in the Faroe Islands. II. Clinical update, transmission, and the nature of MS, *Neurology* **36,** 308, fig. 1.]

Medical Facilities

Færø amt has, of course, been part of the Danish medical system. Its first hospital opened at Tórshavn in 1829. Both Klaksvík Hospital and Tvøroyri Hospital were established in 1904; there was a tuberculosis hospital near Tórshavn from 1908 to 1962. The State Psychiatric Hospital was opened in 1963 at Tórshavn. The first physician was assigned to the Faroes in 1584; the first official government surgeon (*Landkirurgen*) in 1842. In 1943, there were 17 physicians, 1 per about 1500 population, including 1 government physician (*Landslæge*), 8 hospital physicians, and 8 practitioners. In 1980, these numbers were 1, 40, and 20, respectively, equaling 1 per 700 population (Nielsen *et al.*, 1968; Danmarks Statistisk, 1982).

Since medieval times, medical care on the Faroes has been a charge of the Danish government. Danish medical statistics have been perhaps the most accurate and complete of any nation. Their routine hospital recordkeeping has long been outstanding, with each hospital reporting annual discharges by name and diagnosis to The (National) Health Service (*Sundhedsstyrelsen*). The country has had nationwide medical coverage provided by the entire state or the individual counties since 1921.

Faroese patients in need of specialized diagnosis and treatment are entitled to be sent to The National (Royal) Hospital (*Rigshospitalet*) in Copenhagen. Since 1929, this hospital has had a separate Neuromedical Department, although neurologic care was under the Medical Departments beforehand. Faroese are treated there under the "Greenland rules," which require complete assessment of all medical problems regardless of admitting diagnosis.

MULTIPLE SCLEROSIS IN THE FAROES

Case Ascertainment

Critical to our findings and interpretations is that we have found *all* cases of MS that have occurred among Faroese in the 20th century. Therefore, a detailed description of our methods is in order. Obviously, we are constrained by one fact: The person must have been seen medically and neurologic symptoms recorded. But two points argue for completeness: MS clinically is a disorder with repeated or progressive symptomatology over a considerable time, and medical care for Faroese, not constrained by financial factors, is of high quality and well documented.

In 1978–1979, all death certificates for the Faroes from 1900–1977 were searched for any mention of MS or related diagnoses (encephalomyelitis,

myelitis) on any location on the certificate. For every patient with MS whom we identified from any source and who had died, the diagnosis was recorded on the certificate. This is also true of the 1978–1990 deaths.

Hospital records on the Faroes to 1983 were reviewed three times, first from 1900 by a medical secretary, and then from 1920 by a nurse and a Faroese neurology resident, for diagnoses of MS and related diseases. Additionally, Kurtzke and Hyllested personally searched through the files of 1920–1950 for all three hospitals. *Rigshospitalet* records were surveyed twice for MS diagnoses from 1900 to 1983, with an additional review of the Neuromedical Department files. Haslev Hospital, an MS rehabilitation facility outside of Copenhagen, was also the target of a record review; furthermore, the complete hospital diagnosis files of *Sundhedsstyrelsen* were also surveyed, as were the National Disability Compensation files from 1921 to 1977, when this country-wide resource ceased and each county began to maintain its own proceedings.

In the 1940s, Hyllested (1956) performed an extensive nationwide survey of MS in Denmark, with questionnaries to all physicians and hospitals, including the Faroes, and starting with the nationwide MS survey of compensated cases from 1921 to 1933 by Gram (1934). Hyllested's survey led to the formation in 1947 of the Danish MS Registry, which he still heads. All neurologic departments of the Kingdom report any MS suspects to the Registry. The Registry also uses the National Patient and Death Registries. We have repeatedly to this date scanned these files for Faroese cases. In addition, Hyllested studied MS on the Faroes itself in 1957 and was part of the Faroes–Shetland–Ornkey project of 1961–1962 (Fog and Hyllested, 1966).

Furthermore, a special search was made of all 1960–1976 admissions to the three Faroese hospitals by a Faroese neurology resident for all patients with any neurologic signs or symptoms that could possibly reflect MS, regardless of actual diagnosis. This was to determine whether MS was not considered by physicians on the Faroes when it should have been. Upon our review, this yielded no cases even remotely suspicious of MS.

All neurologists at *Rigshospitalet*, and also the other Danish hospitals, have continued since 1975 to alert us to possible cases. On the Faroes, all physicians, and the general public as well, have been aware of our efforts as a result of presentations, radio and television broadcasts, and newspaper reports. An MS Club was founded on the Faroes in 1977, and we remain in close contact with its members.

The Faroes are a rather close-knit community, with knowledge of the health status of neighbors as well as distant relatives. Several friends of patients have on a number of occasions called our attention to possible cases. The cooperation of patients and families has been almost universal. Table I summarizes the means employed to ascertain prospective cases of MS and indicates those that are our current major methods in our continuing search. We have been on the Faroe Islands to examine patients and review resources almost every year since 1974, the last such visit being June 1991.

Case Definition

From whatever source a prospective case was ascertained, we then obtained all medical records from the Faroes and Denmark. We separately read all the charts, of which we each have complete copies. We then jointly examined neurologically each living patient, with special attention to onset dates and symptoms. Where patients had died, relatives were jointly interviewed for the neurologic history. Only after the diagnosis was established to our satisfaction following our case review and exam did we then seek family, travel, and other historical data.

Table I

Case Ascertainment for Faroese Multiple Sclerosis Patients

Faroese death certificates	1900–1977
Faroese hospital (3) records	1900–[a]
Rigshospitalet (RH) records	1900–1983
Sundhedsstyrelsen National Patient Registry	1921–[a]
Disability Compensation Board records	1921–1977
Neuromed Department (RH) records	1929–[a]
All physicians, hospitals in Denmark	1944–1949
Danish MS Registry files	1947–[a]
Faroes survey (by K.H.)	1957
Faroes–Shetland survey (by K.H.)	1960–1962
Neurologic symptoms Faroe hospitals	1960–1976
Haslev Hospital records	1965–[b]
Faroes patients, relatives, friends	1974–[b]
Danish neurologists	1975–[b]
Faroese physicians	1975–[b]
Faroese Multiple Sclerosis Club	1977–[a]
National Registry Causes of Death	1978–[b]

[a] Principal ongoing resources.
[b] Other ongoing resources.

Diagnoses were uniformly agreed to among us all. When a definitive answer could not be given, we reexamined the patient one or more times in succeeding years until the questions could be clarified. We used the diagnostic criteria of the Schumacher Panel (Schumacher *et al.*, 1965) for (clinically definite) MS, except that age at onset was not a bar to inclusion. All patients but two had also been seen by other neurologists, and most of them by some of the most senior neurologists of Denmark. Almost every patient at *Rigshospitalet* had state-of-the-art diagnostic tests appropriate to the time of examination, to include cerebrospinal fluid (oligoclonal bands, IgG), evoked potentials, contrast computed tomographic scanning, and recently in some, magnetic resonance imaging. In most instances, the appropriate abnormalities were found, though we did not rely on laboratory findings for our clinical diagnoses. So far we have autopsy confirmation in two cases: one negative among our "not-MS" suspects, and one positive in the MS group.

Multiple Sclerosis Grouping and Inclusion Criteria

Our study is limited to native-born Faroese with clinical MS. Several non-Faroese MS patients living on the Faroes were ascertained; they are classed as Group D patients.

However, we did need a means of categorizing the Faroese according to their residence history. Throughout the century, many Faroese had spent variable periods living overseas, mostly in Denmark, for educational or occupational purposes. Since the purpose was to investigate the occurrence of MS on the Faroe Islands among Faroese, we then had to exclude those who had been living "too long" off the islands. The reason was so that we could avoid attributing their disease to events on the Faroes when, in actuality, they had acquired the illness elsewhere. Faroese who never left the islands and those who had lived virtually all of their lives overseas posed no problem; the former are included, the latter are not. Because we already knew that MS rarely occurred in Faroese before the 1940s, and because we also knew that overseas travel had not been uncommon, then we could properly conclude that "short" periods overseas were irrelevant to the development of MS.

The question then was what was "short" and "long." For the former, we had decided in 1974 that a total of less than 2 years overseas before clinical onset was highly unlikely to be relevant to the development of MS. We called those patients Group B, having defined Group A as those never living off the Faroes.

Our original 1974 criterion for "long" residence was a total of 3 years or more overseas in a high-risk area before clinical onset. From our findings (see later), two corollaries later arose: only residence intervals from age 11 to onset were relevant, and for exclusion as Group C the "long" intervals must include 2 years of nearly continuous overseas residence (Table II).

Because, as will be seen, MS has been established on the islands, we have recently modified the criteria for a new Group B' (included) and Group C' (excluded) for those exposed to the Faroese MS environment. We thought it necessary in the latter instance to be more restrictive than previously. This decision of 1990 led to our reclassification of all Faroese MS; however, no prior Group C patient needed reassignment on this basis.

The Excluded "Migrant" Multiple Sclerosis

In our basic paper of 1979, we reported the occurrence of MS in 25 native-born resident Faroese up to 1977 as well as the presence of 4 (excluded) Faroese with prolonged foreign residence—and 5 Danish-born patients

Table II

Criteria for Grouping of Cases, Native-Born Faroese Multiple Sclerosis Patients

Original Criteria for Resident Faroese MS	
Acceptance	
1. Group A:	Not off Faroes in high-risk area before CNMS onset, excluding short (≤1 mo) vacations.
2. Group B:	Live off Faroes in high-risk area for a total of <2 years before CNMS onset.
Corollary:	Only period age 11 to CNMS onset relevant.
Rejection	
1. Group C:	Live off Faroes in high-risk area for a total of 3+ years before CNMS onset.
Corollary:	Overseas period of at least 2 years continuous or nearly so: "major period."
Corollary:	Short intervals before "major period" excluded.
	Revised Criteria for Resident Faroese MS
Acceptance	
1. Group A and B:	As previously stated.
2. Group B':	Live off Faroes in high risk area 2+ years before CNMS onset *but* not meet exclusions.
Rejection	
1. Group C':	Foreign residence 6+ years, continuous or nearly so, age 11 to CNMS onset; *or* foreign residence 4+ years, continuous or nearly so, beginning age 11–14; *or* foreign residence period age 11 to CNMS onset equals or exceeds Faroese residence period.
2. Group C:	As previously stated for those age 11 by 1943 or for later residents of no-risk regions of Faroes.

CNMS, clinical neurologic MS.

living on the Faroes (Kurtzke and Hyllested, 1979). In our last published update of the series, there were 41 cases of MS among Faroese who had had clinical onset in this century up to 1986: 32 resident cases and 9 (excluded) Group C (Kurtzke and Hyllested, 1986, 1987).

By the time of the latter papers, we had realized that the Group C cases were not merely "rejects" but, in fact, comprised a group of migrants from a low-risk MS area (Faroes) to a high-risk area (Denmark). So too, were the Group B patients, and their comparison gave us a twofold opportunity: to test whether our inclusion/exclusion criteria appeared correct and, should that be the case, to define the characteristics of the acquisition of MS by yet another low-to-high migrant series.

In Fig. 2, the original Group B and C cases are distributed according to durations from birth to clinical onset, with the times and lengths of foreign

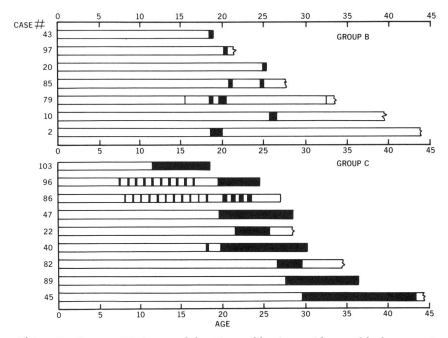

Figure 2   Faroese MS. Ages and durations of foreign residences (black segment of bars) for Group B and C patients. MS clinical onset is the terminus of each patient's bar with its origin at birth; a straight terminal line indicates symptom onset while overseas; a jagged line while in the Faroes. Numbers identify the patients in Kurtzke and Hyllested (1986). [Reproduced, with permission, from J. F. Kurtzke and K. Hyllested, 1986, Multiple sclerosis in the Faroe Islands. II. Clinical update, transmission, and the nature of MS, *Neurology* **36,** 312, fig. 2]

residence specified. Most of the stays began in the second or third decades of life.

In Group B, foreign residence durations summed to between 0.4 and 1.5 years. In Group C, the range was 3–14 years, and six of the nine patients had onset of MS while off the Faroes; their calendar years of onset were 1917–1977. For Group C, ignoring the short childhood visits for two of them, all of the patients had at least 2 years of their stay between age 11 and 31, and 2 years was the minimum period for such stays.

The foreign residences for Group B showed little consistency in time to MS onset. On the other hand, the Group C residences clustered within 10 years or so before clinical onset, and the mean duration from start of major foreign residence to MS onset was 8.6 years. Subtracting 2 years for "exposure" from each patient's overseas residence interval gave an "incubation" period of 6.4 years (range 3–13). The 2-year exposure period was continuous in all patients but one.

From these Group C cases, we concluded that residence in a high-risk MS area by a susceptible, but virgin (as to MS), population for a period of 2 years from age 11+ could result in clinical MS, which would begin after a further period of some 6 years. Additionally, residence need not have been maintained in that interval in the endemic area (patients 22, 82, 45, and 86). In other words, the 6 years is a true incubation or latent interval between disease acquisition and symptom onset.

On the other hand, such residences of less then 2 years duration were not followed by MS in any consistent fashion, and we concluded that residence in a high-risk area for appreciably less than 2 years is not sufficient to acquire MS, even for a previously unexposed individual of the appropriate age.

As of June 1991, the migrant series (Group C, C') comprises 12 cases; the aforementioned findings and conclusions remain unaltered (Kurtzke *et al.*, 1991, in preparation).

The Published Resident Series

By 1986 we ascertained 32 cases of MS among native-born resident Faroese: 25 Group A and 7 Group B. Figure 3 details these patients plus those of Group C according to calendar year of clinical onset. It is clear that, by onset year, Group C differs from the others, but Group B does indeed belong with Group A. Clinical aspects of these cases have been published (Kurtzke and Hyllested, 1979, 1986, 1987, 1988).

As to the resident series, not one single patient had clinical onset of MS in this century until July 1943. Then there were 16 patients with onset in 1943–1949, and another 16 with onset in 1950–1973. To 1987, no further

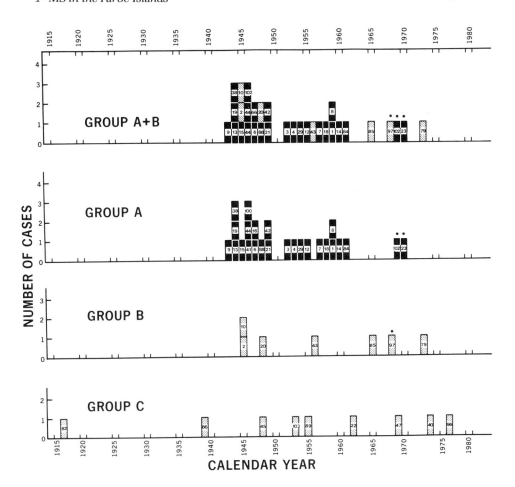

Figure 3 MS in native-born Faroese according to calendar year of clinical onset. Group A (never off Faroes before onset) and B (off Faroes less than 2 years total before onset) comprise the resident Faroese MS series. The Group C (off Faroes 3+ years total before onset) cases are the nonresident series. Numbers identify the patients as cited in Kurtzke and Hyllested (1979, 1986). Asterisks indicate the three patients of postwar birth. [Reproduced, with permission, from J. F. Kurtzke and K. Hyllested, 1988, Validity of the epidemics of multiple sclerosis in the Faroe Islands, *Neuroepidemiology* **7**, 202, fig. 2.]

patients were identified among the native resident Faroese, a period of 14 years in which the population had increased from some 40,000 to over 45,000.

Now, 16 cases occurring in a 7-year interval in a populace of less than 30,000—and none before—does not require a statistical test to meet anyone's criteria for an epidemic. Despite that, formal testing did demonstrate that the appearance at that time was of very high statistical significance (Kurtzke and Hyllested, 1988).

Incidence Rates

The annual incidence rates per 100,000 population showed an early and dramatic rise and fall, followed by two irregular and consecutively lower secondary peaks (Fig. 4, top). The rate exceeded 10 per 100,000 in 1945. The first question was whether this was a single epidemic with a very irregular tail or the incidence rate curve in fact reflected separate epidemics.

Our first approach to that query was to divide the series into two parts, based on whether in 1943 patients were prepubertal or postpubertal. The reason was the evidence considered earlier, that elsewhere MS is in fact acquired between age 10 and 15; and puberty is one obvious and datable event in that interval (Fig. 4, middle).

When this was done, it was clear not only that the first incidence rate peak (Epidemic I) was attributable to the patients postpubertal in 1943, but also that there did still appear to be two later, discrete peaks for the prepubertal patients (Epidemics II and III) (Kurtzke and Hyllested, 1986).

We then referred to the Group C (migrant) experience, where 2 years of

---

Figure 4 MS in native resident Faroese. Annual incidence rates per 100,000 population calculated as 3-year centered moving averages. Top: Rates for patients born after World War II (dashed line) separated from remainder. Middle: Rates for patients postpubertal in 1943 (Epidemic I) versus those then prepubertal or unborn (Epidemics II and III). I, primary epidemic; II, early (secondary) series; III, late (tertiary) series. Bottom: Rates for three epidemics defined by calendar year when patients attained age 11: by 1943 (Epidemic I) or later (Epidemics II and III). Sex and calendar year when patients of Epidemics II and III were age 11 are noted for middle and bottom figures [Modified from J. F. Kurtzke and K. Hyllested, 1986, Multiple sclerosis in the Faroe Islands. II. Clinical update, transmission, and the nature of MS, *Neurology* **36,** figs. 4 and 5; and from J. F. Kurtzke and K. Hyllested, 1987, Multiple sclerosis in the Faroe Islands. III. An alternative assessment of the three epidemics, *Acta Neurol. Scand.* **76,** 324, fig. 5, copyright 1987 Munksgaard International Publishers Ltd., Copenhagen, Denmark.]

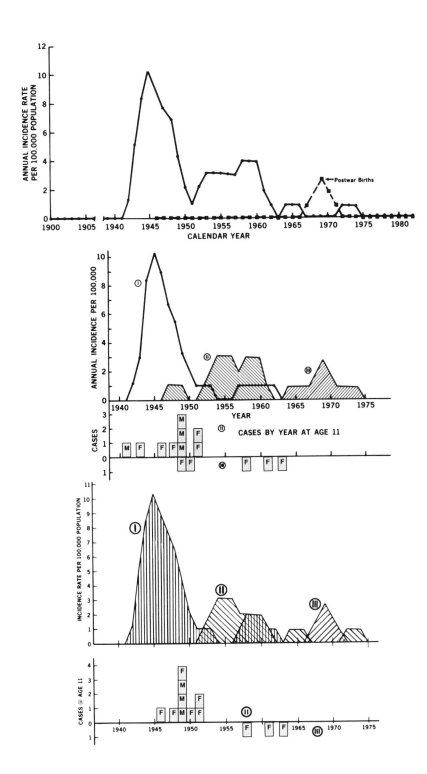

exposure from age 11 were shown to be required to acquire the disease (see earlier). The postpubertal (Epidemic I) resident patients had their age at clinical onset at an average of age 31; the migrants at age 30. Incubation for those residents averaged 5 years from 1943; that for migrants was 6 years. Therefore, we concluded that the residents also required 2 years of exposure before 1943 and, thus, that this exposure was in 1941–1942. In addition, this exposure would then have begun when the patients were at least 11 years of age—also like the migrants.

We then posed the question whether or not in actuality MS was acquired by all Faroese only if they were at least 11 years of age at first exposure, and only if the exposure was then for at least 2 years duration. Hence, we reassessed the Faroese experience by reclassifying the resident series according to the calendar time when the patients had attained age 11. For reasons discussed later, we extended this time from 1941 to 1943 for acceptance as Epidemic I patients, but from that point on, time when age 11 was attained was to determine membership in any later epidemics.

Three Epidemics: An Alternative View

Figure 5 represents the native resident Faroese MS series, showing for all patients their life experience relative to MS from their calendar year of birth (y-axis) to their calendar year of clinical onset (x-axis). It is clear that the series does divide into three parts based on the time when the patients were age 11: by 1941 (1943), or later. Definition either by the pubertal separation or that age 11 was highly significant ($p < 0.001$) in terms of the existence of three discrete groups or epidemics (Kurtzke and Hyllested, 1987).

Epidemic I then comprised all patients age 11+ in 1941 plus those age 11 by 1943 ($n = 20$). Epidemic I accounted for all cases contributing to the

---

Figure 5   MS in native resident Faroese defined by PMSA acquisition in 1943 or at age 13 if later, all after two years exposure (from 1941 or from age 11 if later). Identification of each patient by calendar time when age 11, whether by 1941 or later, and by time of clinical onset. Each patient is represented by a bar, and the number at the end of each bar identifies the patient in Kurtzke and Hyllested (1979, 1986, 1987). The thin portion of each bar represents time and ages for each patient *before* exposure to the primary MS affection (PMSA; see text), and the 2 years of cross-hatching represents the period of PMSA exposure, following which (heavy portion of the bar) the patient is affected but neurologically asymptomatic (the incubation period). Solid circle at terminus of each bar represents time and age of clinical onset. Open circle at the origin of the lower bars represents time of birth for patients born after 1938. The y-axis defines the number of years by each year from 1941 at which time each patient attained age 11, with the calendar

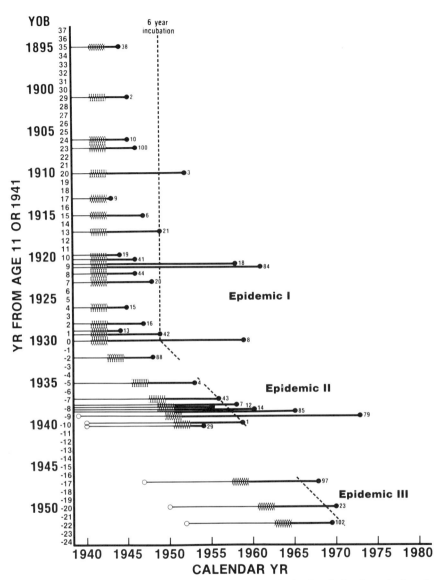

years reflecting their year of birth (YOB) also identified. The dashed vertical and oblique line represents the end of a 6-year incubation period from time of acquisition of PMSA after a 2-year exposure. [Reproduced, with permission, from J. F. Kurtzke and K. Hyllested, 1987, Multiple sclerosis in the Faroe Islands. III. An alternative assessment of the three epidemics, *Acta Neurol. Scand.* **76,** 323, fig. 4. Copyright 1987 Munksgaard International Publishers Ltd., Copenhagen, Denmark.]

first MS incidence rate peak (Fig. 4, bottom). Epidemic II comprised the patients age 11 in 1946–1951; they accounted for the second incidence rate peak ($n = 9$). Epidemic III comprised the patients age 11 in 1958–1963; they accounted for the third incidence rate peak ($n = 3$). This last will need updating; we now have six patients for Epidemic III as of June 1991 (Kurtzke *et al.*, 1991, in preparation).

Age at clinical onset was similar, near age 21, for Epidemics II and III patients, but both were significantly lower than age at onset for Epidemic I cases, age 30. Incubation averaged some 6 years from 1943 or age 13, whichever came later (5, 8, and 6 years for Epidemics I, II, and III, respectively) (Kurtzke and Hyllested, 1987).

The existence of the epidemics on the Faroes has been contested by C. M. Poser *et al.* (1988) and Poser and Hibberd (1988); our detailed response has been published (Kurtzke and Hyllested, 1988).

MULTIPLE SCLEROSIS: INTRODUCTION AND TRANSMISSION

To this date, we have sought any event on the Faroes Islands that took place in 1941–1942 (and later) to explain the appearance of Epidemic I (and later). All we can find is the British occupation.

The British Occupation

As detailed elsewhere (Kurtzke and Hyllested, 1986, 1987), British troops occupied the Faroes from April 1940 to September 1945. At its peak, some 7000 troops were stationed there; throughout 1941–1944, there were at least 1500.

There is no question but that the British occupation was temporally related to the appearance of MS on the Faroes. By our criteria, the exposure period for the Faroese then age 11+ was the 1941 and 1942 interval. In that time, as stated, there were 1500+ British troops stationed on the islands. At least a similar number were also present throughout 1943 and 1944, and thus patients attaining age 11 by 1943 would also have been subject to the British influence. In fact, this added but one patient to the series defined by age 11+ in 1941.

We have searched assiduously for any feature other than the British occupation that could explain the epidemic(s) of MS. We have found nothing that coincided temporally with the appearance of MS—not to mention its abrupt and widespread appearance *and* disappearance. Were there no further relationship found between troops and the Faroese MS patients, we would still be forced to assign a causative role for the latter to the former.

However, the occupation showed not only this strong temporal relationship, but also demonstrated a very strong spatial relationship—for all the patients, regardless of epidemic. In most instances, troops were billeted *within* the Faroese villages. In the major occupation sites, enlisted men (Other Ranks) were quartered in Nissen huts constructed in the "in-mark"—the land area just inshore of the houses—and thus within meters of Faroese homes. Elsewhere, enlisted men were billeted in Faroese houses themselves, as were in general all officers at most occupation sites.

Therefore, we took as the most stringent—and unbiased—measure of contact with British troops the answer to the question whether or not villages with MS patients were the villages with troops quartered there. The answer was clearly in the affirmative with high statistical significance—not only for the patients of Epidemic I, but also for those of Epidemics II and III (Fig. 6). Because we wished also to use a population count, and because the 1943 population was available only by parish, we made similar assessment of the relationship between troops and MS by parish of residence (Table III): the results were similarly positive and again with high statistical significance ($p < 0.01$). An overview of the *populations* of the places where patients lived versus those where troops were stationed is provided in Table IV. The odds ratio of 41 (nearly twice as strong as the relation between heavy cigarette smoking and bronchogenic carcinoma) had a χ^2 value of over 14,000. In 1943, the Faroes comprised 44 parishes, including Tórshavn. There were 16 parishes where any patient with MS lived, containing two-thirds of the 1943 Faroese population, and 96% of the residents of those 16 parishes were living where troops were billeted. Conversely, in the 20 parishes with occupation troops during the war, where three-quarters of the Faroese then lived, 85% of the Faroese of these 20 parishes were living where MS patients, of any epidemic, resided. There was, however, one-quarter of the population living in 21 parishes with neither troops nor MS; we concluded that this proportion of the resident Faroese was not exposed to, and did not acquire, any illness from the British troops and, thus, was not at risk for MS then or later.

Transmission of Multiple Sclerosis and Models Thereof

In our minds, there is no question but that the British troops introduced MS into the Faroe Islands during the occupation of World War II. As already discussed, 1500 asymptomatic British troops, the number present in 1941, must have been sufficient to introduce the disease. Furthermore,

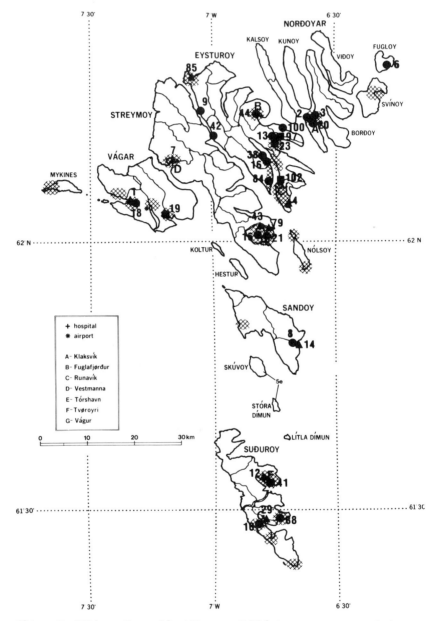

Figure 6 MS in native resident Faroese. British troop encampments (cross-hatched areas) and residence by village of Faroese MS patients in 1943 or at age 11 if then younger, for the three epidemics defined by time when patients attained age 11: Epidemic 1 (circles), Epidemic II (triangles), and Epidemic III

even though it ended in 1945, the occupation was responsible for all three epidemics. The only possible explanations are that the British brought either a persistent toxin or a transmissible infection. A toxin cannot explain three epidemics; therefore, the cause of MS in the Faroes is a transmissible infection.

Because the cumulative risk of MS is such that there would occur only three clinical cases over the lifetime of 2000 healthy British troops (Kurtzke, 1978), a much larger proportion of troops must have been both affected and also able to transmit the disease to Faroese. This means that "MS" exists in a transmissible but neurologically asymptomatic form. It is this state that we have defined as the primary MS affection (PMSA). Like asymptomatic poliomyelitis, PMSA must be common within a population in which clinical MS occurs, but it must only rarely ever produce the neurologic symptoms to which we append the label of clinical neurologic MS (CNMS). The same observation holds for the Faroese: Many more must have been affected (and transmissible) than is evident from the cases comprising the three epidemics. The cases of each successive separate Faroese epidemic must then be the numerator for a ratio whose denominator is a successive separate population cohort of Faroese at risk. How, though, can there be three separate population cohorts over time within the continuum that comprises the total resident population?

We start with the thesis that we are dealing with an infectious agent that was transmitted from the British troops to residents of the Faroes, and among the Faroese in the form of three successive epidemics. To account for the sequence—British to Epidemic I to Epidemic II to Epidemic III—we need three successive population cohorts of Faroese, each cohort being at risk at the appropriate time, duration, and number to account for its respective epidemic. The calendar time for each cohort must encompass the time when the patients were exposed: 1941–1944 for Epidemic I, time age 11 for Epidemics II and III. Duration of exposure, we have said, needs to be 2 years. Duration for transmissibility must therefore be at least 2 years. Over time, this transmissible stage must be intermittent, with nontransmissible intervals separating the transmissible

---

(squares). Numbers identify patients as cited in Kurtzke and Hyllestad (1979, 1986, 1987). Occupation sites where *no* Faroese lived are (1) the southern end of Nólsoy Island, (2) part of the hatched area on the west coast of Vágar Island, (3) the Vágar airport, (4) the western coast of Sandoy Island, and (5) the southern end of Suðuroy Island. [Reproduced, with permission, from J. F. Kurtzke and K. Hyllestad, 1987, Multiple sclerosis in the Faroe Islands. III. An alternative assessment of the three epidemics, *Acta Neurol. Scand.* **76,** 327, fig. 8. Copyright 1987 Munksgaard International Ltd., Copenhagen, Denmark.]

Table III

Faroe Islands Parishes and Populations[a]

Map key	Parish	Population	Troops	MS by epidemic		
				I	II	III
1a	Fugloy	241	−	6[b]	—	—
1b	Svínoy	230	+	—	—	—
1c+d	Viðoyar	483	−	—	—	—
1e	Klaksvík	1805	+	2, 3, 20	—	—
1f	Kunoy	197	−	—	—	—
1g	Mikladalur	139	−	—	—	—
1h	Húsar	176	−	—	—	—
2a+b	Oyndarfjørdur	400	−	—	—	—
2c	Fuglafjørdur	902	+	44	—	—
2d	Leirvík	443	−[c]	100	—	—
2e	Gøta	584	+	13	—	23, 97
2f+g	Nes	1438	+	—	4	102
2h+i	Sjógv	1000	+	16, 38, 84	—	—
2j+k	Eidi	933	+	9, 42	85	—
2l+m	Funningur	434	+	—	—	—
3a	Haldarsvík	427	−	—	—	—
3b	Saksun	42	−	—	—	—
3c+d	Hvalvík	452	−	—	—	—
3e	Kollafjørdur	439	−	—	—	—
3f	Kvívík	494	−	—	—	—
3g	Vestmanna	844	+	—	7	—
3h	Kaldbak	118	−	—	—	—
3i	Tórshavn Uttanb.	322	−	—	—	—
3j	Kirkjubøur	114	−	—	—	—
3k	Hestur	131	−	—	—	—
3l	Nólsoy	258	+	—	—	—
4a	Sandavágur	570	+	—	—	—
4b	Midvágur	666	+	19	—	—
4c	Sørvágur	755	+	18	1	—
4d	Bøur	113	+	—	—	—
4e	Mykines	144	+	—	—	—
5a	Sandur	645	+[d]	—	—	—
5b	Skopun	376	−	—	—	—
5c	Skálavík	217	−	—	—	—
5d	Húsavík	240	−	8[e]	14	—
5e	Skúvoy	168	−	—	—	—
6a	Hvalbøur	819	−	—	—	—
6b	Frodbøur	1939	+	41	12	—
6c	Fámjin	228	−	—	—	—
7a	Hov	209	−	—	—	—
7b	Porkeri	436	+	88	—	—
7c	Vágur	1406	+	10	29	—

continues

Table III *Continued*

Map key	Parish	Population	Troops	MS by epidemic		
				I	II	III
7d	Sunnbøur	775	+	—	—	—
E	Tórshavn	3440	+	15, 21	43, 79	—

[a] 1943 population with presence of British troop encampments and residence of MS patients identified by case number in Kurtzke and Hyllested (1979, 1986, 1987).

[b] Patient in Tórshavn 1/2 year each year throughout the war.

[c] Pier for ferry Eysturoy to Klasksvík used throughout the war.

[d] Troops not stationed in any village.

[e] Claimed extensive contact with troops in his village throughout the war.

[Reproduced, with permission, from J. F. Kurtzke and K. Hyllested, 1988, Validity of the epidemics of multiple sclerosis in the Faroe Islands, *Neuroepidemiology* 7, 213, Table IX.]

Table IV

Faroese Population Distribution[a]

Parishes with troops	Population proportions		
	Parishes with:		
	MS+	MS−	Total
+	0.617	0.104	0.721
−	0.035	0.243	0.279
Total	0.652	0.348	1.000
			($N = 26,232$)

Odds ratio = 41.190

[Modified from J. F. Kurtzke and K. Hyllested, 1987, Multiple Sclerosis in the Faroe Islands. III. An alternative assessment of the three epidemics, *Acta Neurol. Scand.* 76, 328, table IIX. Copyright 1987 Munksgaard International Publishers Ltd., Copenhagen, Denmark.]

Note: (65%) 2/3 population lived in 16 parishes with MS, of whom 96% lived where troops were stationed. (72%) 3/4 population lived in 20 parishes with troops, of whom 85% lived where any MS lived. (24%) 1/4 lived in 21 parishes with neither troops nor MS.

[a] 1943 distribution by parishes with and without MS residents and with and without British troops stationed.

periods responsible for each epidemic. This intermittency can be explained either by taking an arbitrary period of years for transmissibility (for which we have no basis) or by taking an arbitrary age limit beyond which transmissibility would not occur. Lastly, we need an appropriate number. If 1500 young Britons were sufficient to bring in the disease, then 1500 young Faroese would, we can conclude, also be sufficient to carry it on. But this does not give us any minimum. Because the chronic interchange in location of Danes and Faroese over the years did not result in MS on the Faroes, then a "small" number of persons affected is not sufficient for transmissibility. We have in our models, therefore, arbitrarily taken figures of both 1000 and 500 persons as being the minimum number required for effective transmission.

Now the proportion of the total population cohort at risk that was actually affected with our disease among the British or the Faroese is obviously unknown (but need be appreciable), although it clearly cannot exceed 100% of the population groups considered. In our models, then, we used the total actual population numbers, whether for British or Faroese. As to the epidemics, however, the potential Faroese population first affected by the British would not be the total 26,232 living there in 1943 but, rather, the 0.757 of 26,232 who geographically were actually at risk (see earlier). If, as expected, the ages of the clinically symptomatic MS patients define the age limits of susceptibility to this disease, then this number is reduced further to 0.757 those age 13–47 in 1943. Their illness would have been acquired in the 2 prior years 1941 and 1942. We must also add 0.757 those age 11 and 12 in 1943 since they too were exposed to the troops for two years, and thus the total cohort of Faroese affected by the British during World War II would have been 0.757 the Faroese population cohort age 13–49 in 1945, or nearly 11,000 persons. This is called the F1 cohort (F for Faroese, 1 for first), which was exposed (F1 E) to the British for 2 years before being affected (F1 A) with PMSA. Age 49 is then the upper limit for the affected Faroese, and the F1 A cohort was at its maximum size in 1945 with the British departure. That proportion of the F1 A cohort that was transmissible is labeled F1 A+T, and it transmitted PMSA to the next population cohort. This second cohort of Faroese exposed to the F1 A+T cohort is called F2 E and comprised (0.757 of the total) Faroese attaining age 11 each year from 1945 to the end of F1 A+T input.

Were the entire age 13–49 F1 A cohort thereafter transmissible, it would have provided continuing transmission of PMSA well into the 21st century. And this, like a toxin, cannot explain two later epidemics. Thus, not all the F1 A cohort could be F1 A+T.

Now, if we know anything about MS, it is that clinically affected patients do *not* transmit this disease. Therefore, the PMSA-affected would not likely be able to transmit PMSA once they were at (or near) the age of symptom onset in CNMS. Taking age 27 as the average age of clinical onset, then the transmissibility period should be limited to no more than the time age 13–26 or so. Therefore, we defined the F1 A+T cohort—and its successors for F2 and F3—as comprising the F1 A subjects age 13–26. In this manner, the F1 A+T cohort, numbering near 5500 persons in 1945, would have decreased each year by the loss of those then attaining age 27, and it would have disappeared totally by the end of 1958, with cutoffs about a year earlier, respectively, for each of the previously mentioned transmission minima of 500 and 1000 persons.

Recalling the need for 2 years of exposure to PMSA, the F2 E cohort ceased its growth 2 years before the effective end of F1 A+T, and, with the end of F1 A+T, it became the F2 A+T cohort for transmission to the F3 cohort.

Similar considerations define F3 E and the F3 A+T cohort for an F4 E cohort (Figure 7).

The Fourth Epidemic

One point seemed apparent by 1986: The Faroe Islands were behaving as a geographic isolate insofar as MS was concerned. Despite the markedly increasing traffic with other lands and a progressively growing influx of tourists over the years, no evidence whatsoever indicated that the disease was later brought into the islands at any time after the war. The second and third epidemics, respectively, could logically only be attributed to transmission from the affected populace of the first epidemic, who had acquired the disease from the British, and then from that second cohort (including the second epidemic) to the cohort containing the third epidemic.

The major question in 1986 was whether or not the disease had by that time disappeared from the islands. We then had had no case of CNMS since 1973, and the calculated risk estimates for CNMS were progressively lower as we went from Epidemic I to III (Kurtzke and Hyllested, 1987). Even adding the three new cases more recently included in Epidemic III did not negate that decline, because our population denominators had in fact been undercounted by retaining the World War II fraction for the proportion living within the 23 parishes of 1943 where MS cases or British troops resided; this proportion too has grown, from the 76% of the 1943 population to some 84% at present.

This was the situation in 1986: MS was not endemic on the islands. But were the epidemics over or was there to be an Epidemic IV?

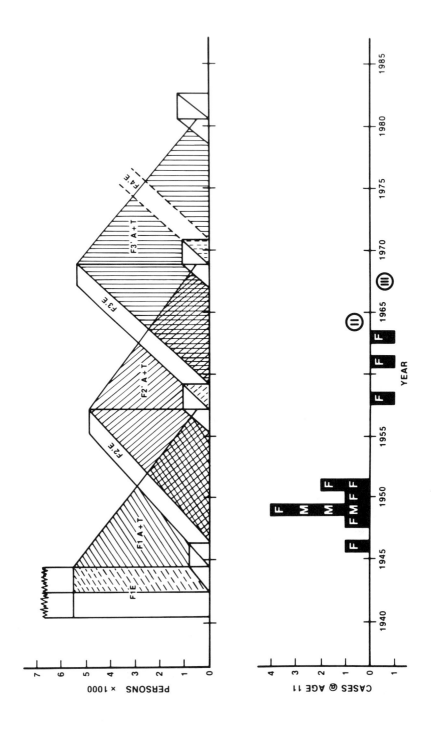

By 1990, however, the situation had clearly changed. We may recall that we have kept the islands under continued surveillance for later cases of MS since 1974 in both Denmark and the Faroes and, with our own visits and examinations, almost every year in that interval. In May 1990, we documented five cases of clinically definite MS with onset 1982–1989.

As of June 1991, we have ascertained a total of seven patients with CNMS with onset 1984–1989 who had attained exposure age in 1973–1980. Therefore, we clearly do have Epidemic IV on the Faroes. One might say that this epidemic was predicted by our transmission models, and that it therefore provides a validation of not only our models, but also our views as to the nature of MS (Kurtzke *et al.*, 1991, in preparation).

THE NATURE OF MULTIPLE SCLEROSIS

It may perhaps now be clear why we are so intrigued with the Faroese saga and why we persist in our efforts there. To end this chapter, we shall present our thinking as of this date in the form of two summary lists, without further elaboration.

Figure 7   MS transmission in Faroese, Model 1 alternate (time when patients age 11). The population cohort of Faroese first *exposed* to the primary MS affection (PMSA) from British troops in 1941–1942 is called the F1 E cohort (open vertical block above upper x-axis). Only that portion of this cohort age 11–45 in 1941 was to become *affected* with PMSA (F1 A), to which are added the newly exposed Faroese age 11 or 12 in 1943 (broken diagonal-lined block). Only the affected under age 27 are *transmissible* (F1 A+T), and this cohort is thus maximal in size in 1945 with the British departure, decreasing each year thereafter by those then attaining age 27 until the time that it reaches the arbitrary minimum number below which transmission will not occur (upward diagonal-lined area ending at heavy vertical line). Transmission is to F2 E, the next cohort of Faroese, comprising those attaining age 11 each year from 1945 (the first open rising parallelogram); after 2 years, this becomes the F2 A cohort, maximal in size when F1 A+T ceases input. The F2 A+T cohort (downward diagonal-lined area) in like manner transmits PMSA to F3 E, which becomes the F3 A+T cohort (vertical-lined area) for transmission to F4 E. Sex and times when CNMS patients of Epidemics II or III attained age 11 are noted above or below the lower x-axis. [Reproduced, with permission, from J. F. Kurtzke and K. Hyllested, 1987, Multiple sclerosis in the Faroe Islands. III. An alternative assessment of the three epidemics, *Acta Neurol. Scand.* **76,** 337, appendix, fig. 2. Copyright 1987 Munksgaard International Publishers, Ltd., Copenhagen, Denmark.]

Multiple Sclerosis in the Faroes: Summation

1. CNMS did not exist among resident Faroese before 1943.
2. PMSA was introduced into the Faroes by British troops in 1941–1944.
3. This introduction led to a point source epidemic of CNMS (Epidemic I) within the cohort of Faroese who were affected with PMSA (F1 A) after 2 years of exposure (F1 E).
4. Only Faroese age 11–45 at onset of exposure were affected with CNMS and, hence, PMSA.
5. Those affected Faroese age 13–26 (F1 A+T) transmitted PMSA to a second cohort of Faroese (F2 E), comprising those attaining age 11 while F1 A+T existed.
6. The F2 A+T cohort included the CNMS of Epidemic II and was the source of PMSA in the F3 cohort with its Epidemic III of CNMS.
7. The F3 A+T cohort similarly has produced Epidemic IV within the F4 cohort with PMSA.

The Nature of Multiple Sclerosis from the Faroese Experience

1. There is a specific, widespread but unidentified infection we call the primary multiple sclerosis affection, or PMSA.
2. PMSA is a persistent infection transmitted person to person.
3. A small proportion of persons with PMSA will later develop clinical neurologic multiple sclerosis, or CNMS.
4. Prolonged exposure (2 years) is needed to acquire PMSA.
5. PMSA acquisition follows first adequate exposure.
6. Susceptibility to PMSA is limited to age 11–45 at start of exposure.
7. Transmissibility of PMSA is limited to a period under the usual age of CNMS onset.
8. Existence of PMSA can now only be inferred from existence of CNMS.

References

Allison, R. S. (1963). Some neurological aspects of medical geography. *Proc. R. Soc. Med.* **56,** 71–76.

Danmarks Statistisk. (1982, 1990). Statistisk Årbog 1982, 1990. København.

Fog, M., and Hyllested, K. (1966). Prevelance of disseminated sclerosis in the Faroes, the Orkneys and Shetland. *Acta Neurol. Scand.* **42**(suppl. 19), 9–11.

Gram, H. C. (1934). Den disseminerede skleroses forekomst i Danmark. *Ugeskr. Laeg.* **96,** 823–825.

Hyllested, K. (1956). "Disseminated Sclerosis in Denmark. Prevalence and Geographical Distribution." DBK, Copenhagen.

Kurtzke, J. F. (1977). Multiple sclerosis from an epidemiological viewpoint. *In* "Multiple Sclerosis. A Critical Conspectus" (E. J. Field, ed.), pp. 83–142. MTP Press, Lancaster, England.

Kurtzke, J. F. (1978). The risk of multiple sclerosis in Denmark. *Acta Neurol. Scand.* **57**, 141–150.

Kurtzke, J. F. (1980a). Epidemiologic contributions to multiple sclerosis—An overview. *Neurology* **30**(pt. 2), 61–79.

Kurtzke, J. F. (1980b). Multiple sclerosis—An overview. *In* "Clinical Neuroepidemiology" (F. C. Rose, ed.), pp. 170–195. Pitman Medical Publishing, London.

Kurtzke, J. F. (1983). Epidemiology of multiple sclerosis. *In* "Multiple Sclerosis. Pathology, Diagnosis, and Management" (J. F. Hallpike, C. W. M. Adams, and W. W. Tourtellotte, eds.), pp. 47–95. Chapman and Hall, London.

Kurtzke, J. F. (1985). Epidemiology of multiple sclerosis. *In* "Handbook of Clinical Neurology. Vol. 3, rev. Deyelinating Diseases" (P. J. Vinken, G. W. Bruyn, and H. L. Klawans, eds.), pp. 259–287. Elsevier, Amsterdam.

Kurtzke, J. F. (1988). Risk factors, course, and prognosis of multiple sclerosis. *In* "Virology and Immunology in Multiple Sclerosis: Rationale for Therapy" (C. L. Cazzullo, D. Caputo, A. Ghezzi, and M. Zaffaroni, eds.), pp. 87–109. Springer-Verlag, Berlin.

Kurtzke, J. F. (in press). The epidemiology of multiple sclerosis. *In* "Multiple Sclerosis," 2nd ed. (J. F. Hallpike, C. W. M. Adams, W. W. Tourtellotte, eds.). Chapman and Hall, London.

Kurtzke, J. F., and Hyllested, K. (1975). Multiple sclerosis: An epidemic disease in the Færoes. *Trans. Am. Neurol. Assoc.* **100**, 213–215.

Kurtzke, J. F., and Hyllested, K. (1979). Multiple sclerosis in the Faroe Islands: I. Clinical and epidemiological features. *Ann. Neurol.* **5**, 6–21.

Kurtzke, J. F., and Hyllested, K. (1986). Multiple sclerosis in the Faroe Islands. II. Clinical update, transmission, and the nature of MS. *Neurology* **36**, 307–328.

Kurtzke, J. F., and Hyllested, K. (1987). Multiple sclerosis in the Faroe Islands. III. An alternative assessment of the three epidemics. *Acta Neurol. Scand.* **76**, 317–339.

Kurtzke, J. F., and Hyllested, K. (1988). Validity of the epidemics of multiple sclerosis in the Faroe Islands. *Neuroepidemiology* **7**, 190–227.

Kurtzke, J. F., Hyllested, K., and Heltberg, A. (1991). Multiple sclerosis in the Faroes: Epidemic IV. *Ann. Neurol.* **30**, 313 (abstr.).

Nielsen, N., Skautrup, P., Mathiassen, T., and Rammussen, J. (eds.). (1968). "J. P. Trap. Danmark, Femte Udgave. Færøerne. Bind. XIII," pp. 133–149. GEC GADS Forlag, Copenhagen.

Poser, C. M., and Hibberd, P. L. (1988). Analysis of the 'epidemic' of multiple sclerosis in the Faroe Islands. II. Biostatistical aspects. *Neuroepidemiology* **7**, 181–189.

Poser, C. M., Hibberd, P. L., Benedikz, J., *et al.* (1988). Analysis of the 'epidemic' of multiple sclerosis in the Faroe Islands. I. Clinical and epidemiological aspects. *Neuroepidemiology* **7**, 168–180.

Rutherford, G. K., and Taylor, C. E. B. (1982). Location and general description. *In* "The Physical Environment of the Faroe Islands," pp. 3–12. Dr. W. Junk Publisher, The Hague.

Schumacher, G. A., Beebe, G. W., Kibler, R. F., *et al.* (1965). Problems of experimental trials of therapy in multiple sclerosis: Report by the Panel on the Evaluation of Experimental Trials of Therapy in Multiple Sclerosis. *Ann. N.Y. Acad. Sci.* **122**, 552–568.

Sutherland, J. M. (1956). Observations on the prevalence of multiple sclerosis in northern Scotland. *Brain* **79**, 635–654.

Young, G. V. C. (1979). "From the Vikings to the Reformation. A Chronicle of the Faroe Islands up to 1538." Shearwater Press, Douglas, Isle of Man, United Kingdom.

2

The Epidemiology of
Alzheimer's Disease in
the People's Republic of China

Elena Yu • Robert Katzman • William T. Liu • Ming-Yuan Zhang
Zheng-Yu Wang • Paul Levy • David Salmon • Guang-Ya Qu

In a number of countries, Alzheimer's disease (AD) is one of the major disorders of the elderly, ranking in importance only behind heart disease, stroke, and cancer. However, earlier reports from China had indicated that AD and dementia were relatively uncommon (Chen *et al.*, 1987, Li *et al.*, 1988). Because the identification of a community in which AD is infrequent might lead to the identification of important risk factors, as has been the case in cardiovascular and cancer epidemiology, a symposium was organized and held in China in 1984 to explore the issue of possible research collaborations. A 16-member team of professors and researchers[1] from the United States interested in the general topic of aging and mental health was invited by China to present their research at two symposia: one held at the Beijing Medical College and the other at the Shanghai Institute of Mental Health. As a result of these two symposia, three institutions joined forces to study cognitive impairment and dementia among older adults in Shanghai: the Shanghai Institute of Mental Health at the Shanghai Mental Health Center in China, the Pacific/Asian American Mental Health Center (formerly housed at the University of Illinois at Chicago and now at California State University at San Marcos), and the Alzheimer Disease Research Center (ADRC) at the University of California at San Diego.

---

[1]The team was led by William T. Liu and Ethel Shanas. Members of the group included (in alphabetic order): Jacob Brody, (the late) Ernest Gruenberg, Mary Harper, Robert Katzman, Nancy Katzman, (the late) Soon D. Koh, Tong-He Koh, Lester Steve Perlman, Harold Sheppard, Conrad Taueber, Dorothy Taueber, Gary Tischler, Mrs. Tischler, Salley Yeh, and Elena Yu.

The Shanghai Survey of Alzheimer's Disease and Dementia (SSADD) was launched in 1987 after 3 years of preparatory work that included travel to China by the U.S. team, affirmation of research objectives, discussion of sampling design and fieldwork management, solicitation of cooperation from appropriate levels of the Shanghai bureaucracy, formation of an external advisory committee, selection and construction of research instruments, translation of selected U.S. instruments, modification of culture-inappropriate items, back-translations, revisions, pretests in both Chicago ($n = 159$) and Shanghai ($n = 150$), a pilot study in Beijing, and the training of interviewers and data-entry perons.

The purpose of this paper is to report the results of the 1987–1989 collaborative study SSADD and to present our working hypothesis concerning the risk factors for dementia and AD in Chinese populations.

BACKGROUND

Between 1958 and 1981, a total of 61 psychiatric epidemiologic investigations were conducted in the People's Republic of China (Lin and Kleinman, 1981). None focused specifically on the elderly population, although data on types of disorders were sometimes presented by age. Between 1981 and 1986, two large-scale psychiatric epidemiologic studies were conducted in China in collaboration with researchers from Europe and the United States (Yang and Lu, 1988; Wang *et al.*, 1992). They were important because they marked the beginning of Chinese psychiatrists' experience with the use of semistructured [in the case of the Present State Examination (PSE)] and fully structured [in the case of the Diagnostic Interview Schedule (DIS)] *diagnostic* instruments developed in the West in community-based research of mental disorders in China.

To our knowledge, the first survey of cognitive disorders in the elderly in the People's Republic of China was conducted in 1981 using an unspecified interview method (Kuang and Zhao, 1984). That study was followed in 1983–1984 by the first large-scale survey of mental disorders among elderly Chinese using the PSE (Chen *et al.*, 1987). The latter, conducted in the West-City District of Beijing, showed strikingly low rates of Alzheimer-type dementia (0.38% of the 8740 surveyed who were 60 years or older), multiinfarct dementia (0.43%), and other organic brain syndrome (0.46%). The absence of detailed information on the criteria adopted by the interviewers in determining caseness makes it difficult to evaluate the reported rates. More recent data collected in the same district, by the same team of investigators but using the Mini-Mental State Examination continue to report low rates of dementia and AD (Li *et al.*, 1988). The SSADD uncovered different rates when they used a probability sample of Chinese elderly in a classic epidemiologic two-stage screening procedure and applied diagnostic criteria for dementia and AD similar to those used in the United States. Preliminary figures on the prevalence of dementia and AD have been published in a recent paper (Zhang *et al.*, 1990). In what follows, we report additional findings on the epidemiology of dementia and AD that have not yet been reported and speculate on some possible hypotheses that might account for the findings. We begin by briefly describing our research methodology.

METHODS

Age 55 years and older is China's definition of *the* elderly population. Jing-An, 1 of 12 districts that made up the City of Shanghai, was designated as the research site for SSADD. As of 1985, it had a population of 497,657.

Sample

A random sample of adults 55 years and older, chosen to represent Jing-An and at the same time yield a nearly equal number of persons ($n = 1500$) in each of three age groups (55–64 years, 65–74 years, and 75 years and older) was drawn by means of a variation of the single-stage cluster sampling method developed by Paul Levy (Levy *et al.*, 1989). Using the Household Registry System managed by Shanghai's Bureau of Public Security, neighborhoods (*jumin xiaozu*), each consisting of 10–100 households, were randomly selected such that in one-third of all neighborhoods everyone 55-years or older was to be included in the survey, in another third only those 65 years and older were selected, and in the last third those 75 years and older were targeted (Table I).

Table I
Age Groups Sampled in Each Cluster Type

Cluster type	Age Group		
	55–64 years old	65–74 years old	75+ years old
1	1961	1384	669
2	—	1348	634
3	—	—	638

Completion Rate

A total of 6634 persons were identified as being eligible for our study by means of the preceding sampling procedure. Of these, 79.5% ($n = 5271$) completed the interview. Reasons for not completing the remaining 1363 targeted interviews were (a) prolonged travel or vacation outside of the city or district ($n = 1202$ persons, or 88.2% of 1363), (b) change of address to another district ($n = 85$ persons, or 6.2%), (c) death ($n = 34$ persons, or 2.5%), (d) serious illness ($n = 18$ persons, or 1.3%), (e) refusal ($n = 21$ persons, or 1.5%), and (f) "empty household registers" ($n = 3$ persons, or 0.2%).

Data Collection

The SSADD involved three phases of data collection, of which the first two phases are pertinent to the objectives of this paper.

Phase 1: Screening

Screening was conducted from January to May of 1987. The purpose of the Phase 1 survey was to identify individuals with likely cognitive impairment who would undergo an intensive clinical evaluation in Phase 2. Of the 5271 respondents who completed the Phase 1 interview, 5055 were able to take the Chinese Mini-Mental State Examination (CMMSE)—the screening instrument used to detect likely symptoms of cognitive impairment. Direct testing could not be performed on the remaining 216 respondents (4.1%) because of the following reasons: 73.6% were deaf, 7.9% were visually impaired, 7.9% were paralyzed and had trouble speaking, 1.4% were seriously ill, 3.2% were diagnosed as having psychosis, and 1.8% showed advanced symptoms of dementia. The remaining nine persons (4.2%) had other reasons.

Only those who scored *above* a broadly defined cutoff score (of 20 or below on the CMMSE) were interviewed directly—immediately following the screening, using a structured sociological interview schedule covering a variety of topics. These included self-reported health status; health practices; Acitvities of Daily Living (ADL), Center for Epidemiologic Studies Depression (CES-D) Scale; social interaction; leisure activities; and lay conceptions of dementia and depression. For those who scored below the predefined cutoff score, the caregiver closest to the sampled elderly was interviewed about the elderly's health and his or her perceptions of dementia symptoms. We also sought information on the caregiver.

The interviewers were psychiatrists and psychiatric nurses who had more than 2 years of clinical experience, either at the Shanghai Mental

Health Center or at the Jing-An Psychiatric Hospital, and had undergone a 14-day training session, including videotapes of such interviews and practice live interviews with Chinese-speaking U.S. members (W.T.L. and E.Y.) of this research collaboration.

Completed interview booklets submitted by the interviewers were checked by two independent teams of supervisors. The first team provided visual inspections of protocols to detect missed questions or erroneous skipping of questions, illegible codes, and illogical, inconsistent, or ambiguous responses. The second team performed computer-automated controls on the quality of interviewing by applying a PC data entry and validation software developed in the United States specifically for this study.

Phase 2: Case Identification

Case identification, conducted from December 1987 to March 1988, involved a clinical evaluation of all persons who were screened "positive" (i.e., below the prespecified cutoff score) for symptoms of dementia during Phase 1 ($n = 510$), and a random sample of 5% of the 5055 elderly, stratified by age and sex, who were screened "negative" (i.e., above the cutoff) based on their performance on the CMMSE ($n = 241$).

Of the 751 respondents targeted for reevaluation in Phase 2 of the study, exactly 643 were able to complete the full battery of diagnostic procedures and clinical evaluations required as part of the present study. For the remaining 108 persons, evaluation was either not conducted or not completed because of the following reasons: 51 persons died before all the evaluation procedures could be completed in Phase 2, and 57 persons refused to continue to be interviewed, moved out of Shanghai, were traveling, or had been admitted to a hospital. Clinical diagnoses of these 108 persons were arrived at using the best judgment based on all the procedures completed up to the time they died or when contact was severed and including, in some cases, additional information based on visits to their homes and interviews with key informants on the respondent.

The clinical evaluation was conducted by a team of experienced clinical psychiatrists recruited from among those who had attended an intensive month-long seminar on AD developed specifically for this research project. They had worked at the Shanghai Center for an average of 10 years and had received at least 3 months of intensive training in neurology. Visits were also made to China by the U.S. investigators. Many of the forms and tests used were Chinese adaptations of forms and tests administered regularly to patients at the ADRC at the University of California at San Diego (under Robert Katzman's directorship). Instruction and experience in their use involved two-way exchange of investigators between Shanghai and San Diego. The psychiatrists who participated in the clinical evaluation for the purpose of case identification during Phase 2 were not informed of any of the respondents' CMMSE test scores in the Phase 1 survey. They compiled the case history of each respondent by paying close attention to the evidence of dementia symptomatology as well as by probing for history of major illnesses that might result in cognitive and functional impairments.

Diagnostic Criteria and Procedures

The differential diagnosis of AD was based on the National Institute of Neurological and Communicative Disorders and Stroke (NINCDS)–Alzheimer's Disease and Related Disorders Association (ADRDA) criteria (McKhann *et al.*, 1984). The diagnosis of vascular dementia utilized the Hachinski score (Hachinski *et al.*, 1974) and *Diagnostic and Statistical Manual of Mental Disorders*, 3rd ed. (DSM-III; American Psychiatric Association, 1980), criteria. Diagnoses of depression or other psychiatric disorders was based on the psychiatric interview, the Diagnostic Interview Schedule (DIS) Depression Section, and the CES-D Scale. Other causes of dementia were sought based on the medical history and clinical examination. Although we have specific clinical diagnoses on all patients made by the initial examiner, we have chosen to group subjects with a diagnosis of dementia other than AD or vascular dementia as "other dementia."

For the diagnosis of dementia, we required that there be changes on one or more of the functional scales as well as below education-determined cutoff[2] performance on two or more cognitive tests. Our purpose was to ensure that we were diagnosing a dementing illness and not longstanding retardation or poor test performance. To meet explicitly the DSM-III criteria that the cognitive impairment be sufficient to interfere with social or occupational performance, the examiners obtained responses to a dementia history questionnaire, the Pfeffer functional questionnaire (Pfeffer *et al.*, 1982), and the ADL scale. The diagnostic procedures also included physical and neurological examinations and psychiatric interviews. The Hasegawa (1974) dementia rating scale was also administered. Neuropsychological tests included Chinese versions of the Fuld Object Memory Test (Fuld, 1981), the Verbal Fluency

---

[2]The cutoff scores for the CMMSE are 17 or less for those with no education (formal or informal), 20 or less for those with elementary or less education, and 24 or less for those with education beyond the elementary school level. These cutoff scores were determined by the best sensitivity and specificity distribution of the CMMSE (obtained in Phase 1) against the clinical diagnosis of dementia (obtained in Phase 2).

Test (Butters *et al.*, 1987), Block Design (Wechsler, 1974), and Digit Span (Wechester Adult Intelligence Scale-Revised Chinese version by Gong, 1982). These neuropsychological tests were selected for several reasons. First, these tests provided a relatively brief examination that assessed several cognitive domains including memory (Fuld Object Memory Test), attention (Digit Span), language (Verbal Fluency Test), and visuospatial and constructional abilities (Block Design). Second, these tests appeared to be less influenced by cultural and educational factors than other neuropsychological tests that were piloted in earlier subject samples. Finally, the selected tests were relatively easy to administer and perform and there was good subject compliance on these tests during pilot testing.

The clinical diagnosis of dementia was made independently by three psychiatrists. If the clinicians' diagnoses were not concordant, a research diagnosis was reached after thorough discussion by the research team. In turn, these diagnoses and the pertinent data on which they were based were reviewed by a senior clinical neurologist (Robert Katzman) and an experienced neuropsychologist (David Salmon). Nineteen diagnoses required a second round of consultation, due mostly to the "bouncing" cognitive state of the elderly respondents across time and measures.

RESULTS

Altogether, we diagnosed 159 cases of dementia, using DSM-III criteria for dementia, and exactly 64.7% of these met the NINCDS–ADRDA clinical criteria for the diagnosis of AD. Twenty-seven percent were classified as vascular dementia, including multiinfarct dementia. Besides these two major kinds of dementia, a few cases of dementia apparently associated with parkinsonism, head injury, physical illness, alcholism, or depression were found in our clinical evaluations.

Table II shows the prevalence of dementia by age and gender weighted by the age and gender distribution of older adults in the Jing-An District of Shanghai. The prevalence of dementia is estimated at 2.57% in persons 55 years and older, 4.61% in those 65 years and older, 12.33% in those 75 years and older, and 24.29% in the oldest age group, 85 years and older—roughly doubling every 10 years. The prevalence of dementia is greater in females than in males: 3.67% versus 1.21% in the age group 55 years and older, 6.62% versus 1.97% in the group 65 years and older, 16.51% versus 5.81% in the group 75 years and older, and 27.30% versus 17.24% in the "oldest old" group of 85 years and older. One notes with interest that the female : male sex ratio in dementia is smallest at the

Table II

Prevalence of Dementia and Alzheimer's Disease, in Percentage, by Age Groups and Gender[a]

Age group (years)	Female	Male	Both sexes	Female : male ratio
Dementia				
55 years and older	3.67	1.21	2.57	3.03
65 years and older	6.62	1.97	4.61	3.36
75 years and older	16.51	5.81	12.33	2.84
85 years and older	27.30	17.24	24.29	1.58
Alzheimer's disease				
55 years and older	2.15	0.62	1.46	3.47
65 years and older	4.03	1.26	2.83	3.20
75 years and older	10.57	4.08	8.04	2.59
85 years and older	22.18	13.79	19.67	1.61

[a] Weighted to represent Jing-An District, Shanghai, People's Republic of China.

oldest cumulative age group and becomes increasingly larger at younger cumulative age groups, where it hovers around 3:1.

Table II also shows the prevalence of AD in Shanghai. In the age group 55 years and older, the prevalence is 1.46%, increasing to 2.83% in the group 65 years and older, 8.04% in the group 75 years and older, 19.67% in the group 85 years and older. The sex ratios in AD by age are quite similar to those found for the diagnosis of dementia, as one would expect.

Table III shows the age-specific prevalence of dementia stratified by age, education, and gender. In both men and women, the prevalence varies with the level of education. At any given age-and-education category, proportionally more women than men had dementia. The effect of gender on the prevalence of dementia was especially apparent among the respondents aged 65–74 and 75–84. Why this is so is far from clear.

To determine whether or not the age, gender, and education effects were independent factors, a stratified analysis using the Mantel–Haenzel test and a logistic regression analysis were employed. These analyses showed that the effects of age, gender (female), and lack of education are each highly significant ($p < 0.001$) and independently related to the prevalence of dementia.

The age-specific prevalence for AD is shown in Table IV. No male AD cases in the 55–64-year-old age group were uncovered in the survey. The prevalence is low for the age group 65–74 years old and begins to increase only for the age group 75–84 years old. With the oldest old group, the

Table III

Age-Specific Prevalence of Dementia by Age, Education, and Gender[a]

Age group Education	Female	Male	Both sexes	Female : male ratio
55–64 years old	0.46	0.47	0.47	0.98
Middle high+[b]	0.68	0.48	0.55	1.42
Elementary[c]	0.56	0.53	0.55	1.06
No education	—	—	—	—
65–74 years old	1.42	0.40	0.96	3.55
Middle high+[b]	0.38	—	0.13	—
Elementary[c]	0.68	1.00	0.84	0.68
No education	2.65	—	2.23	—
75–84 years old	14.33	4.36	10.27	3.29
Middle high+[b]	3.96	3.37	3.57	1.18
Elementary[c]	12.64	3.16	8.04	4.00
No education	18.07	9.18	16.39	1.97
85 years and older	27.30	17.24	24.29	1.58
Middle high+[b]	18.75	12.00	15.14	1.56
Elementary[c]	22.22	18.75	20.99	1.19
No education	32.27	23.53	30.87	1.37

[a] Weighted to represent Jing-An Shanghai, People's Republic of China.

[b] Defined as having more than 6 years of education (i.e., equivalent to middle high school education or higher).

[c] Defined as having had 6 years or less of education, including informal education such as *si-shu* or *saumangban*.

— indicates that no case was found in the survey.

most dramatic difference is between males without any education (8.16%) and those with no more than 6 years of education (1.37%). In the oldest old group (85 years and older), the most dramatic break in prevalence is observed between those who had middle-school or higher education (8%) and those who had only an elementary education or less (18.75%). For women, age by age, the largest difference in AD prevalence is between the elementary education and the no education group. The sex ratios by education show inconsistent results, particularly for the two oldest age groups.

All in all, 96 of the 159 clinically diagnosed dementia cases died as of September 30, 1991, an astonishing mortality rate over a 4-year period. This finding indicates that if we are to do longitudinal studies of dementia and AD, follow-ups should be conducted at fairly short intervals, possibly less than 1 year apart.

Table IV
Age-Specific Prevalence of Alzheimer's Disease by Age, Education, and Gender[a]

Age group Education	Female	Male	Both sexes	Female : male ratio
55–64 years old	0.12	—	0.06	—
Middle high+[b]	—	—	—	—
Elementary[c]	0.28	—	0.17	—
No education	—	—	—	—
65–74 years old	0.59	0.10	0.37	5.9
Middle high+[b]	0.38	—	0.13	—
Elementary[c]	0.23	0.25	0.24	0.92
No education	1.02	—	0.86	—
75–84 years old	8.22	2.86	6.04	2.87
Middle high+[b]	0.99	1.92	1.60	0.52
Elementary[c]	4.27	1.37	2.86	3.12
No education	12.38	8.16	11.58	1.52
85 years and older	22.18	13.79	19.67	1.61
Middle high+[b]	12.50	8.00	10.09	1.56
Elementary[c]	14.81	18.75	16.21	0.79
No education	28.61	17.65	26.85	1.62

[a] Weighted to represent Jing-An Shanghai, People's Republic of China.
[b] Defined as having more than 6 years of education (i.e., equivalent to middle high school education or higher).
[c] Defined as having had 6 years or less education, including informal education such as *si-shu* or *saumangban*.
— indicated that no case was found in the survey.

DISCUSSION

Questions have been raised as to whether the low rates of dementia and AD reported earlier for China by other investigators are indeed accurate or merely a function of the different research methodologies and assessment criteria used in China compared to those of other countries. In the Shanghai survey, we have used the same screening procedure and identical clinical evaluation methods as those used at the ADRC in the United States. We found that age and sex are significantly associated with dementia and AD, a finding consistent with studies reported outside of China.

An unexpected finding in the Shanghai survey, however, is that lack of education is a major risk factor for, and a major determinant of, the prevalence of dementia. The importance of low education in the interpretation of mental status test data in community surveys has been addressed by a number of investigators (Gurland, 1981; Folstein *et al.*, 1985). There has been a concern as to whether low as well as no education is a confounder or lack of education actually increases prevalence of demen-tia. Our data indicate that there is indeed increased prevalence of demen-tia associated with lack of education. Similar results have been obtained in recent community surveys by Rocca *et al.* (1990) in Italy and Evans *et al.* (1989) in East Boston.

Although it is possible that low or no education is a surrogate for the lifelong effects of illiteracy or for some sort of deprivation (e.g., nutrition or other socioeconomic factors) acting early in life, we hypothesize that it is likely that the biological basis of education as a risk factor may be quite different from that of other risk factors and may in fact be due to a difference in *brain reserve.* Now, strong evidence indicates that the degree of dementia in AD is a function of the *loss of synapses* (Hamos *et al.*, 1989; DeKosky and Scheff, 1990). For example, Terry *et al.* (1991) found that a high correlation of midfrontal and inferior parietal synapse density, measured with an antibody to synaptophysin (Masliah *et al.*, 1989), corre-lates with the score on a mental status test with a correlation coefficient of 0.74. Also, cases with a number of neuritic plaques typical of AD without cognitive changes during life have higher-than-normal brain weights and numbers of large neurons, suggesting that the neuronal reserve protected those individuals from manifesting the clinical signs of dementia. If lack of education or other difficulties in early development or throughout life led to a lower reserve of synapses, or to a reduction in the ability to "repair" synapses damaged by an injury of some sort, then there might be an earlier expression of symptoms if AD were developing. Because of the steep age dependence of dementia and AD, an onset of clinical symp-toms 3 years earlier in the course of AD would give rise to more than a 50% increase in prevalence among persons in their 80s.

Gender has been found to be a risk factor for AD by a number of investigators (Jorm *et al.*, 1987; Katzman *et al.*, 1989). The effect of gender on the prevalence of dementia and AD was especially apparent among the elderly in the Shanghai survey. For historical reasons, the age group that was 65 years and older in 1987 had vastly different opportunities to receive education compared to those younger than 65 years (see Appen-dix). In addition to this age difference in educational opportunities, there is also a differential access by sex. Whereas the 75-year-olds or older persons were born no later than 1912 (during the reign just before and including that of the "Last Emperor" in the Ching Dynasty), the 65–74-year-olds were born after Sun Yat Sen's establishment of the Republic in 1911. The questioning of women's roles in family and society, the need to give women formal education opportunities, and the recommendation to modify Chinese verbal communication from formal classical language into the more understandable vernacular form were openly debated in

China in what is now called the May 4th Movement of 1919, which continued until 1921. That era marked a turning point in Chinese history in general and Chinese women's history in particular—especially in large cities like Beijing and Shanghai. Thus, persons who were 65–69 years old specifically (and, therefore, born during 1918–1922) were the beneficiaries of the May 4th Movement in that society's attitudes toward education for the masses, and, in particular, the *educability* of women had begun to change significantly. Likewise, the age group that was 70 years and older in 1987 shared some of the societal advantages that the 65–69-year-old group had when they were young because of the sequence of events that developed in China since 1911, which made it possible for a larger number of persons to have an education. Under these circumstances, however, it is also possible that the gender gap in education actually widened when education was within the reach of the commoners compared to an earlier era where men and women outside of the gentry class were almost equally likely to be uneducated because the school system was simply not developed for the commoners. If so, this may explain why the sex differences in educational attainment are greater when modern school systems were developing in China—precisely because large segments of the female population still did not have the opportunities to receive education when the males did. The Shanghai survey suggests that the key to a better understanding of the prevalence of dementia is to do incidence studies. When designing incidence surveys, we will also need to be able to assess *literacy* rather than just ask questions about the educational level of the elderly. The method of education and the educational system in modern China varied tremendously by time and place so that literacy and lower levels of education (under 6 years) may *not* be highly associated, particularly for older adults. An old Chinese could be literate but not educated (i.e., not have had formal education). We have not yet developed a test in Chinese that can provide graded levels of literacy and that would systematically allow us to measure declines in cognitive functioning, an early marker for dementia.

Because prevalence is a function of incidence times duration, from an epidemiologic viewpoint, the observed prevalence of dementia in Shanghai is most likely a function of differential incidence, by literacy, of dementia and AD, rather than a function of the longer duration from onset to death for the illiterate compared to the literate. This is because it is quite unlikely that the less educated in China have better health care after onset of the disease or live longer than the better educated. On the contrary, sociological data tend to suggest just the opposite. Earlier onset of dementia and AD in the illiterate compared to the literate could account for the expected higher incidence of the disease in our uneducated group.

From the preceding inference about the important role of incidence in contributing to the observed prevalence of dementia, a number of questions come to mind immediately.

1. Is the effect of education on the prevalence and incidence of dementia *an artifact of the use of the CMMSE?*

2. Is the effect of education on the prevalence of dementia due to differences in *later-life cognitive activities* or to the educational process per se in early adulthood?

3. Is the effect of education on the prevalence and incidence of dementia primarily due to the *effect of primary education* or the lack thereof in early childhood?

4. Is the effect of education on the prevalence of dementia *a surrogate for other childhood deprivations* (besides lack of education) or for deprivations throughout the life course?

5. Is the lack of education simply a *surrogate of occupational and/ or environmental exposures?* Or does lack of education increase *host susceptibility (possibly due to loss of synapses)* in the face of exposure to AD-causing agent(s)—whatever it or these may be?

6. Is lack of education a proxy measure of *lower social class?* Or is lack of education a *comorbid factor* rather than an etiologic agent?

7. What roles do certain events (e.g., head injury) or *unattended chronic diseases* (e.g., diabetes, hypertension, stroke, other small blood-vessel damages over a lifetime) play in the development of AD and dementia?

8. Knowing as we do now that these events or diseases are also risk factors for dementia and AD, how are they *moderated by literacy?* Does the lack of education make it harder to develop new synapses once the damage has occurred, thereby increasing the risk for dementia and AD through irreparable loss of synapses and neurons?

Given the findings we have presented, the question also arises as to whether the incidence of AD is constant throughout China or might there be communities where the rates are different from those reported for Jing-An, Shanghai. For example, might a study of a rural community outside of Shanghai, where the number of persons who are uneducated are even *higher* than those found for the city of Shanghai, be informative in increasing our understanding of the etiology and course of AD and dementia? The epidemiologic study conducted in Italy by Rocca *et al.* (1990) suggests that rural rates for dementia might actually be higher than urban rates.

Another important epidemiologic study design issue is the following: In future longitudinal studies of dementia and AD, should we not use a different sampling scheme (e.g., sampling by education or literacy levels instead of *just* oversampling by age alone)? We believe there is value in doing such a study because it would allow us to examine a potentially high-risk population (low-educated persons) compared to a low-risk population (highly educated persons), if indeed lack of education is a major risk factor for dementia and AD. Likewise, future longitudinal or prospective studies should capture a younger age group of adults who are in the preretirement stage of their life, if we are to understand the effects of education on a persons' cognitive development and decline. By conducting our study in China, we have shed light on the ethnic and racial differences of dementia and AD between China and the United States. From the perspective of epidemiology, it is essential that the distribution of the disease by geography be explored as well within China.

In what follows, we propose an explanatory model as a possible working hypothesis to guide our future research. The ideas were first suggested by one of us (W.T.L.).

The significance of *lack of* education in the course of developing dementia or AD lies in the fact that symbolic communication through the written language is a powerful stimulus that can operate in one's mind in the absence of direct contacts. The written words are helpful aids to short-term as well as long-term memory recall. Even after an event or experience is forgotten, a literate person can return to it symbolically through the written language. Thus, being able to read and write enables the literate to make "mental notes" of experiences and feelings of things *past and present.* Illiteracy makes it impossible to record the experiences of life itself beyond what the mind can remember at a given point in time; it also probably generates a special kind of "selective nonperception" of one's surroundings because of the absence of written words to describe what is perceived. Because the human mind is constantly bombarded with events, the amount of information that an illiterate person can register without the aid of characters is inevitably limited in clarity, quantity, volume, and time span. Thus, we suspect that illiteracy makes it necessary to depend on *direct* sense perceptions to stimulate the brain, especially when the experiences and feelings of living are constantly interrupted over the short term because the illiterate is incapable of communicating through the written language. Could this have any influence on the stimulation of synapses in the brain? If so, it is logical to assume that illiteracy drastically reduces the mind's ability to solve complex problems that require several sequential stages precisely because the character symbols required to register multiple events may not exist for the illiterates, or the structure of events stored in one's memory can easily become fuzzy with no lasting record to check its completeness or accuracy and, hence, no chance for memory validation? Do the illiterate habitually register events and experiences—if they must be remembered for reasons of survival—in terms of the actual physical appearance of the objects themselves (i.e., through sensual communication rather than symbolic communication with written characters)? A mind that is not accustomed to solving complex and sequential problems may be encouraged to avoid remembering these tasks when presented with situations requiring memory retention. Might this not have consequences on the development of synapses in the brain? The cumulative and continuous lack of stimulation that is associated with illiteracy could possibly have adverse biological impact on brain reserve or perhaps induce the loss of synapses. Might it be possible that the illiterate have less practice with short-term interrupted recalls than the educated—and over a lifetime of 65 years or longer, might not such inability to register mental notes with characters serve as a promoting agent of AD in the presence of a risk factor for dementia? Or, might it be that psychosocial conditioning as a result of prolonged deprivation of symbolic character stimulation—associated with one's occupation throughout life—deprives the brain of its ability to develop fully its capacity for short-term interrupted recalls, a major marker for cognitive impairment and dementia of the Alzheimer type? Other things being equal, illiterate people in pre-1949 China probably had to rely heavily on others for their jobs, and they probably had jobs that were monotonous, repetitive, mentally unrewarding, and perhaps even hazardous to their physical and mental health. Thus, illiteracy most likely impacted the illiterates' life courses and occupational careers. In addition, might this possibly have biological consequences in the memory functions of, and synapse development in, the brain?

In regard to other risk factors, genetic factors are certainly of major importance (Farrer *et al.*, 1989; Heston *et al.*, 1981; Mohs *et al.*, 1987; Mortimer, 1990). Down's syndrome patients almost invariably develop neuritic plaques containing β-amyloid and neurifibrillary tangles past the age of 40 (Burger and Vogel, 1973). In some families, an autosomal dominant form of AD with early onset (before age 55) has been found to be associated with a familial Alzheimer's disease (FAD) gene located near the centomere of chromosome 21 (St. George-Hyslop *et al.*, 1987), although other families, typically with onset of symptoms at a somewhat later age, do not carry this gene locus but may have a FAD gene on chromosome 19 (Roses *et al.*, 1990). Thus, even the genetic studies indicate heterogeneous factors predisposing to AD, a supposition consistent with the finding that concordance of AD in identical twins has been reported variously between 50 and 75%, never 100% (Jarvik *et al.*, 1980; Cook *et al.*, 1981). Mortimer (1990) has calculated the attributable risk due to a family history of a first-degree relative with the disease at about 26%.

Recent findings have drawn attention to head trauma (Amaducci *et al.*, 1986; French *et al.*, 1985; Heyman *et al.*, 1984) and myocardial infarct (Aronson *et al.*, 1990) as important environmental factors for AD. Graves *et al.* (1990) note in their review that there has been striking consistency in regard to the strength of association between head injury and AD among case-control studies, whereas much lower ratios were found in one retrospective (Chandra *et al.*, 1987) and one prospective (Katzman *et al.*, 1989) study. The issue arises as to whether recall bias can account for the increase in history of head trauma in the case-control studies where the concerned informant or next of kin may have reflected "harder" on past events in contrast to controls or control families. Perhaps in prospective community studies, such recall bias would be less important than in case-control studies.

Questions on head injury were not included in the Shanghai survey; however, we are planning a 1992 follow-up survey of those 65 years and older who were studied in 1987 and will include questions on head injury in the prospective study. We hope also to perform a small number of autopsies, if permission is granted, to help confirm some of our hypotheses. A multidisciplinary approach, combined with a prospective or longitudinal study design, would be extremely productive in answering some of the questions we have encountered in our research on dementia and AD in China.

Acknowledgment

We gratefully acknowledge the following funding agencies for their support of this study: the Shanghai Department of Public Health in China, the National Institute of Mental Health in a grant (MH 36408-07) to the University of Illinois, the National Institute on Aging (1 RO1 AG 10327-01) in a grant to San Diego State University and another grant (AG5131) to the Alzheimer Disease Research Center at the University of California, San Diego. We also thank Anthony Graham-White for his helpful comments on an earlier draft of this paper.

Appendix

Major Life Events of Chinese Persons Aged 65–69 in 1987

Years	Their age then	Major life events
1918–1922	Birth–4 years	May 4th Movement, 1919–1921. Major change in Chinese culture; introduction of the vernacular into literary writings; women's roles questioned; the traditional structure of the Chinese family challenged; the Western concept of "love" and "democracy" introduced; importance of science in education stressed; a call for giving women equal educational opportunities as men made; etc. Founding of the Chinese Communist Party in 1921.
1923–1927	5–9 years	Well-to-do families started to provide female children with opportunities for formal or informal education (through private tutors); significant changes in education: curriculum content now includes arithmetic and other subjects, not just rote memory of classic poetries and Confucian teachings. Feudal warlords became quite evident through parts of China. Collapse of the rural economy; rapid rural-to-urban migration compounded urban poverty problems. Sun Yat Sen died in 1925. Internal rift between the Chinese Communist Party and the Kuomintang Party.
1928–1932	10–14 years	Feudal warlordism continued. Chiang Kai-Shek victorious in his Northern Expedition; civil war between the Chinese Communist Party and the Kuo-Mintang Party. Increasing Japanese militarism in China from 1927 to 1937; Japan invaded southern Manchuria in 1931.
1933–1937	15–19 years	Sino-Japanese War began in 1937. The communists and the Kuomintang united to fight the Japanese; Japanese occupation of Manchuria from 1935 to 1936.
1938–1942	20–24 years	Sino-Japanese War continued for 8 years.
1943–1947	25–29 years	Sino-Japanese War ended and Japan surrendered in 1945. World War II; Chinese Communist Party took over major cities in north China, having military bases in 19 provinces controlling a population of around 100,000,000.
1948–1952	30–34 years	Establishment of People's Republic of China in 1949. Most glorious period in Chinese Communist regime of China. The Chinese primary and higher educational system changed to the Soviet model. Chiang Kai-Shek retreated to Taiwan. Korean War.

continues

APPENDIX *Continued*

Years	Their age then	Major life events
1953–1957	35–39 years	"Let a Hundred Flowers Bloom" campaign heralded a series of Anti-Rightist movements targeted at artists, writers, and intellectuals in general. Great Leap Forward 1957–1959. Soviets withdrew technical assistance completely from China; many projects halted.
1958–1962	40–44 years	Great Leap Forward, 1957–1959, proved to be a failure, followed by 3 years of famine and other natural calamities (droughts, floods, storms, food shortages, and famines). China's economy suffered severe setbacks from 1959–1962. 1960–1962: Serious split between Mao Zedong's leftist faction and his opponents; economic depression in the country.
1963–1967	45–49 years	1966: Cultural Revolution began. Attack against academics, educated, and intellectuals were openly encouraged; house searches, physical assaults; illegal detention at workplace; some smashing of cultural artifacts in public places.
1968–1972	50–54 years	Cultural Revolution continued. The educated ridiculed, imprisoned, sent to the countryside or labor camps. Age at which the women we interviewed in 1987 were required to retire (50-year-olds).
1973–1977	55–59 years	Nixon visited China in 1973. Cultural Revolution ended October 1976. Age at which the men we interviewed in 1987 were required to retire (55-year-olds)
1978–1982	60–64 years	United States and China established diplomatic relations in December 1979.
1983–1987	65–69 years	Opening of China to foreign trade and investments. Our first Survey of Dementia and Alzheimer Disease conducted in Shanghai, in 1987.
1988–1992	70–74 years	Beijing Incident on June 4, 1989. Our 1992 follow-up survey.

References

Amaducci, L. A., Gratiglloni, L., Rocca, W. A., Freschi, C., Livrea, P., Pedone, D., Bracco, L., Lippi, A., Gandolfo, C., Bino, G., Prencipe, M., Bonatti, M. L., Girotti, F., Carella, F., Tavolato, B., Ferla, S., Lenzi, G. L., Carolei, A., Gambi, A., Grigoletto, F., and Shoenbert, B. S. (1986). Risk factor for clinically diagnosed Alzheimer's disease: A case control study of an Italian population. *Neurology* **36**, 922–931.

American Psychiatric Association. (1980). "Diagnostic and Statistical Manual of Mental Disorders," 3rd ed. American Psychiatric Association, Washington, D.C.

Aronson, M. K., Ooi, W. L., Morgenstern, H., Hafner, A., Masur, D., Crystal, H., Frishman, W. H., Fisher, D., and Katzman, R. (1990). Women, myocardial infarction and dementia in the very old. *Neurology* **40,** 1102–1106.

Burger, P. C., and Vogel, F. S. (1973). The development of the pathologic changes of Alzheimer's disease and senile dementia in patients with Down's syndrome. *Am J. Pathol.* **73,** 457–476.

Butters, N., Granholm, E., Salmon, D., Grant, I., and Wolfe, J. (1987). Episodic and semantic memory: A comparison of amnesic and demented patients. *J. Clin. Exp. Neuropsychol.* **9,** 479–497.

Chandra, V., Kokmen, E., and Schoenberg, B. S. (1987). Head trauma with loss of consciousness as a risk factor for Alzheimer's disease using prospectively collected data. *Neurology* **37**(suppl.), 152 (abstr.).

Chen, X. S., Zhang, J. Z., Jiang, Z. N., Zhu, Z. H., Liu, X. H., Wang, L. H., Xia, Y. H., Li, X. Q., Ma, G. Q., Shen, Z. C., Liu, T. F., Xu, L., Chan, S. W., Wang, Q., and Yu, S. X. (1987). A psychiatric epidemiological survey on elderly in Beijing city. *Chin. J. Neurol. Psychiatry* **20,** 145–148 (in Chinese).

Cook, R. H., Schenck, S. A., and Clark, D. B. (1981). Twins with Alzheimer's disease. *Arch. Neurol.* **38,** 300–301.

Dekosky, S. T., and Scheff, S. W. (1990). Synapse loss in frontal cortex biopsies in Alzheimer's disease: Correlation with cognitive severity. *Ann. Neurol.* **27,** 457–464.

Evans, D. A., Funkenstein, H., Alvert, M. S., Scherr, P. A., Cook, N. R., Chown, M. J., Herbert, L. E., Hennekens, C. H., and Taylor, J. O. (1989). Prevalence of Alzheimer's disease in a community population of older person. *JAMA* **262,** 2551–2556.

Farrer, L. A., O'Sullivan, D. M., Cuppies, L. A., Growdon, J. H., and Meyers, R. H. (1989). Assessment of genetic risk for Alzheimer's disease among first-degree relatives. *Ann. Neurol.* **25,** 485–493.

Folstein, M. F., Anthony, J. C., Parhat, I., Duffy, B., and Gruenbert, E. (1985). The meaning of cognitive impairment in the elderly. *J. Am. Geriatric Soc.* **33,** 228–235.

French, L. R., Schoman, L. M., Mortimer, J. A., Hutton, J. T., Boatman, R. A., and Christians, B. (1985). A case-control study of dementia of the Alzheimer type. *Am. J. Epidemiol.* **121,** 414–421.

Fuld, P. A. (1981). "The Fuld Object Memory Evaluation." Stoelting Instrument, Chicago.

Gong, Y. X. (1982) "Manual of Modified Wechesler Adult Intelligence Scale (WAIS-RC)." Junan Med College, Changsha, China (in Chinese).

Graves, A. B., White, E., Koepsell, T. D., Reifier, B. V., Belle, G. V., Larson, E. B., and Raskind, M. (1990). The association between head trauma and Alzheimer's disease. *Am. J. Epidemiol.* **131,** 491.

Gurland, B. J. (1981). The borderlands of dementia; the influence of sociocultural characteristics on rates of dementia occurring in the senium. *In* "Clinical Aspects of Alzheimer's Disease and Senile Dementia: Aging," Vol. 15 (N. E. Miller and G. D. Cohen, eds.), pp. 61–84. Raven Press, New York.

Hachinski, V. C., Lessen, N. A., and Marshall, J. (1974). Multiinfract dementia—A cause of mental deterioration in the elderly. *Lancet* **July 27,** 207–210.

Hamos, J. E., DeGennaro, L. J., and Drachman, D. A. (1989). Synaptic loss in Alzheimer's disease and other dementias. *Neurology* **39,** 355–361.

Hasegawa, K., Inoue, K., and Moriya, K. (1974). An investigation of dementia rating scales for elderly. *Selsin Igaku* **16,** 965–969.

Heston, L. L., Mastri, A. R., Anderson, V. E., White, J. (1982). Dementia of the Alzheimer type. Clinical genetics, natural history, and associated conditions. *Arch. Gen. Psychiatry* **38,** 1085–1990.

Heyman, A., Wilkinson, W. E., Stafford, J. A., Helms, M. J., Sigmon, A. H., and Weinberg, T. (1984). Alzheimer's disease: A study of epidemiological aspects. *Ann. Neurol.* **15,** 335–341.

Jarvik, L. F., Ruth, V., and Matsuyama, S. S. (1980). Organic brain syndrome and aging. A six-year follow-up of surviving twins. *Arch. Gen. Psychiatry* **37,** 280–286.

Jorm, A. F., Korten, A. E., and Henderson, A. S. (1987). The prevalence of dementia: A quantitative integration of the literature. *Acta Psychiatr. Scand.* **76,** 464–479.

Katzman, R., Aronson, M., Fuld, P. A., Kawas, C., Brown, T., Morgenstern, H., Frishman, W., Gidez, L., Eder, H., and Ooi, W. L. (1989). Development of dementia in an 80-year-old volunteer cohort. *Ann. Neurol.* **25,** 317–324.

Kuang, P. G., and Zhao, C. D. (1984). A sampling survey of geriatric mental disturbances at Wuhan in 1981. *Chinese J. Epidemiol.* **5,** 95–98 (in Chinese).

Levy, P. S., Yu, E. S. H., Liu, W. T., Wong, S. C., Zhang, M. Y., Wang, Z. Y., and Katzman, R. (1989). Single stage cluster sampling with a telescopic respondent rule: A variation motivated by a survey of dementia in elderly resident of Shanghai. *Statistics Med.* **8,** 1537–1544.

Li, G., Shen, Y. C., Chen, C. H., Li, S. R., Zao, Y. W., Liu, M., Xu, L., Wang, L. X., and Wang, Q. (1988). The test of MMSE in urban community elderly. *Chinese J. Mental Health* **2,** 13–18 (in Chinese).

Lin, K., and Kleinman, A. (1981). Recent development of psychiatric epidemiology in China. *Culture, Med. Psychiatry* **5,** 135–143.

Masliah, E., Terry, R. D., DeTeresa, R., and Hansen, L. A. (1989). Immunohistochemical quantification of the synapse related protein synaptophysin in Alzheimer disease. *Neurosci. Lett.* **103,** 234–238.

McKhann, G., Drachman, D., Folstein, M., Katzman, R., Price, D., and Stadian, E. M. (1984). Clinical diagnosis of Alzheimer's disease: Report of the NINCDS–ADRDA Work Group under the auspices of Department of Health and Human Services Task Force on Alzheimer's disease. *Neurology* **34,** 939–944.

Mohs, R. C., Breitner, J. C. S., Silverman, J. M., and Davis, K. L. (1987). Morbid risk in first degree relatives of persons with Alzheimer's disease. *Arch. Gen. Psychiatry* **44,** 405–408.

Mortimer, J. A. (1990). Epidemiology of dementia: Cross-culture comparisons. *Adv. Neurol.* **51,** 27–33.

Pfeffer, R. I., Kurosaki, T. T., Harrah, C. H., Chance, J. M., and Filos, S. (1982). Measurement of functional activities in older adults in the community. *J. Gerontol.* **37,** 323–329.

Rocca, W. A., Banaiuto, S., Lippi, A., Luciani, P., Turtu, F., Caverzeran, F., and Amaducci, L. (1990). Prevalence of clinically diagnosed Alzheimer's disease and other dementing disorders: A door-to-door survey in Appignano, Macerata Province, Italy. *Neurology* **40,** 626–631.

Roses, A. D., Pericak-Vance, M. A., Clark, C. M., Gilbert, J. R., Yamaoka, L. H., Haynes, C. S., Speer, M. C., Gaskell, P. C. Hung, W. Y., Trofatter, J. A., Earl, N. L., Lee, J. E., Alberts, M. J., Dawson, D. V., Bartlett, R. J., Siddique, T., Vance, J. M., Conneally, P. M., and Heyman, A. L. (1990). Linkage studies of late-onset familial Alzheimer's disease. *Adv. Neurol.* **51,** 185–196.

St. George-Hyslop, P. H., Tanzi, R. E., Polinsky, R. J., Haines, J. L., Nee, L., and Watkins, P. C. (1987). The genetics defect causing familial Alzheimer's disease maps on chromosome 21. *Science* **235,** 885–890.

Terry, R. D., Masliah, E., Salmon, D. P., Butters, N., DeTeresa, R., Hill, R., Hansen, L. A., and Katzman, R. (1991). Physical basis of cognitive alterations in Alzheimer disease: Synapse loss is the major correlate of cognitive impairment. *Ann. Neurol.* **30,** 572–580.

Wang, C. H., Liu, W. T., Zhang, M. Y., Yu, E., Xia, Z. Y., Fernandez, M., Lung, C. T., Xu, C. L., and Qu, G. Y. (1992). Alcohol use, abuse, and dependency in Shanghai. *In* "Cross-National Studies of Alcoholism" (J. Helzer and G. J. Camino, eds.). Oxford University Press, London.

Wechsler D. (1974). "Manual: Wechsler Intelligence Scale for Children-Revised (WISC-R)." Psychological Corp., New York.

Yang, J. S., and Lu, Y. X. (1988). A survey of physical and mental health among 1229 elderly over 65. *Chinese J. Neurol. Syst. Mental Dis.* **14,** 85–87 (in Chinese).

Zhang, M. Y., Katzman, R., Salmon, D., Jin, H., Cai, G., Wang, Z. Y., Qu, G. Y., Grant, I., Yu, E., Levy, P., Klauber, M. R., and Liu, W. T. (1990). The prevalence of dementia and Alzheimer's disease in Shanghai, China: Impact of Age, Gender, and Education. *Ann. Neurol.* **27,** 428–437.

3

An Update of the Epidemiology of Western Pacific Amyotrophic Lateral Sclerosis

Leonard T. Kurland • *Kurupath Radhakrishnan*

Amyotrophic lateral sclerosis (ALS), the major form of motor neuron disease, is a progressive and fatal illness characterized by upper and lower motor neuron degeneration (Kurland *et al.*, 1968; Kurtzke and Kurland, 1983). On the basis of epidemiologic and genetic features, three forms of ALS are recognized: the classic or sporadic form, which accounts for about 90% of patients in the United States; the relatively rare Western Pacific form occurring in geographic isolates, often in association with a parkinsonism–dementia complex (PDC), and the familial, presumably hereditary form, which accounts for about 10% of the cases (Kurland *et al.*, 1968; Kurtzke and Kurland, 1983; Armon and Kurland, 1990). The remarkable incidence of fatal neurologic disease among the indigenous Chamorro population of Guam and Rota (southern islands of the Marianas Archipelago in the Western Pacific Ocean; Fig. 1) has prompted detailed epidemiologic studies of ALS–PDC since World War II. This chapter provides a review of recent developments in the epidemiology of Western Pacific ALS. The etiologic and pathogenetic implications of these recent developments will be emphasized in our effort to build on, rather than duplicate, previous data descriptions and reviews of this subject (Koerner, 1952; Kurland *et al.*, 1961; Reed and Brody, 1975; Rodgers-Johnson *et al.*, 1986; Kurland and Mulder, 1988; Lavine *et al.*, 1991).

Western Pacific ALS is a prototypic neurodegenerative disorder found among the Chamorro people of Guam and Rota (Mariana Islands), residents of the Kii Peninsula, Honshu Island (Japan), and the Auyu and Jakai linguistic groups of Irian Jaya (western New Guinea) (Fig. 1). The Western Pacific form of ALS has aroused interest over the past 40 years, not only

Neuroepidemiology:
Theory and Method

· **73** ·

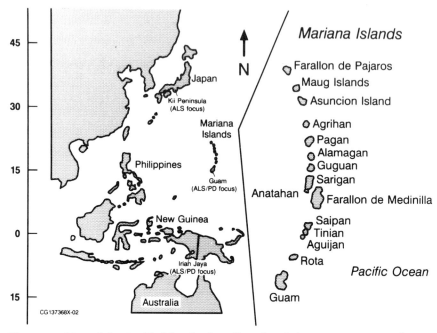

Figure 1 Map of the Pacific islands, the Kii Peninsula in Japan, Guam, and Irian Jaya in western New Guinea. Inset shows the Mariana Islands.

because of its distinctive characteristics, but also because the incidence, prevalence, and mortality rates when first identified were 50–100 times those of the sporadic form in the continental United States, and the male:female ratio approximated 2:1. The median age at onset was 44 years compared to 65 years reported in the study of the population of Rochester, Minnesota (Yoshida *et al.*, 1986).

From the standpoint of epidemiologic research, the distinction between these investigator-identified geographic isolates (Kurland, 1978) and community-identified clusters (Armon *et al.*, 1991) is important. Other than the way these foci were identified, two major differences from community-identified clusters are the extreme excess occurrence (50-fold or more rather than just a fewfold greater than the expected number) and especially the persistence of this excess over time. The use of epidemiologic data to generate or test hypotheses of causation or etiology is not a self-evident process. It is derived from a basic premise or axiom that disease does not occur randomly but, rather, in patterns that reflect the operation of underlying causes (Fox *et al.*, 1970). It is these concepts that

fuel the expectation that the study of Western Pacific ALS may demonstrate genetic or ecologic associations that have not been observed or
appreciated through the study of the sporadic form, and that these will
provide clues to the etiology of the sporadic form. With the realization that
PDC is also endemic in these foci, this concept is extended to Parkinson's
disease, Alzheimer's disease, and progressive supranuclear palsy as members of a spectrum of neurodegenerative diseases that the studies on
Guam suggest may be due to a single causative process.

The lower and upper motor neuron degeneration in Western Pacific
ALS is similar to that of sporadic ALS, with the additional histologic feature
of an excess of neurofibrillary tangles and intracytoplasmic inclusion
(granulovacuolar) bodies, particularly in the nerve cells of the hippocampus and other subcortical areas (Hirano et al., 1961, 1966; Malamud et al.,
1961). The specificity of the neurofibrillary tangles in Western Pacific ALS
and PDC is unclear because an excess of such tangles has also been found
in a large proportion of Chamorros who died apparently free of these
conditions (57% of people aged 40–59 years and 95% of people aged ≥60
years (Chen, 1981). ALS–PDC is also referred to as *lytico-bodig* on Guam.
Lytico, from paralytico, is the Chamorro term for ALS, and *bodig*, or *raput*
(slowness or laziness), is the parkinsonian variant of this disease. The
neurofibrillary tangles occurring in Chamorros, both with and without
recognized ALS–PDC, have been shown to be similar to those of Alzheimer's disease by immunocytochemical characterization techniques
(Shankar et al., 1989; Ito et al., 1992). The histopathologic features of Guam
ALS and PDC have been described in detail by Hirano and colleagues
(Hirano et al., 1961, 1966; Malamud et al., 1961) and are beyond the scope
of this chapter.

EPIDEMIOLOGIC DATA FROM GUAM AND THE MARIANA ISLANDS

Evidence indicates that the incidence of ALS among the Chamorro population of Guam was excessive as early as 1815 (Kurland, 1957). Frequent
reports of "lytico" and "paralytico" have been found in the earliest death
certificates, dating back to the early 1900s. The clinical and pathologic
features were thought initially to be those of classic ALS. Early reports by
Zimmerman (1945), Koerner (1952), Arnold et al. (1953), and Tillema and
Wynberg (1953) were confirmed in surveys by Kurland and Mulder (1954),
who showed that ALS was 50–100 times more prevalent among the
Chamorros of Guam than in the population of the continental United
States.

ALS was also prevalent in the Chamorros on the nearby island of Rota and among those who had moved to California in the previous 40 years (Lavine *et al.*, 1991). It was less common among the Chamorros on Saipan, and there was some uncertainty about whether or not an atypical form of motor neuron disease characterized by a slowly progressive paraparesis with fasciculations and minimal muscle atrophy was occurring among the Carolinians on Saipan, who had partly adopted Chamorro customs. In the Caroline Islands to the south, neither ALS nor PDC was found (Kurland and Mulder, 1954).

On Guam, the highest prevalence rate of ALS has been and continues in the southern village of Umatac (Fig. 2). However, ALS alone is encountered less frequently now than in the 1950s; most cases of "ALS" occur as

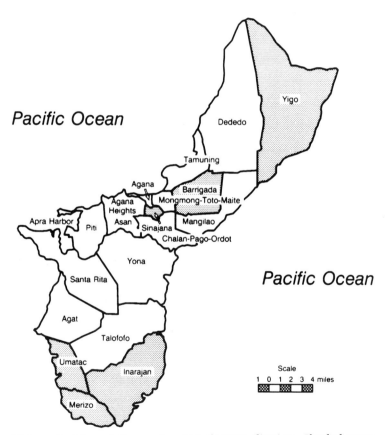

Figure 2 Map of Guam showing election districts. Shaded areas represent high prevalence for ALS.

a component of the ALS–PDC symptom complex. A genetic explanation for the observed familial aggregation was initially proposed (Kurland, 1957), but it has been displaced by the realization that some exogenous factor(s) unique to the geographic foci offers the best explanation as to cause.

During the first surveys by Kurland and Mulder (1954), patients were encountered with what was first regarded as postencephalitic parkinsonism. Japanese B encephalitides had been reported on Guam in the 1940s. It became evident that this combination of parkinsonism and dementia was in fact a new entity, which had been well recognized by the native population as *bodig* or *raput*, meaning slowness or laziness. The intensive clinical, pathologic and familial studies that were carried out suggested that PDC was a clinical variant of the local form of ALS, often coexisting with it (Hirano *et al.*, 1961; Malamud *et al.*, 1961; Kurland *et al.*, 1968). Cases of presenile dementia without parkinsonism or ALS are referred to as Marianas dementia; their relationship to Alzheimer's disease is under intensive study. Such cases, which have become prevalent in recent years, were not described in the 1950–1960 surveys. It cannot be determined at this stage whether such patients were indeed absent or they were missed because their symptoms were overshadowed by the ALS–PDC with its striking pathology.

The unusual concentration of individuals with neurologic disease on Guam led to the establishment of a National Institute of Neurologic Disease and Stroke (NINDS) research center registry, which recorded incident cases of neurodegenerative disease from 1945 to 1985. However, the reports based on review of that registry at 10-year intervals (Reed *et al.*, 1966; Reed and Brody, 1975; Rodgers-Johnson *et al.*, 1986) showed a steady decline in the annual incidence of ALS, reportedly down to only 2–3 times the rate found on the mainland so that, by 1982, it was concluded that the high incidence of ALS–PDC on Guam had "disappeared" (Garruto *et al.*, 1985). It was this apparent disappearance of neurodegenerative disease from Guam that led to the reduction of staff in 1982 and, finally, the closure of the NINDS research center registry in 1985. Similarly declining rates of ALS have also been observed in the other two geographically and genetically distinct high-incidence foci in the Western Pacific region: in Hobara and Kozagawa of the Kii Peninsula of Japan (Uebayashi, 1980) and in villages among the Auyu and Jakai people of Irian Jaya (western New Guinea) (Fig. 1) (Gajdusek and Salazar, 1982).

There was, however, reason to doubt the completeness of case ascertainment within the NINDS research center registry as compared to that attained with the earlier surveys by Mulder and Kurland (1954). This difference was due not only to the methodologic shortcomings of passive versus active surveillance, but also to the existence of financial disincentives for patients to be registered: The legislation providing for free care for ALS and PDC patients at the Guam Memorial Hospital was linked to the revocation of the medical insurance entitling them to private care. This may have served as a disincentive for both patients and local practitioners to report cases.

Reed *et al.* (1987) followed a large cohort of ALS and PDC patients and unaffected family members on Guam that had been identified in 1968, and in 1987 they reported that the incidence rate of ALS was decreasing but that of PDC continued to be high. Active ascertainment of neurodegenerative disease in three villages in southern Guam was therefore undertaken (Lavine *et al.*, 1991). These villages were chosen for survey because they had high prevalence rates of ALS in previous surveys and had maintained a traditional Chamorro life-style. These surveys showed that the prevalence of ALS in these villages continued to be high, 50 times greater than that of Rochester, Minnesota, and for those over 55 years old, 70 times greater than in Rochester, Minnesota (Yoshida *et al.*, 1986). Furthermore, the age of onset of both ALS and PDC had increased, on average, about 10 years since the 1950s. A case was reported as ALS if lower motor neuron disease was present with or without evidence of parkinsonism and/or dementia. Prevalence of parkinsonism was 5 times that of Parkinson's disease in Rochester, Minnesota (Rajput *et al.*, 1984), whereas dementia in PDC or Marianas dementia was about 4 times greater than the prevalence of Alzheimer's disease in Rochester, Minnesota (Kokmen *et al.*, 1989).

In the continental United States, ALS, Parkinson's disease, and Alzheimer's disease tend to occur as single diseases in patients, although as many as one-third of those with Parkinson's disease will develop cognitive impairment. However, on Guam, a combination of two or all three of these disorders (ALS, parkinsonism, and dementia) frequently occur in the same patient. When one, two, or all three conditions are considered and the number of persons affected rather than the number of syndromes is counted, the prevalence rate on Guam is 2.8 times greater than that of Rochester, Minnesota. The reason for this dramatic difference in relative risks between the individual diseases and the number affected is that almost all patients on Guam have more than one component of the ALS–parkinsonism–Marianas dementia complex.

New patients with ALS–PDC have been identified on Guam by intense village surveys of recent years. During the University of Guam–Mayo Clinic surveys conducted March 1990 through February 1991 among the residents who were 55 years and older of Rota, Tinian, and Yigo on Guam (Fig. 1 and 2), a high prevalence of PDC and Marianas dementia was found on Rota, no definite cases of ALS or PDC were observed in Tinian, and an increased prevalence of ALS–PDC was found in Yigo. This pattern was similar to that reported after World War II, which suggests that the distribution of the etiological agent(s) has not changed significantly in four decades. A case registry established at the University of Guam–Mayo Clinic Center identified 77 Chamorros with definite (47) or suspected (30) ALS–PDC and 20 Filipinos with ALS, PDC, or both.

Furthermore, in the course of these surveys, supranuclear disturbances of ocular motility, usually mild, were noted in a majority of the patients with ALS–PDC (Lepore *et al.*, 1988). These comprised saccadic and pursuit paresis, nystagmus, conjugate gaze limitation, abnormal convergence, optokinetic nystagmus, and vestibuloocular reflex cancellation (Lepore *et al.*, 1988). There is thus the suggestion that the spectrum of neurodegenerative disease on Guam is broader than previously suspected and includes features of ALS, Parkinson's disease, Alzheimer's disease, and progressive supranuclear palsy. Compared to the survey in 1953, the mean age at onset for ALS and PDC has increased by about 10 years; however, the male : female ratio continued to be 2:1. In the southern villages, dementia alone or in association with early parkinsonism was noted predominantly in older women; this may reflect their selective survival.

Observations that at present are of uncertain significance are the collagen changes in the skin of about 50% of patients with ALS–PDC (Fullmer *et al.*, 1960) as well as in patients in the continental United States with sporadic ALS; these changes have not been seen in a small number of patients with spinal muscular atrophy (Ono *et al.*, 1988, 1989). Another recent discovery that is under investigation is a pigmentary retinopathy resembling posterior ophthalmomyiasis interna seen in 26 of 49 Chamorros with ALS–PDC as well as in 16% of neurologically asymptomatic individuals aged 50 and over (Cox *et al.*, 1989). It is estimated that there may be as many as 1000 cases of this asymptomatic retinopathy on Guam. In contrast to published case reports of ophthalmomyiasis interna posterior (Gass and Lewis, 1976; Syralden *et al.*, 1982), the pathology in the fatal neurological cases from Guam shows no evidence of a parasite. The picture of this pigmentary retinopathy, as seen by ophthalmoscopy, is characterized by hypopigmented subretinal tracks, which crisscross in a random fashion and at times form loops. There is focal degeneration of the retinal pigmented epithelium with the formation of macromelanosomes similar to that seen with experimental intracarotid injection of MPTP (Personal communication, R. Nick Hogan, M.D., June 1, 1992). But the cause and mechanism are unknown at this date. As far as we are aware, a similar pigment retinopathy has not been described in patients with either ALS or Parkinson's disease in other geographic sites. Since 1986, more than 100 Guamanian Chamorros have been identified with this retinopathy, but it has been detected in only one non-Chamorro patient, an elderly Filipino and a resident of the island for 50 years (Campbell *et al.*, 1992).

The persistence of a high prevalence of ALS–PDC on Guam suggests the continued presence of an etiologic mechanism, although the long latent period suggests that exposure may have occurred decades earlier. The change in types and age at onset of disease over time may reflect improved case ascertainment or differences in the interaction between the environmental factors and susceptible individuals. One mechanism that could explain the observed changes would be exposure to an environmental toxin that peaked during World War II and has declined but not disappeared. Individuals exposed to higher doses of that toxin might develop ALS at a relatively early age with or without associated PDC. Individuals exposed to a lesser dose might develop, at a later date, ALS with or without PDC, PDC alone, or dementia alone. Additional surveys on Guam and careful review of ecologic and life-style factors within case-control studies may help to identify the factor(s) responsible for the changing prevalence of neurodegenerative diseases on Guam.

PATTERNS OF DISTRIBUTION AND ETIOLOGIC IMPLICATIONS

Familial aggregation of ALS–PDC on Guam was recognized in the first published reports (Koerner, 1952; Arnold *et al.*, 1953; Kurland and Mulder, 1954). This pattern has persisted to date, with the result that some families are considered "afflicted" and, possibly, their members may be perceived as less than ideal candidates for marriage. However, the pattern of putative inheritance within "afflicted families" has not followed simple Mendelian patterns. Questions of parenthood should be resolved with modern tissue typing techniques. The possibility of mitochondrial inheritance predisposing to ALS–PDC is also being pursued. The presence of excessive neurofibrillary tangles and the loss of odor identification in asymptomatic Chamorros suggests a predisposition to neurodegenerative disorders; these features are also under intensive study. In the present study, asymptomatic Chamorros who have shown none of the features of ALS or PDC have been examined and will be reexamined periodically; autopsies on such well-documented asymptomatic individuals are expected to provide a much needed neuropathologic reference, against which the findings in affected individuals can be compared.

The following factors suggest that genetics alone does not account for the high prevalence of ALS–PDC among Chamorros on Guam and the other Western Pacific foci: (1) three apparently different populations are involved, (2) an excess of ALS or PDC appears among Filipinos who settled in Guam as young adults (Garruto *et al.*, 1981), and (3) the shift in the ratio of ALS to PDC and the remarkable increase in age at onset of ALS and PDC in the southern villages of Guam over the past 30 years (Lavine *et al.*, 1991).

Thus, while strong consideration should be given to genetic predisposition in the development of Western Pacific ALS–PDC, that explanation alone cannot account for the changing clinical features and its pattern of distribution.

ENVIRONMENTAL CONSIDERATIONS

The cumulative epidemiologic data strongly incriminate an environmental factor as the cause of ALS–PDC in the geographic isolates. Two types of environmental hypotheses have been proposed to account for Western Pacific ALS–PDC. One is the presence of an exogenous toxin common to the three affected areas, and the other is the absence of essential minerals.

The leading candidate as the source of an exogenous toxin has been the seed of the false sago palm, *Cycas circinalis*. *Cycas circinalis* is a member of the order cycadeles, the palmlike evergreens that flourish in subtropical and tropical climates. The seeds of *C. cicinalis* have been known to be highly toxic for humans since ancient times. Some populations learned how to process the seeds for food so that the acute toxicity could be avoided. Among the Chamorros of Guam, a ritual of prolonged soaking developed, and during times of famine, especially following hurricanes and in times of conflict such as World War II, cycad became an important source of carbohydrate in the diet. The husk of the nut was sometimes used as a chew, and the freshly ground cycad seed was also used as a medicinal, particularly in the form of a poultice applied to ulcers and other lesions of the skin. The cycad seed was identified as a potential cause of ALS on Guam as a result of Marjorie Whiting's (1963) observation during the field studies in Umatac and Yigo. Two toxins have now been identified in *C. circinalis.* One is cycasin [methylazoxymethanol (MAM) β-D-glucoside], a major component of the cycad seed (2–4%). Cycasin is metabolized by plant and animal β-glucosidases to MAM, a potent cytotoxin and carcinogen. The neurotoxicity of cycasin may be related to the intracellular production of the potent alkylating agent, MAM, a chemical with the ability to alter cell function irreversibly and progressively long after exposure has ceased (Polsky *et al.*, 1972, Matsumoto, 1985). This toxin can be removed by adequate soaking when the seeds are prepared for consumption. However, in periods of stress and hunger, as in the Japanese occupation of Guam during World War II, water for soaking and time (several days, as recommended) were often not available, so the exposure to the toxin was increased. A second water-soluble toxin that has been identified is α-amino-β-mehtylaminopropionic acid, or β-N-methylamino-L-alanine (BMAA), as described below.

Muscle atrophy and weakness and degeneration of motor neurons in the brain and spinal cord was described by Dastur (1964) in one of the four rhesus monkeys fed 1 g of washed cycad flour daily for 8 months. Subsequently, Dastur, 1964; Dastur *et al.* (1990) reported early motor neuron changes in pathologic specimens of additional animals who had been fed cycad but who had not developed clinical disease. When another toxin from the cycad seed, BMAA, was isolated in the late 1960s (Vega and Bell, 1967; Polsky *et al.*, 1972), its etiologic relevance to ALS was uncertain because its only apparent acute effects were convulsions and paralysis in mice that received high doses. But interest in cycad continued (Kurland and Molgaard, 1982; Kurland and Mulder, 1987). A renewed impetus for the cycad hypothesis has been given by Spencer and Schaumburg (1983), who suspected that there might be parallels between the toxin responsible for lathyrism, β-N-oxalylamino-L-alanine (BOAA), and the BMAA from cycad. Both of these chemicals have structures similar to glutamic acid. The neurotoxicity of BOAA and of BMAA has been demonstrated when applied to explants of the central nervous system (Nunn *et al.*, 1987; Weiss *et al.*, 1989). Using large doses of a purified synthetic L-isomer of BMAA, Spencer reported that monkeys developed an illness with skeletal muscle weakness as in human ALS and possibly parkinsonism–dementia (Spencer *et al.*, 1986, Spencer, 1987).

Spencer has further reported that unwashed cycad had been used as a medicinal in the other foci of Western Pacific ALS, namely, the Irian Jaya focus in western New Guinea (as a poultice) and the Kii Peninsula of Japan (as a "tonic" made from dried seeds of *Cycas revoluta*) (Spencer *et al.*, 1987a,b). The feeding experiment in monkeys by Spencer has not been replicated; others have made efforts to feed monkeys various preparations of cycad, but they have failed to reproduce Spencer's findings (Garruto *et al.*, 1988). However, these apparently negative findings raise questions of the potency of the cycad used in those studies, because one would expect hepatic toxicity to cycasin in the monkeys fed a substantial quantity of fresh unwashed cycad. The absence of such a toxic response suggests that the cycad may have been modified by long storage or some handling procedure. Furthermore, it is unclear whether or not the monkeys who showed no apparent neurological disease were fed BMAA in quantities corresponding to Spencer's experiment. Seawright *et al.* (1990) recently reported a cerebellar neurotoxic effect with pathologic confirmation in rats fed BMAA.

In a recent study, Kisby *et al.* (1992) found that the traditionally processed (washed) cycad flours obtained from Chamorro residents of Guam still retained variable quantities of cycasin. The residual cycasin was approximately 10 times that of residual BMAA. On the basis of the cycasin content, the ingestion of such flour would result in an estimated human exposure to milligram amounts of cycasin per day. Kisby and Spencer (1989) have suggested that MAM, the aglycone of the cycad carcinogen, cycasin, may react with naturally occurring amino acids to produce derivatives that have neurotoxic properties similar to those of the glutamate agonist, *N*-methyl-D-aspartate, as demonstrated in cortical organotypic cultures. A compound such as BMAA was produced when monkey serum was incubated with MAM under physiologic conditions (Kisby and Spencer, 1989). While the experimentally induced primate disorder has some clinical and neuropathological features reminiscent of ALS–PDC, it lacks neurofibrillary pathology and fails to progress once dosing has ceased. Studies of the central nervous system uptake, distribution, and metabolism of BMAA and MAM are needed to clarify their role in the human disease.

Another possible mechanism that could account for cycad toxicity is that of the pollen of *C. circinalis*, which has recently been found to contain both cycasin and BMAA. Cycad pollens from other parts of the world studied to date contain smaller quantities of BMAA but no cycasin. It is postulated that the pollen could transport these toxins to the nasal mucosa and thereby to the nerve fibers, which could carry them to the neurons of the olfactory bulb. From there, it is conceivable that the toxin could spread to the entorhinal cortex, the amygdala and hippocampus, and other areas of the central nervous system. This transport mechanism could explain the serious loss of neurons with neurofibrillary tangle degeneration in the olfactory bulb as well as the hippocampus and other parts of the brain. The loss of the odor identification in a high proportion of patients with early PDC and some with early ALS on Guam apparently reflects cell loss in the olfactory nucleus. Studies are underway by Seawright (University of Queensland) and Kurland to test this hypothesis that the nasal mucosa may serve as another portal of entry for the cycad toxins.

An alternative hypothesis to cycad toxicity has been that the absence or excess of essential minerals is related to Western Pacific ALS. Low levels of calcium and magnesium in the soil and water have been proposed as culprits (Gajdusek *et al.*, 1980; Yase, 1977). However, recent studies on Guam have shown an adequate calcium and magnesium content of water and foods grown in the soil of areas such as Umatac, where ALS and PDC are particularly prevalent (Zolan and Ellis-Neill, 1986; D. R. McLachlan, personal communication). Garruto (1987) has demonstrated deposition of aluminum in affected neurons, and more recently he has shown that a low-calcium, high-aluminum diet may induce motor neuron pathology in cynomolgus monkeys (Garruto *et al.*, 1989).

It remains to be seen whether or not either of these hypotheses, that of an exogenous toxin in cycad or the depletion of calcium and magnesium causing an increase in aluminum uptake, can explain the etiology of Western Pacific ALS–PDC. To us, cycad remains the primary candidate; others believe that more than one mechanism may be acting, perhaps on a genetically susceptible population. Although a causal relationship between cycad exposure and ALS–PDC has yet to be established, the consumption of food containing agents (cycasin, BMAA) with multifarious toxic potential would seem to be contraindicated. Reduction in the use of cycad medicinally has apparently accompanied the reduction in ALS from the disease epicenters of the Kii Peninsula in Japan and Irian Jaya on the island of New Guinea. Comparably, if the incompletely detoxified cycad flour is a major etiologic factor for ALS–PDC on Guam, cessation of cycad use should result in the eventual disappearance of the unique form of this disease.

References

Armon, C., and Kuland, L. T. (1990). Classic and Western Pacific amyotrophic lateral sclerosis: Epidemiologic comparisons. *In* "Amyotrophic Lateral Sclerosis: Concepts in Pathogenesis and Etiology" (A. J. Hudson, ed.), pp. 144–165. University of Toronto Press, Toronto.

Armon, C., Daube, J. R., O'Brien, P. C., Kurland, L. T., and Mulder, D. W. (1991). When is an apparent excess of neurologic cases epidemiologically significant? *Neurology* **41,** 1713–1718.

Arnold, A., Edgren, D. C., and Palladino, V. S. (1953). Amyotrophic lateral sclerosis: Fifty cases observed on Guam. *J. Nerv. Ment. Dis.* **117,** 135–139.

Campbell, R. J., Steele, J. C., Cox, T. A., Loerzel, A. J., Belli, M., Belli, D. D., and Kurland, L. T. (1992). Pathologic findings in the retinal pigment epitheliopathy associated with the amyotrophic lateral sclerosis/parkinsonism dementia complex of Guam. *Ophthalmology* (in press).

Chen, L. (1981). Neurofibrillary change on Guam. *Arch. Neurol.* **38,** 16–18.

Cox, T. A., McDarby, J. V., Lavine, L., Steele, J. C., and Calne, D. B. (1989). A retinopathy on Guam with high prevalence in lytico-bodig. *Opthalmology* **96,** 1731–1735.

Dastur, D. K. (1964). Cycad toxicity in monkeys: Clinical, pathological, and biochemical aspects. *Fed. Proc.* **23,** 1368–1369.

Dastur, D. K., Palekar, R. S., and Manghani, D. K. (1990). Toxicity of various forms of cycas circinalis in rhesus monkeys: Pathology of brain, spinal cord and liver. *In* "Amyotrophic Lateral Sclerosis: New Advances in Toxicoloty and Epidemiology (F. C. Rose, and F. H. Norris, eds.), pp. 129–141. Smith Gordon & Co., London.

Fox, J. P., Hall, C. E., and Elveback, L. R. (1970). Epidemiology: Man and Disease. Macmillan (Collier-Macmillan), London, p. 185.

Fullmer, H. M., Siedler, H. D., Krooth, R. S., and Kurland, L. T. (1960). A cutaneous disorder of connective tissue in amyotrophic lateral sclerosis: A histochemical study. *Neurology* **10,** 717–724.

Gajdusek, D. C., and Salazar, A. M. (1982). Amyotrophic lateral sclerosis and parkinsonism syndromes in high incidence among the Auyu and Jakai people of West New Guinea. *Neurology* **32,** 107–126.

Gajdusek, D. C., Garruto, R. M., and Salazar, A. M. (1980). Ecology of high incidence foci of motor neuron disease in Eastern Asia and Western Pacific and the frequent occurrence of other chronic degenerative neurological diseases in these foci. Tenth International Congress on Tropical Medicine and Malaria, Manila, Philippines, November 9–15, p. 382.

Garruto, R. M. (1987). Neurotoxicity of trace and essential elements: Factors provoking the high incidence of motor neurone disease, parkinsonism and dementia in the Western Pacific. *In* "Motor Neurone Disease: Global Clinical Patterns and International Research" (M. Gourie-Devi, ed.), pp. 73–82. Oxford and IBH Publishing, New Delhi.

Garruto, R. M., Gajdusek, D. C., and Chen, K.-M. (1981). Amyotrophic lateral sclerosis and parkinsonism–dementia among Filipino migrants to Guam. *Ann. Neurol.* **10,** 341–350.

Garruto, R. M., Yanagihara, R., and Gajdusek, D. C. (1985). Disappearance of high-incidence amyotrophic lateral sclerosis and parkinsonism–dementia on Guam. *Neurology* **35,** 193–198.

Garruto, R. M., Yanagihara, R., and Gajdusek, D. C. (1988). Cycads and amyotrophic lateral sclerosis/parkinsonism dementia. *Lancet* **ii,** 1079.

Garruto, R. M., Shankar, S. K., Yanagihara, R., Salazar, A. M., Amyx, H. L., and Gajdusek, D. C. (1989). Low calcium, high aluminum diet-induced motor neuron pathology in cynomolgus monkeys. *Acta Neuropathol.* **78,** 210–219.

Gass, J. D. M., and Lewis, R. A. (1976). Subretinal tracks in ophthalmomyiasis. *Arch. Ophthalmol.* **94,** 1500–1505.

Hirano, A., Malamud, N., and Kurland, L. T. (1961). Parkinsonism–dementia complex, an endemic disease on the island of Guam. II. Pathological features. *Brain* **84,** 662–679.

Hirano, A., Malamud, N., Elizan, T. S., and Kurland, L. T. (1966). Amyotrophic lateral sclerosis and parkinsonism–dementia complex on Guam. *Arch. Neurol.* **5,** 35–51.

Ito, H., Hirano, A., Yen, S.-H., and Kato, S. (1991). Demonstration of β amyloid protein-containing neurofibrillary tangles in parkinsonism–dementia complex on Guam. *Neuropathol. Appl. Neurobiol.* **17,** 365–373.

Kisby, G., and Spencer, P. S. (1989). Neurotoxic amino acids from the cycad carcinogen methylazoxymethanol. *Intl. ALS·MND Update* **2Q89,** 27–28(abstr.).

Kisby, G. E., Ellison, M., and Spencer, P. S. (1992). Content of the neurotoxins cyasin (methylazoxymethanol β-D-glucoside) and BMAA (β-2N-methylamino-L-alanine) in cycad flour prepared by Guam Chamorros. *Neurol.* **42,** 1336–1340.

Koerner, D. R. (1952). Amyotrophic lateral sclerosis on Guam: A clinical study and review of the literature. *Ann. Intern. Med.* **37,** 1204–1220.

Kokmen, E., Beard, C. M., Offord, K. P., and Kurland, L. T. (1989). Prevalence of medically diagnosed dementia in a defined United States population: Rochester, Minnesota, January 1, 1975. *Neurology* **39,** 773–776.

Kurland, L. T. (1957). Epidemiologic investigations of amyotrophic lateral sclerosis. 3. A genetic interpretation of incidence and geographic distribution. *Proc. Staff Meet. Mayo Clin.* **32,** 449–462.

Kurland, L. T. (1978). Geographic isolates: Their role in neuroepidemiology. *In* "Neurological Epidemiology: Principles and Clinical Applications" (B. S. Schoenberg, ed.). *Adv. Neurol.*, Vol. 19, pp. 69–82. Raven Press, New York.

Kurland, L. T., and Molgaard, C. A. (1982). Guamanian ALS: Hereditary or acquired? *In* "Human Motor Neuron Diseases" (L. P. Rowland, ed.), pp. 165–171. Raven Press, New York.

Kurland, L. T., and Mulder, D. W. (1954). Epidemiologic investigations of amyotrophic lateral sclerosis: 1. Preliminary report of geographic distribution, with special reference to the Mariana Islands, including clinical and pathologic observations. *Neurology* **4,** 355–378, 438–448.

Kurland, L. T., and Mulder, D. W. (1987). Overview of motor neurone diseases. *In* "Motor Neurone Disease: Global Clinical Patterns and International Research" (M. Gourie-Devi, ed), pp. 31–44. Oxford and IBH Publishing, New Delhi.

Kurland, L. T., and Mulder, D. W. (1988). Recent epidemiologic developments in the context of earlier observations on ALS: Geographic isolates in the Marianas and other islands of the Western Pacific. *In* "Amyotrophic Lateral Sclerosis: Recent Advances in Research and Treatment" (T. Tsubaki, and Y. Yase, eds.), pp. 3–9. Elsevier Science Publishers (Biomedical Division), Amsterdam.

Kurland, L. T., Hirano, A., Malamud, N., and Lessell, S. (1961). Amyotrophic lateral sclerosis on Guam. *Clin. Neurol.* **1,** 301–306.

Kurland, L. T., Choi, N. W., and Sayre, G. P. (1968). Implications of incidence and geographic patterns on the classification of amyotrophic lateral sclerosis. *In* "Motor Neuron Diseases: Research on Amyotrophic Lateral Sclerosis and Related Disorders" (F. H. Norris and L. T. Kurland, eds.), pp. 28–50. Grune & Stratton, New York.

Kurtzke, J. F., and Kurland, L. T. (1983). The epidemiology of neurologic disease. *In* "Clinical Neurology," Vol. 4, Ch. 66 (R. J. Joynt, ed.), pp. 1–143. J. B. Lippincott, Philadelphia.

Lavine, L., Steele, J. C., Wolfe, N., Calne, D. B., O'Brien, P. C., Williams, D. B., Kurland, L. T., and Schoenberg, B. S. (1991). Amyotrophic lateral sclerosis/parkinsonism–dementia complex in southern Guam: Is it disappearing? *In* "Amyotrophic Lateral Sclerosis and Other Motor Neuron Diseases" (L. P. Rowland, ed.). *Adv. Neurol.*, Vol. 56, pp. 271–285. Raven Press, New York.

Lepore, F. E., Steele, J. C., Cox, T. A., Tillson, G., Calne, D. B., Duvoisin, R. C., Lavine, L., and McDarby, J. V. (1988). Supranuclear disturbances of ocular motility in lytico-bodig. *Neurology* **38,** 1849–1853.

Malamud, N., Hirano, A., and Kurland, L. T. (1961). Pathoanatomic changes in amyotrophic lateral sclerosis on Guam: Special reference to the occurrence of neurofibrillary changes. *Arch. Neurol.* **5,** 401–415.

Matsumoto, H. (1985). Cycasin. *In* "CRC Handbook of Naturally Occurring Food Toxicants" (M. Rechcigl, ed.), pp. 43–61. CRC Press, Boca Raton, Florida.

Mulder, D. W., and Kurland, L. T. (1954). Amyotrophic lateral sclerosis in Micronesia. *Proc. Staff Meet. Mayo Clin.* **29,** 666–670.

Nunn, P. B., Seelig, M., Zagoren, J. C., and Spencer, P. S. (1987). Stereospecific acute neuronotoxicity of "uncommon" plant amino acids linked to human motor-system diseases. *Brain Res.* **410,** 375–379.

Ono, S., Toyokura, Y., Mannen, T., and Ishibashi, Y. (1988). "Delayed return phenomenon" in amyotrophic lateral sclerosis. *Acta Neurol. Scand.* **77,** 102–107.

Ono, S., Mannen, T., and Toyokura, Y. (1989). Differential diagnosis between amyotrophic lateral sclerosis and spinal muscular atrophy by skin involvement. *J. Neurol. Sci.* **91,** 301–310.

Polsky, F. I., Nunn, P. B., and Bell, E. A. (1972). Distribution and toxicity of α-amino-β-methylaminopropionic acid. *Fed. Proc.* **31,** 1473–1475.

Rajput, A. H., Offord, K. P., Beard, C. M., and Kurland, L. T. (1984). Epidemiology of parkinsonism: Incidence, classification, and mortality. *Ann. Neurol.* **16,** 278–282.

Reed, D. M., and Brody, J. A. (1975). Amyotrophic lateral sclerosis and parkinsonism–dementia on Guam, 1945–1972: I. Descriptive epidemiology. *Am. J. Epidemiol.* **101,** 287–301.

Reed, D. Plato, C., Elizan, T., and Kurland, L. T. (1966). The amyotrophic lateral sclerosis/parkinsonism–dementia complex: A ten-year follow up on Guam. I. Epidemiologic studies. *Am. J. Epidemiol.* **83,** 54–73.

Reed, D., Labarthe, D., Chen, K.-M., and Stallones, R. (1987). A cohort study of amyotrophic lateral sclerosis and parkinsonism–dementia on Guam and Rota. *Am. J. Epidemiol.* **125,** 92–100.

Rodgers-Johnson, P., Garruto, R. M., Yanagihara, R., Chen, K.-M., Gajdusek, C. D., and Gibbs, C. J. (1986). Amyotrophic lateral sclerosis and parkinsonism–dementia on Guam: A 30-year evaluation of clinical and neuropathologic trends. *Neurology* **36,** 7–13.

Seawright, A. A., Brown, A. W., Nolan, C. C., and Cavanaugh, J. B. (1990). Selective degeneration of cerebellar cortical neurons caused by cycad neurotoxin, L-β-methylaminoalanine (L-BMAA), in rats. *Neuropathol. Appl. Beurobiol.* **16,** 153–169.

Shankar, S. K., Yanagihara, R., Garruto, R. M., Grundke-Iqbal, I., Kosik, K. S., and Gajdusek, D. C. (1989). Immunocytochemical characterization of neurofibrillary tangles in amyotrophic lateral sclerosis and parkinsonism–dementia of Guam. *Ann. Neurol.* **25,** 146–151.

Spencer, P. S. (1987). Guam ALS/parkinsonism–dementia: A long-latency neurotoxic disorder caused by 'slow toxin(s)' in food? *Can. J. Neurol. Sci.* **14,** 347–357.

Spencer, P. S., and Schaumburg, H. H. (1983). Lathyrism: A neurotoxic disease. *Neurobehav. Toxicol. Teratol.* **5,** 625–629.

Spencer, P. S., Nunn, P. B., Hugon, J., Ludolph, A., and Roy, D. N. (1986). Motor neuron disease on Guam: Possible role of a food neurotoxin. *Lancet* **i,** 965.

Spencer, P. S., Palmer, V. S., Herman, A., and Asmedi, A. (1987a). Cycad use and motor neurone disease in Irian Jaya. *Lancet* **ii,** 1273–1274.

Spencer, P. S., Ohta, M., and Palmer, V. S. (1987b). Cycad use and motor neurone disease in the Kii Peninsula of Japan. *Lancet* **ii,** 1462–1463.

Syralden, P., Nitter, T., and Mehl, R. (1982). Opthalmomyiasis interna posterior: Report of case caused by the reindeer warble fly larva and review of previous reported cases. *Brit. J. Ophthalmol.* **66,** 589–593.

Tillema, S., and Wynberg, C. J. (1953). 'Endemic' amyotrophic lateral sclerosis on Guam: Epidemiological data, preliminary report. *Doc. Med. Geogr. Trop.* (*Amsterdam*) **5,** 366–370.

Uebayashi, Y. (1980). Epidemiological investigation of motor neuron diseases in the Kii Peninsula, Japan, and on Guam: The significance of long survival cases. *Wakayana Med. Rep.* **23,** 13–27.

Vega, A., and Bell, E. A. (1967). α-amino-β-methylaminopropionic acid, a new amino acid from seeds of cycas circinalis. *Phytochemistry* **6,** 759.

Weiss, J. H., Koh, J.-Y., and Choi, D. W. (1989). Neurotoxicity of BMAA and BOAA on cultured cortical neurons. *Brain Res.* **497,** 64–71.

Whiting, M. G. (1963). Toxicity of cycads. *Econ. Bot.* **17,** 271–302.

Yase, Y. (1977). The basic process of amyotrophic lateral sclerosis as reflected in Kii Peninsula and Guam. *Excerpt Med. Intl. Cong. Ser.* **434,** 413–427.

Yoshida, S., Mulder, D. W., Kurland, L. T., Chu, C.-P., and Okazaki, H. (1986). Follow-up study on amyotrophic lateral sclerosis in Rochester, Minn., 1925 through 1984. *Neuroepidemiology* **5,** 61–70.

Zimmerman, H. M. (1945). Monthly Report to Medical Officer in Command, U.S. Naval Medical Research Unit No. 2.

Zolon, W. J., and Ellis-Neill, L. (1986). University of Guam Technical Report No. 64.

4

The Epidemiology of Stroke-Related Disability

Craig Anderson • Konrad Jamrozik

After a long period of neglect, there is now fresh interest in the epidemiology of cerebrovascular disease. This arises in part from the advent of sophisticated, noninvasive diagnostic technology, in part from a desire to compare and contrast explanations for the downward trends in mortality from stroke and ischemic heart disease now established in many Western countries, and in part from the need to plan health services for an elderly population that is growing quickly in both absolute and relative terms.

Previous studies that have considered more than short-term case-fatality after a stroke have mostly reported only the physical function of surviving patients. However, a complete evaluation of the outcome of stroke must also include the patient's psychological and social function because physical independence in the activities of daily living does not necessarily equate with a return to full health.

Data are presented for the follow-up over 1 year of patients registered during the first 10 months of operation of the Perth Community Stroke Study (PCSS). The protocol for this study includes use of multiple sources of ascertainment to identify all episodes of acute cerebrovascular disease affecting a geographically defined population in Perth, Western Australia; follow-up of all patients at 4 and 12 months after the onset of their symptoms; application of well-standardized instruments at baseline and follow-up assessments; and formal review by a psychiatrist at 4 months poststroke.

The results show that the cumulative incidence of depression in a truly representative series of stroke survivors is lower than that previously reported from selected cases, that as many patients suffer incapacitating anxiety as develop significant depression, and that household and social activities continue to be regained over the whole of the first year following

Neuroepidemiology:
Theory and Method

a stroke. Because mortality was highest among those who were not living in their own homes when their stroke occurred, the absolute demand for dependent accommodation actually fell during the year after stroke.

INTRODUCTION

Compared to ischemic heart disease and certainly cancer, the epidemiology of cerebrovascular disease is greatly underdeveloped. Many factors contribute to this situation. To begin with, even now the accepted definitions of both stroke (Hatano, 1976) and transient (cerebral) ischemic attack (TIA; Warlow and Morris, 1982) refer to diagnoses by exclusion of other than vascular explanations for the symptoms and clinical signs. By contrast, the microscope, essential for the histological confirmation of neoplastic disease, has been available for more than 200 years, whereas the electrocardiograph, central to the diagnosis of acute myocardial infarction, was invented just after the turn of this century. It is only with the advent of computerized tomography (CT) scanners in the last two decades that the diagnosis of stroke could be absolutely and positively confirmed in most living patients. The same instrument has also finally made it possible to distinguish among the different pathological subtypes of stroke, rather than relying on correlation of the symptoms and signs with the findings at necropsy in the selected subset of patients for whom the latter data become available. The attending neurologist can now differentiate hemorrhagic from thrombotic cerebrovascular disease with the same confidence that a cardiologist can distinguish inferior from anterior myocardial infarction, or the oncologist primary from secondary hepatic malignancy.

Even with suitable diagnostic technology at hand, epidemiological research into cerebrovascular disease is still very challenging. There is not yet a satisfactory method for distinguishing TIAs from other fleeting neurological problems. In addition, whereas most patients with acute myocardial infarction or cancer other than nonmelanocyctic skin cancer are usually admitted to the hospital for investigation or treatment, a sizable proportion of patients with stroke are not, making studies of its descriptive epidemiology difficult and costly.

Another factor that may have contributed to the relative epidemiological neglect of cerebrovascular disease is that mortality from stroke has been falling steadily in many industrialized countries for at least four decades (Dobson *et al.*, 1981; Bonita *et al.*, 1984; Whisnant, 1984; National Heart Foundation of Australia, 1990). Despite this fact, it remains prominent as a cause of death, accounting for 10.1% of all deaths in Australia in 1989

(National Heart Foundation of Australia, 1990) and is a major cause of permanent and severe disability. Yet, there has probably been a perception among researchers that it is more important to study problems that are still with us rather than to explore the epidemiology of one that may be disappearing.

Finally, thinking about the etiology of stroke has long been dominated by the influence of hypertension, and considerable effort has also been spent on the far less common problem of atrial fibrillation as a risk factor for stroke. It is remarkable that major randomized controlled trials of the management of hypertension such as the Hypertension Detection and Follow-Up Program (Hypertension Detection Follow-Up Program Cooperative Group, 1982), the Australian Therapeutic Trial (Australian National Blood Pressure Study Management Committee, 1980), and the British Medical Research Council Trial (Medical Research Council Working Party, 1985) were designed, conducted, analyzed, and reported before cigarette smoking received anything like appropriate attention as a risk factor for stroke, given the size of the risk it carries and the frequency of the behavior.

The situation today is that there are still very few well-designed population-based studies of stroke available (Malmgrem *et al.*, 1987) and that only now are questions being asked as to whether or not the decline in mortality from stroke might represent selective disappearance of one pathological subtype and whether or not the risk factors for hemorrhagic stroke are different from those for thrombotic stroke. Renewed interest in the epidemiology of cerebrovascular disease can be traced to several sources. Obviously, the advent of accurate, noninvasive diagnostic techniques has been important, while the evolution of epidemiological methods also has to be taken into consideration. Second, recent efforts to explain a remarkable downturn in mortality from ischemic heart disease, seen first in the non-European English-speaking countries, appear to have carried over into a belated investigation of the older, and even more marked, downward trend in mortality from stroke. Third, escalating costs of medical investigation and treatment, combined with a failure to develop any specific treatment for acute stroke, have led to a reopening of the question of stroke prevention. Finally, the rapid relative and absolute growth of the elderly population in industrialized countries has prompted systematic consideration of the medical problems of the elderly and a fear that available economic and medical resources will, in the foreseeable future, be overwhelmed by the needs for long-term care of a large and growing number of disabled elderly, many of whom have been victims of a stroke.

Malmgren *et al.* (1989) combined detailed demographic projections with data on the incidence and outcome of first-ever stroke to show that, in fact, a very rapid expansion in the number of "handicapped" stroke survivors in the community was unlikely, despite the growing numbers of elderly. Even so, considerable resources will probably continue to be used to provide acute hospital care and rehabilitation services for patients who suffer an acute stroke, despite controversy surrounding the role, organization, and effectiveness of such treatment (Wade and Langton Hewer, 1985; Reding and McDowell, 1989; Dobkin, 1989). The prospect for successful recovery from stroke is not an unrealistic goal for many patients, but if a significant proportion of the patients who suffer a stroke remain permanently disabled, this will have important implications for family caregivers and community services, from whom practical and other help will be sought. Clearly, accurate data on the magnitude and pattern of disability arising from stroke is needed to plan services. In addition, epidemiological information on the natural history of stroke is important for the evaluation of preventive and therapeutic measures.

METHODOLOGICAL ISSUES

Previous assessments of the outcome from stroke have been largely restricted to selected patients, such as those admitted to hospital or referred for rehabilitation. An accurate assessment of the total burden of stroke borne by the community requires the inclusion of patients with more severe strokes who may not survive beyond the first few days, as well as those patients with mild strokes, for whom referral for rehabilitation might not be warranted. Other methodological problems such as differences in the timing of follow-up and in criteria for outcome, and the use of measurement instruments whose validity and reliability have not been established, make comparisons among studies difficult (Gresham, 1986; Jongbloed, 1986). Mobility and self-care activities of daily living (ADL) have been the major outcome measures of disability following stroke, and the few community-based studies available suggest that 52–87% of surviving patients are independent in walking and 43–68% are independent in ADL (Wade and Langton Hewer, 1987). While ADL scales effectively identify those patients in most need and show where assistance is required, they fail to identify the effects of mild functional losses or other problems associated with disability (Kay, 1989). Successful recovery from disability requires more than being able to move about and take care of one's basic needs independently. Few studies have assessed how patients actually manage once back at home, where satisfactory recovery of social activities and other aspects of general life are the hallmarks of truly successful rehabilitation (Searle and Davies, 1987).

In the early 1970s, data were collected on stroke survivors and an equal number of matched controls in the Framingham Heart Study cohort (Gresham *et al.*, 1975, 1979). In a later paper (Labi *et al.*, 1980), the same authors highlighted the high frequency of psychosocial disability even among those patients with good levels of physical restoration, social activities outside the home and hobbies or interests being particulary affected. However, it is difficult to determine from this study how much psychosocial disability was related to an individual's emotional problems or cognitive impairment, on the one hand, and to environmental factors, on the other.

Over the last decade, the amount of research devoted to the study of emotional changes following stroke has expanded rapidly. Most attention has focused on depression in the belief that it is very common and a major unmet need of patients. Studies based on hospitalized patients suggest that almost one-half of all stroke survivors suffer from depression, with a prevalence of major depression ranging from 20 to 30% (Starkstein and Robinson, 1989). In addition, knowledge of the emotional changes that follow stroke may shed some light on our understanding of the structural correlates and biological basis of behavior; in particular, some researchers have claimed that depressive illness following stroke is associ-ated with anterior lesions in the left hemisphere (Robinson *et al.*, 1984; Sinyor *et al.*, 1986), but this is disputed by others (House *et al.*, 1990). The importance of depression is that, if recognized early and treated effectively, then this may not only help the individual and his or her family but might also reduce demand on health and other services. However, the considerable conceptual and methodological problems associated with many of these studies make it difficult to draw firm conclusions from the findings (House, 1987). Few studies have detailed the longitudinal course of depression following stroke (House *et al.*, 1991; Wade *et al.*, 1987; Robinson *et al.*, 1987; Morris *et al.*, 1990), and the frequency and importance of other emotional disorders, particularly anxiety, have been ignored by researchers until recently (House *et al.*, 1991).

THE EPIDEMIOLOGICAL STUDY OF CEREBROVASCULAR DISEASE IN AUSTRALIA

In Australia, little has been written on the subjects of stroke epidemiology or the rehabilitation of stroke survivors. Wallace (1967) conducted the first published incidence study in the country town of Goulburn, Victoria, in the 1960s, and he demonstrated the role that general practitioners have in community studies of stroke. This was followed by Christie's landmark studies on the incidence, prevalence, and sequelae of stroke, in Melbourne over 10 years ago (Christie, 1981a,b). Since then, there have only been several audits or reviews based on patients referred for rehabilitation (Flicker, 1989) and a study of all admissions to hospital with stroke in Brisbane, Queensland (Shah and Bain, 1989).

Although, worldwide, there have been few attempts to determine for a defined population the total number of patients receiving or requiring rehabilitation and community services (Dombovy *et al.*, 1987; Legh-Smith *et al.*, 1986), these studies are not readily applicable to health care planning in Australia. Australia is a physically vast country of 17 million people, but, in contrast to its pastoral image, nearly 90% of the population is concentrated in urban areas, usually located near the coastline (Neutze, 1981). Even though Australia has never experienced the massive movement of people from rural to urban areas, which dislocated family ties in Europe and America, strong preferences for institutional care are rooted in a British colonial past (Kendig, 1988). In addition, Australia has experienced a massive postwar migration and is now slowly moving toward a distinctive multicultural nation (Jamrozik and Hobbs, 1989). The structure and availability of hospital and other health services, both public and private, share certain similarities with those of both Britain and the United States but are identical with neither. For example, a universal health insurance scheme, Medicare, was introduced in 1984, but 43% of the population still has private hospital insurance (Willcox, 1991). All of these factors are reasons why lessons learned overseas about services for the care and rehabilitation of patients with stroke cannot necessarily be applied to the Australian scene, despite the fact that the Australian community is undergoing the same rapid demographic changes as those occurring in other developed countries.

THE PERTH COMMUNITY STROKE STUDY

Aims and Methods

The PCSS is a community-based study of acute cerebrovascular disease events in a representative segment of the population of Perth, Western Australia. The four specific aims of the study are

1. to determine the incidence of stroke and its pathological subtypes in a defined population,
2. to determine the relationship between the subtypes of stroke and defined risk factors,
3. to determine the outcome of stroke in terms of survival, physical disability, medical care, and use of services, and

4. to determine the etiology and sequelae of psychiatric disturbance following stroke.

The remainder of this chapter reports preliminary results on the recovery profile over the first year poststroke among consecutive stroke survivors registered in the 10-month period beginning on February 20, 1989. The dimensions of physical disability, emotional problems, social activities, and place of residence are considered in turn.

Ascertainment of Cases

The compilation of the stroke register is based on methods that have been described in full elsewhere (Ward *et al.*, 1988) and that were developed and refined during a pilot phase conducted in 1986. Briefly, all episodes of possible acute cerebrovascular disease between February 20, 1989 and August 19, 1990, inclusive, occurring within a geographically defined area of Perth were registered with the study. The study area is bounded by the Swan River to the south and east, a major arterial road on the west, and the metropolitan boundary to the north and covers eight complete post code districts and part of a ninth. Based on the National Census, conducted in 1986, the projected population of the study area in 1989 was 138,708, these residents being slightly older and less likely to have moved over the previous 10 years than those of the remainder of Perth, but otherwise representative of the city. A variety of overlapping sources of ascertainment of cases was used, including notifications from general practitioners; scrutiny of attendances at and admissions to all acute hospitals, rehabilitation centers, and nursing homes; coroner's reports and death registrations; and surveillance of computerized hospital discharge statistics. All patients were seen as soon as possible after an event by a physician (CA), who conducted a standardized interview and physical examination. Information obtained included data on associated illnesses, risk factors, and the patterns of disability, social activity, and behavior in the premorbid period. If a patient was unconscious or otherwise unassessable, information was obtained from the patient's spouse or another reliable proxy. Standard definitions were used for stroke (Hatano, 1976) and TIA (Warlow and Morris, 1982), and patients were classified as having had either first-ever or a recurrent stroke, or TIA. CT scanning, magnetic resonance imaging, or necropsy was performed in almost 90% of cases.

Follow-Up Schedule

Patients for whom a final diagnosis of the index episode was a stroke and who were not known to have died were contacted again by the same investigator at 4 and 12 months following the initial event. They were usually interviewed in their place of residence, the only patients being seen in the hospital were those who were inpatients at the time of follow-up. Outcome from stroke was assessed in a two-stage procedure. First, all patients were seen again by the same investigator who had made the assessment at the time of the initial registration. At follow-up, he recorded clinical information and data on physical function, social activities, behavior, and mental status according to published measures. A patient's actual level of function was recorded rather than his or her potential ability, and this information was checked against other available sources. The second stage of the follow-up schedule involved an interview by a psychiatrist who was a member of the study team and who was blind to clinical information about the patient.

Assessment Instruments

Physical function or disability status was measured according to the Barthel Index of self-care ADL (Mahoney and Barthel, 1965). This index is a valid and reliable measure of physical function that has been modified to give a score between 0 and 20 in increments of 1 point (Wade and Collin, 1988). These scores can be arbitrarily divided into five categories of disability, with 0–4 signifying severe disability or total dependence, and the top score of 20 implying independence in ADL although not necessarily normality. Previous researchers have shown that these items of ADL represent core dimensions of function, which tend to be lost and regained in a hierarchical sequence (Wade and Langton Hewer, 1987; Katz *et al.*, 1963). Continence and eating are the first functions to recover, whereas showering, dressing, and climbing stairs tend to recover late. Furthermore, equivalent score among groups of patients imply similar disabilities.

Social function was assessed using the Frenchay Activities Index (FAI) (Holbrook and Skilbeck, 1983; Wade *et al.*, 1985), which is based on the frequency with which a patient performs 15 separate activities (e.g., shopping, reading books, cooking) and gives a score between 15 (no activities) and 60 (full activities). Dysphasia was assessed using a modified token test (De Renzi and Faglioni, 1978) and cognitive impairment was assessed using the Mini-Mental State Examination (Folstein *et al.*, 1975). The chief caregiver of the patient was also interviewed about the patient's recent behavior.

The psychiatric interview involved using the Psychiatric Assessment Schedule (PAS) (Dean *et al.*, 1983). The PAS is a questionnaire for administration in a semistructured interview and consists of sections of the Present State Examination supplemented by additional questions (Wing *et al.*, 1974; Cooper *et al.*, 1977). It allows documentation and measurement of the presence and severity of a wide range of psychiatric symptomatology and can be used to derive a clinical diagnosis of depressive and anxiety disorders according to the standard psychiatric classifications in the *Diagnostic and Statistical Manual*, 3rd ed. (DSM-III; American Psychiatric Association, 1980), and DSM-III, revised (American Psychiatric Association, 1987). Additional questions were also asked about episodes of pathological emotionalism (or alternatively called emotional lability). Only those patients who had a clinically evident psychiatric disorder at 4 months were reassessed by a psychiatrist at 12 months.

Results

During the first 10 months of registration, 225 patients—119 (53%) males—had suffered an acute stroke (first-ever and recurrent). As may be seen from Table I, 7% of patients were less than 54 years old, while 56% were 75 years or older. Of these patients, 106 (48%) were married at the time of their stroke, and about one-fifth were managed outside a hospital during the acute phase. At 4 months after the first registered stroke, 90 (31%) of these patients had died, and by 12 months, another 17 patients had died, so that the cumulative mortality after 1 year was 38%. All patients had a full assessment of their overall disability status but four patients refused or were unavailable for the psychiatric interview.

Physical Disability

Figure 1 shows the distribution of Barthel Index scores before stroke and in survivors at onset and 4 and 12 months after their first registered stroke. At the time of their stroke, 67 (30%) patients were at least mildly dependent in physical function. By 4 months, 75 (48%) patients were totally independent and 13 (8%) totally dependent in ADL. The corresponding figures at 12 months were 78 (56%) independent and 13 (10%) dependent. While

Table I

Age Distribution of Cases of Stroke in the Perth Community Stroke Study

Age group	Number	Percent
<55 years	16	7
55–64 years	27	12
65–74 years	57	25
75–84 years	92	41
85+ years	33	15
Total	225	100

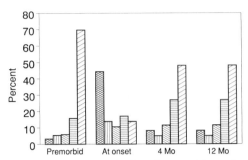

Figure 1   Proportion (%) of patients with stroke dependent in physical function according to the Barthel Index of activities of daily living. ▨ ,0–4, ▥ ,5–9, ▨ ,10–14, ▤ ,15–19, ▨ ,20.

the proportions of patients at the extremes of the scale had remained relatively stable between 4 and 12 months, the number of patients in the intermediate grades, mild to severe disability, fell from 69 (44%) to 48 (34%).

Emotional Disorders

Table II shows the frequency of depression and anxiety disorders among survivors assessed 4 months after their stroke. About one-quarter of survivors of stroke from this population suffered from depression. The prevalence of major depression was 17%, which is much lower than that

Table II

Prevalence of Emotional Disorders 4 Months after Acute Stroke[a]

Emotional Disorder	Number	Percent
Major depression	24	17
Dysthymia	12	9
Emotionalism	11	8
Social/agoraphobia	25	19
Generalized anxiety	12	9
Simple phobia	19	14
Panic disorder	2	1
Not assessable	21	15

[a] Diagnoses based on psychiatric interview and the *Diagnostic and Statistic Manual,* 3rd ed. and rev. ed. Prevalence figures are not mutually exclusive.

reported from series of selected patients. Pathological emotionalism was evident at interview in 8% of patients but many more gave a history of its occurrence soon after the stroke. Varying states of anxiety were just as prevalent as depression, with 25 (19%) patients suffering from social or agoraphobia.

Social Activities

Figure 2 shows the proportions of patients undertaking household activities at the highest frequency recorded by the FAI before stroke and corresponding data for survivors at 4 and 12 months poststroke. At each point, patients either did not perform the activity or did the activity a lot, and some items such as light housework are less affected by a stroke than others, such as cooking and heavy housework. The figure also shows that substantial recovery occurs between 4 and 12 months.

Figure 3 profiles the recovery in outdoor activities. While the relative number of people who did not perform a particular outdoor activity at 12 months remained about the same compared to that at prestroke, the middle categories of frequency increased such that fewer patients were in the category of highest frequency. Figure 4 presents data on leisure and work activities. The interesting observation in these data is that the

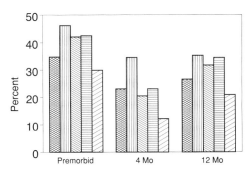

Figure 2 Recovery of household social activities after stroke. Data in the figure are the proportions (%) of patients undertaking the activity with the highest frequency specified by the Frenchay Activities Index, that is, "most days" for cooking and washing dishes and "at least weekly" for washing clothes and light and heavy housework (h-work). ▓ , cooking, ▥ , wash dishes, ▨ , wash clothes, ▤ , light house work, ▨ , heavy house work.

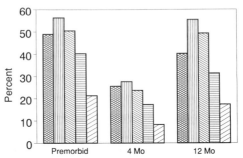

Figure 3 Recovery of outdoor activities after stroke. Data in the figure are the proportions (%) of patients undertaking the activity with the highest frequency specified by the Frenchay Activities Index, that is, "at least weekly" for each activity. ▨ , shopping, ▥ , local visits, ◩ , walking, ▤ , driving, ▧ , travel.

proportion of patients engaged in social outings, either local visits or travel farther afield, increased between 4 and 12 months. This is probably best explained by the selective survival of the most socially active patients, but there may also be a contribution from community support

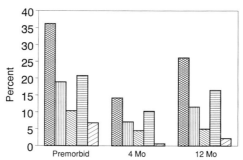

Figure 4 Recovery of leisure and work activities after stroke. Data in the figure are the proportions (%) of patients undertaking the activity with the highest frequency specified by the Frenchay Activities Index, that is, "at least weekly" for reading and hobby, "all necessary" for gardening and household maintenance, and "more than 30 hr per week" for paid work. ▨ , hobby, ▥ , gardening, ◩ , maintenance, ▤ , reading, ▧ , paid work.

services such as day centers. Fifteen patients were in full-time employment before their stroke, but, at 12 months, only three had returned to work.

Place of Residence

Residence is a well-defined measure that is useful for planning purposes, but it is also a good surrogate measure of dependence. The residence of patients before stroke and at 12 months is given in Table III. Among survivors at 1-year poststroke, 12% were in institutional care. When mortality is compared to place of residence, the 12-month case-fatality for those living home at the time of their stroke was 31% compared to 100% for those living in institutional care at onset. Thus, the majority of patients living in a nursing home 12 months after a stroke are newly admitted individuals who had previously lived in their own homes, and the absolute number of subjects living in an institution fell from 40 at the time of onset of the stroke to 27 at 1-year follow-up.

Discussion

The PCSS overcomes many of the shortcomings in previous studies of the outcome from stroke because it is based on a completely representative group of patients and uses multidimensional measures of outcome, stan-

Table III

Residence at the Time of Stroke and 12 Months Aferward

Residence at time of stroke	Status at follow-up									
	Own home		Lodge or hostel		Nursing home		Hospital		Dead	
	n	%	n	%	n	%	n	%	n	%
Own home ($n = 175$)	105	60.0	4	2.3	9	5.1	3	1.7	54	30.9
Lodge or hostel ($n = 21$)	0	0	4	19.0	6	28.6	0	0	11	52.4
Nursing home ($n = 13$)	0	0	0	0	0	0	0	0	13	100.0
Hospital ($n = 1$)	0	0	0	0	0	0	0	0	1	100.0
Other ($n = 5$)	2	40.0	0	0	1	20.0	0	0	2	40.0
Total ($n = 215$)	107	49.8	8	3.7	16	7.4	3	1.4	81	37.7

dardized techniques for psychiatric diagnosis, and uniform timing of assessments linked to the onset of stroke.

As reported in other community-based studies of stroke, at least 50% of long-term survivors of a stroke are independent in physical function as measured by ADL. One important limitation of ADL scales is that they have both floor and ceiling effects; that is, they have limited sensitivity to changes at the extremes of the scale. However, even when this factor is considered, our data suggest that, for some patients, recovery continues over 12 months after a stroke, so that patients tend to diverge into two distinct groups of physical function. One year after their illness, survivors of stroke from this population are generally either completely independent (or at most only mildly disabled) or totally dependent in physical function. This can partly be explained on the basis that those patients already severely disabled at the time of their stroke, as well as those patients who suffer the most severe strokes, have the greatest risk of early death.

Another limitation of ADL scales is that they are silent about etiology. Disability after stroke often relates to nonstroke pathology, such as arthritis or vascular disease, the latter being more common in those patients who suffer a stroke. An interesting finding was that several patients had worsening symptoms of their angina or intermittent claudication over the months subsequent to their stroke. Other studies have shown that when these comorbid factors are eliminated from the analysis, the difference in functional loss between survivors of stroke and matched controls appears less dramatic (Gresham *et al.*, 1979).

Emotional problems following stroke are an important cause of failure to regain social activities and of reduced quality of life and must also be considered if the evaluation of rehabilitation and outcome is to be complete. The prevalence of major depression (17%) in this study is lower than in series of selected patients but higher than the figure of 9% recently reported from the Oxfordshire Community Stroke Project among survivors assessed 6 months after a first stroke (House *et al.*, 1991). The number and extent of psychiatric symptoms in the patients from Perth suggested that any major depression tended to be mild. Nevertheless, where it was present, depression was an important cause of distress in both patient and caregiver. At this stage, the relative importance of various etiological factors is unknown, but, as in other studies (Starkstein and Robinson, 1989; House, 1987), the level of physical disability does not appear to be an important factor. However, a history of depression appears to increase the risk of depression following stroke, and several patients actually had a depressive illness at or shortly before their stroke. These factors have not been adequately considered in previous studies of depression after stroke.

Pathological emotionalism is a disorder that has been included under the category of depressive illness, although its presence does not necessarily imply that a patient is depressed (for a review of this phenomenon, see Allman, 1991). It can be defined as "an easy susceptibility to tearfulness, crying or laughter" and is better termed "emotionalism" rather than "emotional lability," because "lability" suggests a degree of spontaneity in mood in either direction, which is inappropriate and unprovoked. The emotionalism seen after a stroke is usually crying and is secondary to an appropriate stimulus. The patient is usually in control of his or her emotions, but if he or she reads or hears something sad or upsetting, then the reaction occurs. This commonly happens when watching the television or reading a book, or if a person expresses love or kindness toward the patient. Emotionalism occurred in about 8% of cases during interview, but many more patients gave a history of its occurrence soon after the stroke. It proved to be particularly distressing and embarrassing for both the patient and family, often leading the patient to avoid social company outside the immediate family.

Varying forms of anxiety were equally important following stroke. Anxiety was greatest in the first few days after the onset of the illness, which is obviously a period of great uncertainty, and also when a patient first returns home. The most frequent anxiety state was social or agoraphobia, which occurred in 19% of patients. Although this category included a heterogeneous range of symptoms, some common features emerged. Female patients and those with predominantly physical disability tended to develop agoraphobia. The fears revolved around leaving the house or being alone, crossing a road, or negotiating physical obstacles such as steps. This loss of confidence in mobility and the fear of falling or injury both inside and outside the home led many patients to rely heavily on friends or family members to do their shopping and banking. The importance of this factor as a cause of "psychosocial" disability and dependency has not previously been emphasized in the literature. Despite being an important early cause of failure to resume social activities, it was encouraging to see that most patients with agoraphobia generally made a spontaneous recovery over several months after their stroke. Patients would gradually increase the distances that they would venture outside the home, but the last major obstacle was usually riding on public transport. This often proved most difficult to overcome for many elderly patients, who then had to rely on community services, taxis, or family members for transport.

Social phobia, on the other hand, tended to occur more frequently among men and those patients with speech disturbance. Crowds or situations where patients would have to meet new people precipitated symptoms of anxiety, often with intense autonomic disturbance, and consequently these patients would avoid these situations. The inability to follow conversation or to express themselves, or the feeling of being different, were often cited by patients as the main reasons for this behavior. In a similar way to the patients with agoraphobia, patients with social phobia gradually made a recovery over the year after their stroke and long after specific rehabilitation therapies had ceased.

Several patients had generalized anxiety states. When the anxiety was associated with severe autonomic disturbance it was classified as a panic disorder. This occurred in two patients. A number of other patients had simple phobias, but these tended to be longstanding and not related to the stroke. Finally, information on mood state could not be obtained in 15% of patients because of severe dementia or aphasia.

The recovery in social activities following stroke is a difficult area to measure accurately. The FAI appears to give a useful, easily administered, and objective measure of actual activities in the recent past among patients who have suffered a stroke (Wade *et al.*, 1985). Unfortunately, the original validation study in a large sample of patients who had suffered a stroke was complicated by a significant proportion of incomplete data, particularly among patients who died in the first 6 months. The FAI has recently been validated in Oxford in a sample of community-dwelling people aged 70 years and over. Although women tended strongly to have higher scores than men, this reflects the emphasis given in the instrument to household activities, and the difference between the sexes was reduced when marital status is taken into account (Cockburn *et al.*, 1990). Lower levels of social activity were found among people with lower levels of cognitive performance, and age did not appear to be a significant independent factor affecting the score attained. One limitation of brief assessment scales such as the FAI is that they do not assess the quality of social activities, contacts, and events, themselves important components of health (Ware, 1987). Despite these limitations, these preliminary data from the PCSS do present an overview of the important area of social recovery after stroke.

Some household activities such as heavy housework and cooking are more affected by stroke than others, such as light housework. Although many patients are able to return to activities such as driving a motor vehicle, the frequency of such activities is reduced. Some activities such as socialization outside the home actually seemed to increase after stroke. While patients may resume a particular activity, the quality of their participation is difficult to measure. For example, many patients were able to return to driving but the distances they would travel, or the time of day at which they would drive, had changed following the stroke. This was often due to an emotional disorder or to a simple lack of confidence among those patients with good restoration of physical function. For Australians, driving is important both as a component of social activities and as a source of independence, and the inability to return to driving, even in a limited capacity, was often cited by patients as an important factor in their reduced quality of life.

These preliminary data relating to a total community present a more optimistic outlook for those patients who survive a stroke than is apparent from series of hospitalized patients. The finding of substantial recovery between 4 and 12 months after a stroke is encouraging. To some degree, this probably reflects differential survival of the fittest, and most socially active individuals as those patients in dependent accommodation at the time of their stroke had a reduced survival compared to those previously living at home. Bonita *et al.* (1988) also found that place of residence at the time of the stroke was a strong independent predictor of long-term survival. The fact that strokes are more likely to kill people who are already dependent is an important argument against the concern that the burden on the community of supporting these patients is likely to increase in the future as the population ages (Malmgren *et al.*, 1989).

CONCLUSION

There is renewed interest in the epidemiology of cerebrovascular disease, at least partly because of fear that a rapid expansion in the size of the elderly population will result in a major increase in the number of disabled survivors of stroke. PCSS, a comprehensive study of stroke in a defined population, confirms that there is a broad spectrum of problems that a patient may have to overcome to make a satisfactory recovery from a stroke. However, despite the high case-fatality of stroke, the majority of patients who survive return home with relatively good levels of physical restoration. Nevertheless, emotional disorders, particularly depression and phobias, are frequent and equally important causes of failure to resume social activities. All of these factors must be addressed by those involved in the care of such patients, and the mixed nature of the problems that may be faced by an individual patient supports the multidisciplinary team approach to rehabilitation.

In the PCSS, the differentially greater mortality of patients who were living in residences other than private homes at the time of the onset of their illness meant that the absolute number of individuals requiring dependent accommodation actually fell during the first year after the stroke occurred. The combination of demographic projections with data on the incidence and case-fatality of stroke may therefore provide a misleading picture of future requirements for health and other services related to cerebrovascular disease.

Acknowledgments

The Perth Community Stroke Study is supported by grants from the National Health and Medical Research Council of Australia, the Australian Brain Foundation, and the Royal Perth Hospital Medical Research Foundation. The Perth Community Stroke Study is a collaborative project involving the following departments: Departments of Neurology (Dr. C. Anderson, Dr. E. Stewart-Wynne) and Radiology (Dr. T. Chakera), at Royal Perth Hospital, and Departments of Medicine (Dr. K. Jamrozik, Mr. F. Gout, Ms. R. Broadhurst), and Psychiatry and Behavioural Science (Professor P. Burvill, Dr. G. Johnson), at the University of Western Australia.

References

Allman, P. (1991). Depressive disorders and emotionalism following stroke. *Int. J. Geriat. Psychiaty* **6,** 377–383.

American Psychiatric Association (1980). "Diagnostic and Statistics Manual," 3rd ed. American Psychiatric Association, Washington, D.C.

American Psychiatric Association. (1987). "Diagnostic and Statistical Mannual of Mental Disorders," 3rd ed., rev. American Psychiatric Association, Washington, D.C.

Australian National Blood Pressure Study Management Committee. (1980). The Australian therapeutic trial in mild hypertension. *Lancet* **i,** 126–127.

Bonita, R., Beaglehole, R., and North, J. D. K. (1984). Event, incidence and case-fatality rates for cerebrovascular disease in Auckland, New Zealand. *Am. J. Epidemiol.* **120,** 236–243.

Bonita, R., Ford, M. A., and Stewart, A. W. (1988). Predicting survival after stroke: A three-year follow-up. *Stroke* **19,** 669–673.

Christie, D. (1981a). Prevalence of stroke and its sequelae. *Med. J. Aust.* **12,** 182–184.

Christie, D. (1981b). Stroke in Melbourne, Australia: An epidemiological study. *Stroke* **12,** 467–469.

Cockburn, J., Smith, P. T., and Wade, D. T. (1990). Influence of cognitive function on social, domestic, and leisure activities of community-dwelling older people. *Int. Disabil. Stud.* **12,** 169–172.

Cooper, J., Nixon, S. A., Mann, A., and Leff, J. (1977). Reliability of the PSE (9th edition) used in a population survey. *Psychol. Med.* **7,** 505–516.

De Renzi, E., and Faglioni, P. (1978). Normative data and screening power of a shortened version of the token test. *Cortex* **14,** 41–49.

Dean, C., Surtees, P. G., and Shashidharan, S. P. (1983). Comparison of research diagnostic systems in an Edinburgh community sample. *Brit. J. Psychiat.* **142,** 247–256.

Dobkin, B. H. (1989). Focussed stroke rehabilitation programs do not improve outcome. *Arch. Neurol.* **46,** 701–703.

Dobson, A. J., Gibberd, R. W., Wheeler, D. J., and Leeder, S. R. (1981). Age-specific trends in mortality from ischaemic heart disease and cerebrovascular disease in Australia. *Am. J. Epidemiol.* **113,** 404–412.

Dombovy, M. L., Basford, J. R., Whisnant, J. P., and Bergstralh, E. J. (1987). Disability and use of rehabilitation services following stroke in Rochester, Minnesota, 1975–1979. *Stroke* **18,** 830–836.

Flicker, L. (1989). Rehabilitation for stroke survivors—A review. *Aust. N. Z. J. Med.* **19,** 400–406.

Folstein, M. F., Folstein, S. E., and McHugh, P. (1975). Mini-mental state—A practical method for grading the cognitive state of patients for the clinician. *J. Psychiat. Res.* **12,** 189–198.

Gresham, G. E. (1986). Stroke outcome research. *Stroke* **17,** 358–360.

Gresham, G. E., Fitzpatrick, T. E., Wolf, P. A., McNamara, P. M., Kannell, W. E., and Dawber, T. R. (1975). Residual disability in stroke survivors: The Framingham study. *N. Engl. J. Med.* **293,** 954–956.

Gresham, G. E., Phillips, T. F., Wolf, P. A., McNamara, P. M., Kannel, W. B., and Dawber, T. R. (1979). Epidemiological profile of long-term stroke disability: The Framingham study. *Arch. Phys. Med. Rehabil.* **60,** 487–491.

Hatano, S. (1976). Experience from a multicentre stroke register: A preliminary report. *Bull. W. H. O.* **54,** 541–553.

Holbrook, M., and Skilbeck, C. E. (1983). An activities index for use with stroke patients. *Age Ageing* **12,** 166–170.

House, A. (1987). Mood disorders after stroke: A review of the evidence. *Int. J. Geriatr. Psychiaty* **2,** 211–221.

House, A., Dennis, M., Hawton, K., Warlow, C., and Molyneux, A. (1990). Mood disorders after stroke and their relation to lesion location: A CT scan study. *Brain* **113,** 113–129.

House, A., Dennis, M., Mogridge, L., Warlow, C., Hawton, K., and Jones, L. (1991). Mood disorders in the year after stroke. *Brit. J. Psychiaty* **158,** 83–92.

Hypertension Detection and Follow-up Program Co-operative Group. (1982). Five-year findings of the hypertension detection and follow-up program. III. Reduction in stroke incidence among persons with high blood pressure. *JAMA* **247,** 633–638.

Jamrozik, K., and Hobbs, M. S. T. (1989). Migrants and medicine—Many challenges. *Med. J. Aust.* **150,** 415–417.

Jongbloed, L. (1986). Prediction of function after stroke: A critical review. *Stroke* **17,** 765–776.

Katz, S., Ford, A. B., Moskowitz, R. W., Jackson, B. A., and Jaffe, M. W. (1963). Studies of illness in the aged. The index of ADL: A standardised measure of biological and psychosocial function. *J. Am. Med. Assoc.* **185,** 914–919.

Kay, D. W. K. (1989). Ageing of the population: Measuring the need for care. *Age Ageing* **18,** 73–76.

Kendig, H. L. (1988). Aging, intergenerational support, and social change in Australia. *In* "Crossroads in Aging" (M. Bergener, M. Ermini, and H. B. Stahelin, eds.), pp. 233–261. Academic Press, London.

Labi, M. L., Phillips, T. F., and Gresham, G. E. (1980). Psychosocial disability in the physically restored long-term stroke survivors. *Arch. Phys. Med. Rehabil.* **61,** 561–565.

Legh-Smith, J., Wade, D. T., and Langton Hewer, R. (1986). Services for stroke patients one year after stroke. *J. Epidemiol. Community Health* **40,** 161–165.

Mahoney, F. I., and Barthel, D. W. (1965). Functional evaluation: The Barthel Index. *Maryland State Med. J.* **14,** 61–65.

Malmgren, R., Warlow, C., Bamford, J., and Sandercock, P. (1987). Geographical and secular trends in stroke incidence. *Lancet* **2,** 1196–1199.

Malmgren, R., Bamford, J., Warlow, C., Sandercock, P., and Slattery, J. (1989). Projecting the number of patients with first ever stroke and patients newly handicapped by stroke in England and Wales. *Brit. Med. J.* **298,** 656–660.

Medical Research Council Working Party. (1985). MRC trial of treatment of mild hypertension: Principal results. *Br. Med. J.* **291,** 97–104.

Morris, P. L. P., Robinson, R. G., and Ralphael, B. (1990). Prevalence and course of depressive disorders in hospitalized stroke patients. *Int. J. Psychiatry Med.* **20,** 349–364.

National Heart Foundation of Australia. (1990). "Heart Facts Report—1989." National Heart Foundation of Australia, Canberra.

Neutze, M. (1981). Urban development in Australia: A descriptive analysis. Allen & Unwin, Sydney.

Reding, M. J., and McDowell, F. H. (1989). Focussed stroke rehabilitation programs improve outcome. *Arch. Neurol.* **49,** 700–701.

Robinson, R. G., Kubos, K. L., Starr, L. B., *et al.* (1984). Mood disorders in stroke patients: Importance of lesion location. *Brain* **107,** 81–93.

Robinson, R. G., Bolduc, P., and Price, T. R. (1987). Two year longitudinal study of post stroke mood disorders: Diagnosis and outcome at 1 and 2 years. *Stroke* **18,** 837–843.

Searle, C., and Davies, P. (1987). Outcome measurement in stroke rehabilitation research. *Int. Disabil. Stud.* **9,** 155–160.

Shah, S. K., and Bain, C. (1989). Admissions, patterns of utilisation and disposition of cases of acute stroke in Brisbane hospitals. *Med. J. Aust.* **150,** 256–260.

Sinyor, D., Jacques, P., Kaloupek, G., *et al.* (1986). Post-stroke depression and lesion location: An attempted replication. *Brain* **109,** 537–546.

Starkstein, S., and Robinson, R. (1989). Affective disorders and cerebral vascular disease. *Brit. J. Psychiaty* **154,** 170–182.

Wade, D. T., and Collin, C. (1988). The Barthel ADL Index: A standard measure of physical disability? *Int. Disabil. Stud.* **10,** 64–67.

Wade, D. T., and Langton Hewer, R. (1985). Hospital admission for stroke: Who, for how long, and to what effect? *J. Epidemiol. Community Health* **39,** 347–352.

Wade, D. T., and Langton Hewer, R. (1987). Functional abilities after stroke: Measurement, natural history, and prognosis. *J. Neurol. Neurosurg. Psychiaty* **50,** 177–182.

Wade, D. T., Legh-Smith, J., and Langton Hewer, R. (1985). Social activities after stroke: Measurement and natural history using the Frenchay Activities Index. *Int. Rehabil. Med.* **7,** 176–181.

Wade, D. T., Legh-Smith, J., and Langton Hewer, R. (1987). Depression after stroke: A community assessment. *Brit. J. Psychiaty* **151,** 200–206.

Wallace, D. C. (1967). A study of the natural history of cerebral vascular disease. *Med. J. Aust.* **1,** 90–95.

Ward, G., Jamrozik, K., and Stewart-Wynne, E. (1988). Incidence and outcome of cerebrovascular disease in Perth, Western Australia. *Stroke* **19,** 1501–1506.

Ware, J. E. (1987). Standards for validating health measures: Definitions and content. *J. Chron. Dis.* **40,** 473–480.

Warlow, C. P., and Morris, P. J. (1982). Introduction. *In* "Transient Ischaemic Attacks" (C. P. Warlow and P. J. Morris, eds.), pp. vii–xi. Marcel Dekker, New York.

Whisnant, J. (1984). The decline of stroke. *Stroke* **15,** 467–469.

Willcox, S. A. (1991). A healthy risk? Use of private insurance, March 1991. The National Health Strategy Background Paper No. 4.

Wing, J., Cooper, J., and Sartorious, N. (1974). "Measurement and Classification of Psychiatric Symptoms." Cambridge University Press, London.

5

The Neuroepidemiology of Human T-Cell Lymphotrophic Virus-I

Stephanie K. Brodine • *Richard J. Thomas*

The human retroviruses, including human immunodeficiency virus (HIV) and human T-cell lymphotrophic virus-I (HTLV-I), are a new class of RNA viruses that are named for their unique feature of "reverse" genetic flow in which a DNA copy is made and inserted into a host chromosome. HTLV-I was the first human retrovirus to be isolated and has been shown to be the etiologic agent of adult T-cell leukemia–lymphoma (ATLL) and the sporadic form of tropical spastic paraparesis (TSP), now termed HTLV-I-associated myelopathy–TSP (HAM/TSP). The recent institution of blood donor screening for HTLV-I and the availability of commercial serologic testing has led to increased awareness and diagnosis of HTLV-I-associated disease. This chapter will focus on the neurologic syndrome associated with HTLV-I, discussing the classification of the tropical myeloneuropathies, the history and epidemiology of HTLV-I, and the disease entity of HAM/TSP.

TROPICAL MYELONEUROPATHIES

The occurrence of chronic neurologic diseases in the tropics, tropical myeloneuropathies, has been reported since the 19th century. Kark *et al.* (1947) alludes to authors such a Kipling, Conrad, and Somerset Maugham, who included descriptions of "tropical deterioration" or a "tropical neurasthenia" in Europeans emigrating to colonial regions. Some of the early reports in the medical literature were from Jamaica, where Strachan (1888, 1897) and Scott (1918) described large series of patients with dramatic neurologic symptoms of ataxia, painful paresthesias, amblyopia, and less commonly spastic paraplegia. Various etiologies including malaria, arsenic poisoning, and malnutrition were proposed. It was not until World War II, with documentation of nutritional deficiency-related neurologic diseases in prisoners of war (POWs), that interest emerged in the Western world (Roman *et al.*, 1985) and the interrelationships of nutrition, environment, infectious agents, and toxins began to be systematically investigated.

There are two major clinical presentations of tropical myeloneuropathies—tropical ataxic neuropathy (TAN) and TSP—although some patients have overlapping features. Patients with TAN have a predominantly sensory disorder with the primary lesion being in the dorsal columns. Patients present with ataxia and painful neuritis of the lower extremities, often accompanied by optic neuropathy, sensorineural hearing loss, and muscle wasting (Montgomery *et al.*, 1964). This is most likely the syndrome that was described by Strachan (1888, 1897) in association with malnutrition and was the most common neurologic disorder of POWs (Denny-Brown, 1947). Although TAN was more prevalent than TSP worldwide, the incidence of TAN in some of the tropical regions such as Jamaica has sharply declined in recent years, probably due to an improvement in the population's socioeconomic and health status (Morgan *et al.*, 1988).

TSP is a pyramidal tract disorder that presents with spasticity, predominantly of the lower extremities, difficulty with micturition, constipation, and minor sensory abnormalities (Montgomery *et al.*, 1964). Two forms of the disease occur: an epidemic form related to ingestion of chickling pea (lathyrus) (Mani *et al.*, 1969) or cassava (Roman *et al.*, 1985) and a sporadic endemic form, which is now known to be associated with HTLV-I infection (Gessain *et al.*, 1985). The epidemic form usually occurs in time of drought and famine with increased dietary intake of cassava and chickling pea. As the cyanogenic glycosides in cassava are normally detoxified with sulfur-containing amino acids, malnutrition and sulfur deficiency increase the frequency and severity of TSP in this setting. Typically, victims have a subacute or abrupt onset of stiffness and spasticity, predominately of the lower extremities, difficulty with micturition, and lumbar pain. In most cases, deficits reach a stable level without progression or improvement. The largest documented outbreak of epidemic TSP was during a drought in Mozambique in 1981, in which more than 1000 cases were reported (Cliff *et al.*, 1985). Chronic ingestion of inadequately processed cassava can result in a TAN-like syndrome (Roman *et al.*, 1985).

The sporadic form of TSP was known to predominate in certain regions such as the Caribbean (Jamaican neuropathy) (Montgomery *et al.*, 1964), Colombia (Pacific spastic paraparesis) (Zaninovic, 1986), and South India (South Indian paraplegia) (Mani *et al.*, 1969) (Fig. 1). The term tropical spastic paraplegia, or TSP, was first proposed by researchers in South India (Mani *et al.*, 1969) to unify these apparently identical syndromes characterized by a slowly progressive paraplegia of unknown etiology.

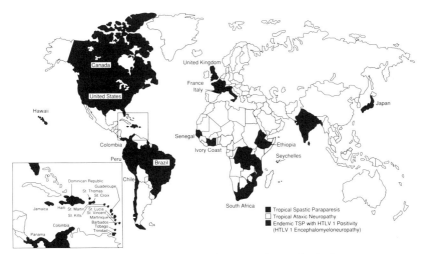

Figure 1 Map of the world showing the areas from which the various types of tropical myelopathies have been reported. Inset shows the Caribbean basin and islands with HTLV-I-positive tropical spastic paraparesis (TSP).

Patients were typically in their third to fourth decade and had an insidious onset of gait stiffness and weakness, low back pain, and bladder dysfunction, which progressed over several months to years. Ultimate disability varied from minor spasticity to a bedridden state. The etiology of these sporadically occurring cases was obscure and could not be linked to nutritional deficits or ingestion of cassava or chickling pea. Autopsy studies revealed a widespread meningomyelitis, particularly in the long tracts of the spinal cord, which raised the possibility of an infectious etiology. In the Jamaican series, the majority of patients had positive treponemal serology, and Montgomery *et al.* (1964) proposed that this represented an atypical form of neurosyphilis or yaws.

HUMAN T-CELL LEUKEMIA VIRUS-I-ASSOCIATED MYELOPATHY

In 1982, the Caribbean basin was shown to be an endemic focus for a human retrovirus, HTLV-I, which had been linked to an aggressive T-cell leukemia in southwestern Japan (Blattner *et al.*, 1982). Gessain *et al.* (1985) conducted a serosurvey in patients in Martinique for evidence of HTLV-I infection and serendipitously noted an association between TSP and HTLV-I. Further study showed 15 of 23 (65%) patients with TSP to be seropositive for HTLV-I compared to 11 of 252 (4.4%) healthy blood donors. This report was followed by similar reports from Jamaica and Colombia (Rodgers-Johnson *et al.*, 1985), the Seychelles (Roman *et al.*, 1987), and Trinidad (Bartholomew *et al.*, 1986). Evidence for a causal relationship between HTLV-I infection and this neurologic syndrome was further provided by viral culture and detection of the viral antigen in cerebrospinal fluid and serum of patients (Bhagavati *et al.*, 1988; Kwok *et al.*, 1988). In southwestern Japan, Japanese investigators documented a previously unrecognized but similar spastic syndrome in patients seropositive for HTLV-I. Because Japan is not "tropical," these investigators coined the term HTLV-I-associated myelopathy, or HAM (Osame *et al.*, 1986).

Initially, differences between the two syndromes TSP and HAM were emphasized (Roman, 1987); however, it is now believed that these are identical syndromes (Roman and Osame, 1988). The current terminology is HAM–TSP. Subsequent studies of patients with TSP in India have shown the majority of these patients in one case series to be seronegative for HTLV (Richardson *et al.*, 1989); however, unusual serologic patterns suggest the possibility that a variant retrovirus or another infectious agent may be involved (Dalgleish *et al.*, 1990).

ISOLATION OF HUMAN T-CELL LYMPHOTROPHIC VIRUS-I

The search for the first human retrovirus began in the early 20th century, gaining impetus as animal retroviruses such as the feline leukemia virus were ultimately isolated and proven to be etiologically linked to malignancy (Gallo, 1986). The possible association of a clinically distinct type of leukemia with an infectious etiology was first proposed by investigators in Japan (Yodoi *et al.*, 1974; Uchiyama *et al.*, 1977). A subset of leukemia patients was described with acute T-cell leukemia with distinctive features of skin involvement, generalized lymphadenopathy, absence of mediastinal adenopathy, and hypercalcemia. Response to chemotherapy was poor, and these patients typically had a progressive, downhill course. A striking feature was the clustering of birthplaces in southwestern Japan and, in particular, on the island of Kyushu. An infectious agent or geographical cofactor was proposed to explain this clustering. The authors concluded that these patients were not a variant of other T-cell leukemias such as Sezary syndrome or mycosis fungoides and proposed the name adult T-cell leukemia (ATL) (Uchiyama *et al.*, 1977).

In the 1970s, two major laboratory breakthroughs were requisite to the ultimate viral isolation of HTLV. Discovery of the enzyme that allows the

RNA virus to make a DNA copy for insertion into the host genome, reverse transcriptase, provided a means to assay retrovirus activity and a biologic explanation for this new class of viruses (Temin and Mizutani, 1970). The discovery of interleukin-2, also called T-cell growth factor, permitted propagation of T-cells in culture (Morgan *et al.*, 1976). HTLV-I was first isolated at the National Cancer Institute from the peripheral lymphocytes and lymph node biopsy specimen of a patient who was presumed to have mycosis fungoides (Poiesz *et al.*, 1980). Subsequently, Japanese researchers were able to demonstrate similar retroviral particles from the MT-1 cell line established from the peripheral blood of an ATL patient, which they named the adult T-cell leukemia virus (ATLV). Using indirect immunofluorescence testing, antibodies to ATLV were detected in 44 of 44 ATL patients and in 32 of 40 patients with a T-cell lymphoma with clinical characteristics similar to ATL (Hinuma *et al.*, 1981). The etiologic link was further strengthened by demonstration of monoclonal integration of the HTLV-I provirus in the malignant cells. Isolates of HTLV-I from the United States and ATLV from Japan were later shown to have the same proviral sequences by Southern blotting techniques (Watanabe *et al.*, 1984). HTLV-I is the current terminology for this type C retrovirus.

Serosurveys in Japan showed an association between areas endemic for ATL and HTLV-I seropositivity in the population. A north–south gradient of increasing HTLV-I seroprevalence was delineated with rates <1% in northern Japan and as high as 37% in the ATL-endemic area of Nagasaki (Hinuma *et al.*, 1982).

Attention was drawn to the Caribbean when British investigators noted the similarities between the ATL cases reported by the Japanese and cases of "T-lymphosarcoma-cell leukaemia" in Blacks who had emigrated to Europe from the West Indies and Guyana (Catovsky *et al.*, 1982). HTLV-I seropositivity was confirmed in these patients and in additional Caribbean population and hospital-based samples. Three communities in St. Vincent had a combined seroprevalence of 3.2% (Blattner *et al.*, 1982). The finding of a 56-year-old Jamaican woman with a spastic neuropathy and HTLV seropositivity in this survey foreshadowed the association between HTLV-I infection and neurologic disease.

HUMAN T-CELL LYMPHOTROPHIC VIRUS-I

The two major diseases linked to HTLV-I are ATL and HAM–TSP. The spectrum of ATL has been expanded to include a non-Hodgkin's T-cell-type lymphoma so that the syndrome is now more properly termed ATLL. The list of disease associations is growing and includes immune dysfunction, bronchopulmonary alveolitis, arthritis, infective dermatitis, and myositis. HTLV-I also may have an indirect role in other malignancies such as B-cell leukemias (Gallo, 1991). The estimated lifetime risk of an infected individual developing disease appears to be low, with estimates ranging from 1 to 4% (Manns and Blattner, 1991).

EPIDEMIOLOGIC PATTERN OF INFECTION

Population serosurveys of HTLV-I, worldwide, have shown this virus to have an unusual pattern of endemicity with foci of infection identified in widely disparate geographical locations. Southwestern Japan and the Caribbean basin are the two best-characterized endemic regions. Other endemic areas that have been identified include parts of Central and South America and sub-Saharan Africa (Blattner, 1990). Representative HTLV-I studies of either general populations or blood donors worldwide are shown in Fig. 2. To explain this divergent geographic pattern of infection, it has been proposed that Africa was the origin of HTLV-I and the virus was spread to the Caribbean and Japan with the slave trade (Gallo

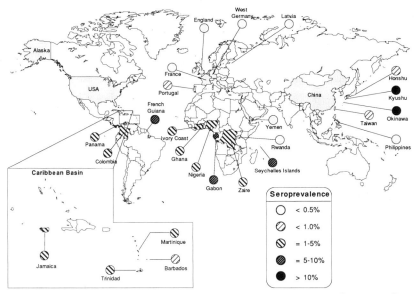

Figure 2   World map showing representative HTLV-I seroprevalence studies. Various types of population studies are displayed including blood donors, clinical patients, and general population studies.

and Sliski, 1983). Although this theory does not completely explain the worldwide distribution of HTLV-I, it is interesting to note that the majority of HAM–TSP cases in the Caribbean, South America, and Africa are of black ancestry (Molgaard *et al.*, 1989). Also, many of the islands that are endemic for HTLV-I (Seychelles, Tobago, Trinidad) were on the African slave trade circuit. No better alternative hypothesis has been proposed to date (Bucher *et al.*, 1990).

The United States is considered a nonendemic area. A survey conducted by the American Red Cross in eight U.S. cities identified 10 seropositive individuals in >39,000 donors for an overall seroprevalence of 0.025% (Williams *et al.*, 1988). There are populations at risk for HTLV-I infection in the United States including persons from endemic areas, intravenous drug abusers, recipients of multiple blood transfusions, and sexual contacts of these risk groups.

Another striking epidemiologic feature of HTLV-I infection is the rising seropositivity rate with age, which occurs in all populations studied. In Okinawa, for example, the seroprevalence rate varies from 1 to 4% in individuals less than 20 years of age to more than 30% in individuals more than 50 years of age (Kajiyama *et al.*, 1986). Three major mechanisms have been hypothesized to explain this: a cohort effect, perinatal infection with delayed seroconversion, and ongoing acquisition of infection during adulthood. No data support the existence of antibody-negative HTLV-I infection (Blattner, 1991). The correlation with age is more likely related to ongoing infection during adulthood, perhaps combined with a cohort effect.

TRANSMISSION OF HUMAN T-CELL LYMPHOTROPHIC VIRUS-I

HTLV-I is now known to be transmitted perinatally, sexually, and parenterally, via blood transfusion or needle sharing among intravenous drug abusers. Milk-borne transmission was suspected with the finding of approximately 1000 infected T-cells per milliliter in the milk of seropositive mothers and confirmed with the successful infection of common marmosets with oral inoculation of carrier mother's milk (Yamanouchi *et al.*, 1985). Prospective studies in Nagasaki, Japan, have shown that approximately 15–20% of infants breastfed by seropositive mothers will seroconvert versus 3% of infants who are bottlefed (Hino *et al.*, 1990).

Parenteral transmission via blood products requires transfusion of cells (i.e., whole blood, packed cells, and/or platelets) with approximately 40–60% of recipients of infected components seroconverting (Okochi *et al.*, 1984; Manns and Blattner, 1991). In Japan, blood donors have been screened for HTLV-I since 1986. This has markedly reduced the number of transfusion-associated HTLV-I infections with an overall seroconversion rate in blood product recipients of 8.3% prior to screening versus 0.15% afterward (Kamihira *et al.*, 1987). The United States began to screen all blood donors in early 1989.

The efficiency of heterosexual transmission is not well defined. Early family studies in Japan suggested that transmission occurred sexually almost exclusively from husband to wife. The calculated transmission rate to males over a 10-year period was 0.4% versus 60.8% to females (Kajiyama *et al.*, 1986).

Since that time, more evidence has accumulated indicating that heterosexual transmission is bidirectional; however, it appears to be more efficient from male to female (Chen *et al.*, 1991; Brodine *et al.*, 1991). This would explain the increased seroprevalence rates observed in females over the age of 40 years, because they are more likely to acquire infection from their seropositive spouse than are the males. The relative inefficiency of heterosexual transmission is presumed to be due to the highly cell-associated nature of HTLV-I. The presence of cofactors such as genital ulcer disease appears to enhance transmission (Murphy *et al.*, 1989).

EPIDEMIOLOGY OF HUMAN T-CELL LYMPHOTROPHIC VIRUS-I-ASSOCIATED MYELOPATHY–TROPICAL SPASTIC PARAPARESIS

In the HTLV-I endemic areas of the world (Fig. 2), such as the Caribbean and Japan, 70–90% of TSP cases are HTLV-I infected. In other areas such as India, where HTLV-I is not endemic, a low percentage of the cases are secondary to HTLV-I. These HTLV-I-negative TSP cases are seemingly identical to HAM–TSP. Another infectious agent, perhaps a variant retrovirus, probably acts to initiate a similar autoimmune process (Roman, 1988).

The pathogenesis of HTLV-I-associated leukemia–lymphoma is thought to require perinatal acquisition of infection. In contrast, there are well-described cases of adult-acquired HTLV-I infection with subsequent development of HAM–TSP. The most convincing examples of adult-acquired HAM–TSP are related to transfusion. Seronegative patients have been documented to seroconvert and develop disease following transfusion of HTLV-I-infected blood (Gout *et al.*, 1990a). In Japan, more than 20% of the

HAM–TSP patients have a history of blood transfusion (Osame *et al.*, 1990b); this percentage has fallen since the institution of HTLV-I and -II screening of blood donors (Kamihira *et al.*, 1987). Isolated cases of HAM–TSP have also been shown to be related to blood-borne transmission in the United States (Kaplan *et al.*, 1991).

Heterosexual transmission can also lead to HAM–TSP. One of the first recorded American cases of TSP was a 42-year-old male whose symptoms began 16 years after marriage to a seropositive Japanese spouse. He had no other risk factors for HTLV-I infection (McFarlin and Koprowski, 1990). Thus, cases of HAM–TSP can occur as a result of HTLV-I infections acquired perinatally, parenterally, and probably sexually. This difference in pathogenesis with perinatal transmission being requisite for ATLL, but not for HAM–TSP, has been used to explain the sex distribution pattern in these two syndromes. Among ATLL cases, sex distribution is equal. Among HAM–TSP cases, there is a predominance of females, which parallels the HTLV-I seroprevalence pattern in many areas and may be due to the increased efficiency of male-to-female heterosexual transmission (Kajiyama *et al.*, 1986).

One of the striking epidemiologic characteristics of HTLV-I infection is latency of the virus. In ATLL, the mean time of presentation after perinatal transmission is 55 years. The incubation period of HAM–TSP is shorter with the mean age of patients being 40 years. Frequently symptoms start during the third decade. A few adolescents have developed HAM–TSP with the youngest recorded case being 11 years old. The latency period is briefer in blood transfusion-transmitted infections, with 50% of the cases occuring within 3 years of the transfusion. A cardiac transplant recipient on immunosuppressants had the onset of symptoms within 4 weeks of HTLV-I seroconversion and was paraplegic within 11 months (Gout *et al.*, 1990a).

Disease expression in HTLV-I is not only delayed but is also variable. The estimated life-time risk of an HTLV-I-infected individual developing disease secondary to the infection is approximately 4%. In HTLV-I-endemic areas, the annual incidence of ATLL is markedly greater than HAM–TSP, and it is estimated that the annual risk of HAM–TSP is 0.025% among HTLV-I-infected persons (Kaplan *et al.*, 1990). This comparatively lower rate is possibly in part due to underdiagnosis of more subtle cases. With the risk of disease being so low, it is proposed that cofactor(s) may be required for development of disease. Emigrants and their offspring from HTLV-I endemic areas to nonendemic areas have a similar presentation of HAM–TSP (Dixon *et al.*, 1990; Gessain *et al.*, 1990a). Thus, environmental cofactors unique to HTLV-I-endemic areas do not appear to be required. The familial clustering of both HAM–TSP and ATLL cases suggests that at least part of the propensity of an infected person to develop disease is inherited (McKhann *et al.*, 1989).

DIAGNOSIS OF HUMAN T-CELL LYMPHOTROPHIC VIRUS-I INFECTION

A major problem in delineating the pattern of HTLV-I seropositivity has been the evolving status of HTLV diagnostics. The diagnosis of HTLV-I infection is made by detection of antibody to the virus. Laboratory assays include a screening HTLV enzyme-linked immunosorbent assay (ELISA), with confirmation via more specific assays including Western blot and radioimmune precipitation assay (RIPA). In 1988, the Food and Drug Administration established serologic criteria for the diagnosis of HTLV infection (Anderson *et al.*, 1990). Sera positive on the ELISA screen require one or more confirmatory assay(s). Antibodies reactive to both the core (p24) and envelope (p46 and/or gp61/68) of the virus must be present. If there is reactivity to only the core or envelope, a specimen is considered "indeterminate." Unlike the situation with another retrovirus, HIV, the Western blot is frequently nondiagnostic, because it is most sensitive for core and relatively insensitive for envelope proteins. Confirmation then requires a RIPA. Many of the previously published surveys' criteria required only p24 for HTLV seropositivity and, therefore, have a potential for inflated infection rates. Some of these previously published series have been duplicated with the more stringent criteria with very different results. For example, a survey completed in 1984 in the Alaskan Eskimo population suggested this to be an endemic area with a 2.7% seropositivity rate (Robert-Guroff *et al.*, 1985). Repeat testing of the same sera and additional specimens showed the true rate to be closer to 0.5% (Davidson *et al.*, 1990).

A second obstacle in HTLV diagnosis is the inability of current serologic tests to differentiate HTLV-I from HTLV-II. This requires detection of the specific viral DNA by polymerase chain reaction (PCR) on fresh lymphocytes (Anderson *et al.*, 1990), a costly and logistically difficult process. Work to develop rapid diagnostic methods to differentiate HTLV-I from HTLV-II is in progress. Many published reports do not include PCR testing. This additional step is particularly important in populations, such as intravenous drug abusers and blood donors, in which both viruses exist. In the absence of PCR testing, HTLV seropositive individuals are best classified as HTLV-I/II.

CLINICAL FEATURES OF HUMAN T-CELL LYMPHOTROPHIC VIRUS-I-ASSOCIATED MYELOPATHY–TROPICAL SPASTIC PARAPARESIS

The majority of patients with HAM–TSP present between the ages of 20 and 60, with a mean age in the early 40s, although childhood cases do occur. There is a female predominance, which in some case series is as marked as 2.7:1 (Rodgers-Johnson *et al.*, 1988). The syndrome is typically insidious in onset with early symptoms of lumbar pain and a stiff, awkward gait. Initially, only one of the lower extremities may be involved, but the disease process is usually bilaterally symmetric within 6 months. As the disease progresses, there is invariably impairment of bladder and anal sphincter control manifested by urinary hesitancy, frequency, and incontinence as well as constipation and fecal incontinence. The majority of patients do not have upper extremity spasticity; however, mild involvement can occur. Sensory symptoms are not usually prominent but can include distal dysthesias, and loss of proprioception and vibratory sense. Mentation is clear without obvious central nervous system disability. Typically, these symptoms progress slowly over several months to years. Disease progression can be shorter, particularly in the setting of transfusion-associated HTLV-I infection. Patients develop progressive disability with the vast majority ultimately bedridden or requiring crutches for ambulation. Other systemic diseases can accompany HAM–TSP and include bronchopulmonary alveolar lymphocytosis, arthritis, myositis, and, rarely, ATLL.

On physical examination, patients are afebrile with no changes in mental status. Abnormalities are generally limited to the neurologic and muscular systems. Neurologic exam demonstrates evidence of spasticity with increased tendon reflexes, clonus, and increased muscle tone of the lower extremities. Although spasticity of the upper extremities occurs infrequently, most patients will have increased tendon reflexes. The Babinski reflex response to plantar reflex, which signifies an upper motor neuron process, is often present. Sensation may be normal, or there may be reduced proprioception and vibration sense distally. The anal sphincter tone may be reduced. Patients with advanced disease will show evidence of muscle atrophy and contractures of the lower extremities (Osame *et al.*, 1990a; Morgan, 1990).

Laboratory studies including complete blood count and serum chemistries are usually normal. On careful peripheral blood smear review, most patients will have a low level ($<1\%$) of circulating atypical lymphocytes

(ATL or "flower" cells), identical in morphology to the malignant cells seen in ATLL. Cerebrospinal fluid (CSF) analysis may be normal or may demonstrate pleocytosis, ATL cells, and, less commonly, increased protein. Requisite to the diagnosis is the presence of HTLV-I antibody in both sera and CSF. Evidence of intrathecal synthesis of HTLV-I antibody can be demonstrated in some patients and oligoclonal bands can be present. Myelography is normal. Radiologic scans of the head, including computed tomographic scanning and magnetic resonance imaging (MRI), are usually normal but may show lesions, particularly in the periventricular white matter and less commonly in the white matter of the cerebrum and cerebellum (McFarlin and Koprowski, 1990).

In 1988, a Scientific Committee appointed by the World Health Organization to study HTLV-I and its disease associations met in Kagoshima and standardized the diagnostic guidelines for HAM–TSP (Osame *et al.*, 1990a). The diagnosis of HAM–TSP can be made if a patient has a compatible clinical presentation in conjunction with HTLV-I antibodies in the sera and CSF. In early disease, there may be a paucity of symptoms or only a single symptom (i.e., lumbar pain, urinary frequency, or mild gait disturbance only). Frequently, a myelogram must be performed to rule out a spinal mass, because this process can also present with low back pain and symmetric spasticity (Bucher *et al.*, 1990). The differential diagnosis also includes multiple sclerosis (MS). Most presentations of MS are distinguished by disseminated neurologic lesions and a clinical course with remissions and relapses and can be easily differentiated from HAM–TSP. More difficult to differentiate is the spinal cord form of MS, particularly because patients with HAM–TSP can have laboratory abnormalities consistent with MS (i.e., periventricular lesions on MRI and oligoclonal banding on CSF analysis). Currently, no direct link betwen HTLV-I and MS is believed to exist, despite early reports to the contrary. Patients with a progressive paraplegia in association with documented HTLV-I infection should be diagnosed as HAM–TSP (Paty, 1990).

Because HAM–TSP is predominantly associated with morbidity and has a low mortality rate, few pathologic specimens have been available for study. To date, autopsy findings have shown degeneration and demyelination with some axonal destruction mainly of the pyramidal tracts of the spinal cord. The dorsal columns, and the white matter of the cerebrum and cerebellum, can also be involved, but to a lesser degree. The histopathology is remarkable for capillary proliferation, astrogliocytic cell proliferation, and the presence of lymphocytic infiltrates in the subarachnoid layer of the meninges with prominent perivascular cuffing. Demyelination with some destruction to the axon is also present (Akizuki *et al.*, 1987).

The marked differences in the two major disease outcomes of HTLV-I infection (leukemia–lymphoma versus a chronic neurologic syndrome) has been the focus of a number of studies. In patients with HAM–TSP, as in asymptomatic carriers of HTLV-I infection, the integration site of the provirus in the host DNA varies from lymphocyte to lymphocyte (polyclonal integration) (Gessain *et al.*, 1990b). In ATLL, a transformation occurs so that only one malignant clone is present (monoclonal integration) (Greenberg *et al.*, 1989). However, the HTLV-I virus appears to be identical in both of these disease states, with 97% homology demonstrated with proviral sequencing (McFarlin and Koprowski, 1990). The difference in disease expression is possibly related to the host response to the virus and, perhaps, the presence of cofactors. There are different HLA haplotypes in patients with ATLL versus those with HAM–TSP, which lends support to the concept that there are genetic differences in the immune response to HTLV-I in these two patient groups. Even more interesting is the observation that lymphocytes from patients with HAM–TSP have a high "hyperimmune" response to HTLV-I, whereas lymphocytes from patients with ATLL have a low "permissive" response (Usuku *et al.*, 1988). Further study of the lymphocyte populations in patients with HAM–TSP have shown that there are subpopulations of cytotoxic lymphocytes that are committed to HTLV-I gene products and thus may be the effector cells of the disease process represented by the inflammatory lymphocytic infiltrates seen on histopathology (Jacobson *et al.*, 1990). All evidence to date supports the concept that HAM–TSP represents an autoimmune disorder.

Based on the precept that HAM–TSP is an autoimmune disorder, the therapeutic approach has been primarily the use of immunosuppressants. Japanese investigators have reported a significant improvement in approximately 90% of their case series with the use of prednisone (Osame *et al.*, 1990a). Others have not been able to duplicate this remission rate (Morgan, 1990).

Additional therapies under investigation include plasmapheresis and intravenous interferon. Antiretroviral therapy with zidovudine was not successful in a small treatment group (Gout *et al.*, 1990b).

OTHER HUMAN T-CELL LYMPHOTROPHIC VIRUSES

Other type C retroviruses similar to HTLV-I have been identified. HTLV-II was isolated from two patients with hairy cell leukemia (Kalyanaraman *et al.*, 1982; Rosenblatt *et al.*, 1986). Further surveys in this group of patients did not confirm an etiologic link (Rosenblatt *et al.*, 1988). This second human retrovirus has been termed the "orphan" virus, because endemic regions and disease associations have not been identified (Blattner, 1990), although more recently, native populations such as the Guayami Indians in Panama have been identified as possible endemic populations for HTLV-II (Lairmore *et al.*, 1990). It is the most common HTLV virus associated with intravenous drug abuse (Lee *et al.*, 1989). Researchers initially thought that the etiologic agent of the acquired immunodeficiency syndrome, or AIDS, was also a type C retrovirus. However, HTLV-III and -IV were reclassified as human immunodeficiency virus types 1 and 2 when DNA sequencing showed these viruses to be more closely related to the lentivirus family (Barre-Sinoussi *et al.*, 1983; Popovic *et al.*, 1984). Italian researchers have recently identified a HTLV-V from the lymphocytes of patients with an ATL-like leukemia. Information about this isolate is still preliminary (Manzari *et al.*, 1990).

CONCLUSION

The sporadic form of TSP is now known to be caused by a retroviral infection with HTLV-I. Identification of the etiology has exciting implications, not only for HAM–TSP but also for further impetus to investigate the etiologies of other neurologic disease processes such as MS and HTLV-negative TSP. Major challenges still exist in providing much needed information regarding the mechanisms of latency and disease expression, treatment for affected individuals, and transmission, particularly sexual transmission.

References

Akizuki, S., Nakazato, O., Higuchi, Y., Tanabe, K., Setoguchi, M., Yoshida, S., Miyazaki, Y., Yamamoto, S., Sudou, S., Sannomiya, K., and Okajima, T. (1987). Necropsy findings in HTLV-I-associated myelopathy. *Lancet* **1,** 156–157.

Anderson, D. W., Epstein, J. S., Pierik, L. T., Lee, T. H., Lairmore, M. D., Saxinger, C., Kalyanaraman, V. S., Slamon, D., Parks, W., Poiesz, B. J., and Blattner, W. A. (1990). Development by the Public Health Service of criteria for serological confirmation of HTLV-I/II infections. *In* "Human Retrovirology: HTLV" (W. A. Blattner, ed.), pp. 391–396. Raven Press, New York.

Araki, K., Shiny, O., Tajima, H., and Gormandizing, M. (1986). Type I HTLV antibody of healthy adults in Okinawa and of Okinawans in Hawaii. *Jap. J. Clin. Hematol.* **27,** 659–663 (in Japanese with English abstr.).

Barre-Sinoussi, F., Chermann, J., Rey, F., Nugeyre, M., Chamaret, S., Gruest, J., Dauguet, C., Axler-Blin, C., Verzinet-Brun, F., Rouzioux, C., Rozenbaum, W., and Montagnier, L. (1983). Isolation of a T-lymphotropic retrovirus from a patient at risk for acquired immune deficiency syndrome (AIDS). *Science* **220,** 868–871.

Bartholomew, C., Cleghorn, F., Charles, W., Ratan, P., Roberts, L., Maharaj, K., Jankey, N., Daisley, H., Hanchard, B., and Blattner, W. (1986). HTLV-I and tropical spastic paraparesis. *Lancet* **1,** 99–100.

Bhagavati, S., Ehrlich, G., Kula, R. W., Kwok, S., Sninsky, J., Udani, V., and Poiesz, B. J. (1988). Detection of human T-cell lymphoma/leukemia virus type-I DNA and antigen in spinal fluid and blood of patients with chronic progressive myelopathy. *N. Engl. J. Med.* **318,** 1141–1147.

Biggar, R., Saxinger, C., Gardiner, C., Collins, W., Levine, P., Clark, J., Nkrumah, F., and Blattner, W. (1984). HTLV-I antibody in urban and rural Ghana, West Africa. *Int. J. Cancer* **34,** 215–219.

Blattner, W. A. (1990). Epidemiology of HTLV-I and associated diseases. *In* "Human Retrovirology: HTLV" (W. A. Blattner, ed.), pp. 251–265. Raven Press, New York.

Blattner, W. A. (1991). Letter. *N. Eng. J. Med.* **325,** 284.

Blattner, W., Kalyanaraman, V., Robert-Guroff, M., Lister, T., Galton, D., Sarin, P., Crawford, M., Catovsky, D., Greaves, M., and Gallo, R. (1982). The human type-C retrovirus, HTLV in Blacks from the Caribbean region, and relationship to adult T-cell leukemia/lymphoma. *Int. J. Cancer* **30,** 257–264.

Brodine, S., Oldfield, E., Corwin, A., Thomas, R., Ryan, A., Holmberg, J., Molgaard, C., Golbeck, A., Ryden L., Benenson, A., Roberts, C., and Blattner, W. (1992). HTLV-I among U.S. Marines stationed in a hyperendemic area: Evidence for female-to-male sexual transmission. *J. AIDS* **5,** 158–162.

Bucher, B., Poupard, J. A., Vernant, J., and DeFreitas, E. C. (1990). Tropical neuromyelopathies and retroviruses: A review. *Rev. Infect. Dis.* **12,** 890–899.

Cardosa, E., Robert-Guroff, M., Franchini, G., Gartner, S., Moura-Nunes, J., Gallo, R., and Terrinha, A. (1989). Seroprevalence of HTLV-I in Portugal and evidence of double retrovirus infection of a healthy donor. *Int. J. Cancer* **43,** 195–200.

Catovsky, D., Greaves, M. F., Rose, M., *et al.* (1982). Adult T-cell lymphoma–leukaemia in Blacks from the West Indies. *Lancet* **1,** 639–643.

Chen, Y. A., Okayama, A., Lee, T. H., Tachibana, N., Mueller, N., and Essex, M. (1991). Sexual transmission of human T-cell leukemia virus type I associated with the presence of anti-tax antibody. *Proc. Natl. Acad. Sci. USA* **88,** 1182–1186.

Cliff, J., Lundquist, P., Martensson, J., Rosling, H., and Sorbo, B. (1985). Association of high cyanide and low sulphur intake in cassava-induced spastic paraparesis. *Lancet* **2,** 1211–1212.

Coste, J., Lemaire, J., Barin, F., and Courouche, A. (1990). HTLV-I/II antibodies in French blood donors. *Lancet* **336,** 1167–1168.

Dalgleish, A. G., Richardson, J. H., Newman, P. K., Newell, A. L., Rangan, G., and Mani, K. S. (1990). HTLV-I, tropical spastic paraparesis, and other neurological diseases in South India. *In* "Human Retrovirology: HTLV" (W. A. Blattner, ed.), pp. 245–250. Raven Press, New York.

Davidson, M., Kaplan, J. E., Hartley, T. M., Lairmore, M. D., and Lanier, A. P. (1990). Prevalence of HTLV-I in Alaska natives. *J. Infect. Dis.* **161,** 359–360.

Delaporte, E., Dupont, A., Peeters, M., Josse, R., Merlin, M., Schruvers, D., Hamano, B., Bedjabaga, L., Cheringou, H., Boyer, F., Brun-Vezinet, F., and Larouze, B. (1988). Epidemiology of HTLV-I in Gabon (Western Equatorial Africa). *Int. J. Cancer* **42,** 687–689.

Denny-Brown, D. (1947). Neurological conditions resulting from prolonged and severe dietary restriction. (Case reports in prisoners-of-war, and general review). *Medicine (Baltimore)* **26,** 41–74.

Dixon, P. S., Bodner, A. J., Okihiro, M., Milbourne, A., Diwan, A., and Nakamura, J. M. (1990).

Human T-lymphotropic virus type-I (HTLV-I) associated myelopathy in Hawaii. *West. J. Med.* **152,** 261–267.

Dolken, G., Bross, K., Chosa, T., Schneider, J., Bayer, H., and Hunsmann, G. (1983). No evidence for HTLV infection among leukaemia patients in Germany. *Lancet* **ii,** 1495.

Fleming, A., Maharan, R., Abraham, M., Kulkarni, A., Bhusnurmath, S., Okpara, R., Williams, E., Akinsete, I., Schneider, J., Bayer, H., and Hunsmann, G. (1986). Antibodies to HTLV-I in Nigerian blood donors, their relatives and patients with leukaemais, lymphomas, and other diseases. *Int. J. Cancer* **38,** 809–813.

Gallo, R. C. (1986). The First Human Retrovirus. *Sci. Am.* **255,** 88–98.

Gallo, R. C. (1991). Human retroviruses: A decade of discovery and link with human diseases. *J. Infect. Dis.* **164,** 235–243.

Gallo, R. C., and Sliski, A., (1983). Origin of human T-cell leukemia–lymphoma virus. *Lancet* **2,** 962–963.

Gessain, A., Barin, F., Vernant, J. C., Gout, O., Maurs, L., Calender, A., and de The, G. (1985). Antibodies to human T-lymphotropic virus type-I in patients with tropical spastic paraparesis. *Lancet* **2,** 407–410.

Gessain, A., Gout, O., Saal, F., Daniel, M. T., Rio, B., Flandrin, G., Sigaux, F., Lyon-Caen, O., Peries, J., and de The, G. (1990a). Epidemiology and immunovirology of human T-cell leukemia/lymphoma virus type-I-associated adult T-cell leukemia and chronic myelopathies as seen in France. *Cancer Res.* **50**(suppl.), 5692s–5696s.

Gessain, A., Saal, F., Gout, O., Daniel, M. T., Flandrin, G., de The, G., Peries, J., and Sigaux, F. (1990b). High human T-cell lymphotropic virus type-I proviral DNA load with polyclonal integration in peripheral blood mononuclear cells of French West Indian, Guianese, and African patients with tropical spastic paraparesis. *Blood* **75,** 428–433.

Gout, O., Baulac M., Gessain, A., Semah F., Saal, F., Peries, J., Cabrol, C., Foucault-Fretz, C., Laplane, D., Sigaux, F., and de The, G. (1990a). Rapid development of myelopathy after HTLV-I infection acquired by transfusion during cardiac transplantation. *N. Eng. J. Med.* **322,** 383–388.

Gout, O., Gessain, A., Saal, F., Daniel, M. T., Bolgert, F., Brunet, P., Cabanis, E., Sigaux, F., de The, G., and Lyon-Caen, O. (1990b). Effects of azidothymidine (AZT) on chronic encephalomyelopathy associated with HTLV-I: A prospective study. 3rd Annual Retrovirology Conference, Makena, Maui.

Greenberg, S. J., Jacobson, S., Waldmann, T. A., and McFarlin, D. E. (1989). Molecular analysis of HTLV-I proviral integration and T-cell receptor arrangement indicates that T-cells in tropical spastic paraparesis are polyclonal. *J. Infect. Dis.* **159,** 741–744.

Hayes, C., Burans, J., and Oberst, R. (1991). Antibodies to human T-lymphotropic virus type-I in a population from the Philippines: Evidence for cross-reactivity with *Plasmodium falciparum. J. Infect. Dis.* **163,** 257–262.

Hino, S., Kubota, K., Doi, H., and Miyamoto, T. (1990). Preliminary follow-up survey of children born to HTLV-I carrier mothers who refrained from breast feeding. 3rd Annual Retrovirology Conference, Makena, Maui.

Hinuma, Y., Nagata, K., Hanaoka, M., Nakai, M., Matsumoto, T., Kinoshito, K., Shirakawa, S., and Miyoshi, I. (1981). Adult T-cell leukemia: Antigen in an ATL cell line and detection of antibodies to the antigen in human sera. *Proc. Nat. Acad. Sci. USA* **78,** 6476–6480.

Hinuma, Y., Komoda, H., Chosa, T., Kondo, T., Kohakura, M., Takenaka, T., Kikuchi, M., Ichimaru, M., Yunoki, K., Sato, I., Matsuo, R., Takiuchi, Y., Uchino, H., and Hanaoka, M. (1982). Antibodies to adult T-cell leukemia-virus-associated antigen (ATLA) in sera from patients with ATL and controls in Japan: A nation-wide sero-epidemiologic study. *Int. J. Cancer* **29,** 631–635.

Jacobson, S., Shida, H., McFarlin, D. E., Fauci, A. S., and Koenig, S. (1990). Circulating CD8+ cytotoxic T-lymphocytes specific for HTLV-I pX in patients with HTLV-I associated neurological disease. *Nature* **348,** 245–248.

Kajiyama, W., Kashiwagi, S., Ikematsu, H., *et al.* (1986). Intrafamilial transmission of adult T-cell leukemia virus. *J. Infect. Dis.* **154,** 851–857.

Kalyanaraman, V. S., Sarngadharan, M. G., Robert-Guroff, M., Miyoshi, I., Golde, D., and Gallo, R. C. (1982). A new subtype of human T-cell leukemia virus (HTLV-II) associated with a T-cell variant of hairy cell leukemia. *Science* **218,** 571–573.

Kamihira, S., Nakasima, S., Oyakawa, Y., *et al.* (1987). Transmission of human T-cell lymphotropic virus type-I by blood transfusion before and after mass screening of sera from seropositive donors. *Vox Sang* **52,** 43–44.

Kaplan, J. E., Osame, M., Kubota, H., Igata, A., Nishitani, H., Maeda, Y., Khabbaz, R. F., and Janssen, R. S. (1990). The risk of development of HTLV-I associated myelopathy/tropical spastic paraparesis among persons infected with HTLV-I. *J. AIDS* **3,** 1096–1101.

Kaplan, J. E., Litchfield, B., Rouault, C., Lairmore, M. D., Luo, C. C., Williams, L., Brew, B. J., Price., R. W., Janssen, R., Stoneburner, R., Ou, C. Y., Folks, T., and De, B. (1991). HTLV-I-associated myelopathy associated with blood transfusion in the United States: Epidemiologic and molecular evidence linking donor and recipient. *Neurology* **41,** 192–197.

Kark, R. M., Aiton, H. F., Pease, W. O., Bean, W. B., Henderson, C. R., Johnson, R. E., and Richard, L. M. (1947). Tropical deterioration and nutrition. *Medicine (Baltimore)* **26,** 1–41.

Kuo, T., Chan, H., Su, I., Eimoto, T., Maeda, Y., Kikuchi, M., Chen, M., Kuan, Y., Chen, W., Sun, C., Shih, L., Chen, J., and Takeshita, M. (1985). Serological survey of antibodies to the adult T-cell leukemia virus-associated antigen (HTLV-A) in Taiwan. *Int. J. Cancer* **36,** 345–348.

Kwok, S., Kellogg, D., Ehrlich, G., Poiesz, B., Bhagavati, S., and Sninsky, J. J. (1988). Characterization of a sequence of human T-cell leukemia virus type-I from a patient with chronic progressive myelopathy. *J. Infect. Dis.* **158,** 1193–1197.

Lairmore, M. D., Jacobson, S., Gracia, F., De, B. K., Castillo, L., Larreategui, M., Roberts, B. D., Levine, P. H., Blattner, W. A., and Kaplan, J. E. (1990). Isolation of human T-cell lymphotropic virus type 2 from Guaymi Indians in Panama. *Proc. Natl. Acad. Sci. USA* **87,** 8849–8844.

Lavanchy, D., Bovet, P., Hollanda, J., Shamlaye, C., Burczak, J., and Lee, H. (1991). High seroprevalence of HTLV-I in the Seychelles. *Lancet* **337,** 248–249.

Lee, H., Swanson, P., Shorty, V. S., Zack, J. A., Rosenblatt, J. D., and Chen, I. S. (1989). High rate of HTLV-II infection in seropositive I.V. drug abusers in New Orleans. *Science* **244,** 471–475.

Lee, H., Swanson, P., Rosenblatt, J., Chen, I., Sherwood, W., Smith, D., Tegtmeier, G., Fernando, L., Fang, C., Osame, M., and Kleinman, S. (1991). Relative prevalence and risk factors of HTLV-I and HTLV-II infection in U.S. blood donors. *Lancet* **337,** 1435–1438.

Maeda, Y., Furukawa, M., Takehara, Y., Yoshimura, K., Miyamoto, K., Matsuura, T., Morishima, Y., Tajima, K., Okochi, K., and Hinuma, Y. (1984). Prevalence of possible adult T-cell leukemia virus-carriers among volunteer blood donors in Japan: A nation-wide study. *Int. J. Cancer* **33,** 717–720.

Maloney, E., Ramirez, H., Levin, A., and Blattner, W. (1989). A survey of human T-lymphotropic virus type-I (HTLV-I) in south-western Columbia. *Int. J. Cancer* **44,** 419–423.

Mani, K. S., Mani, A. J., and Montgomery, D. (1969). A spastic paraplegic syndrome in South India. *J. Neurol. Sci.* **9,** 179–199.

Manns, A., and Blattner, W. A. (1991). The epidemiology of the human T-cell lymphotrophic virus type I and type II: Etiologic role in human disease. *Transfusion* **31,** 67–75.

Manzari, V., Collati, E., Silvestri, I., Modesti, A., Santoni, A., and Frati, L. (1990). Human T-lymphotropic virus V: HTLV-V. *In* "Human Retrovirology HTLV" (W. Blattner, ed.), pp. 143–145, Raven Press, New York.

McFarlin, D. E., and Koprowski, H. (1990). Neurological disorders associated with HTLV-I. *Curr Top. Microbiol. Immunol.* **160,** 99–119.

McKhann II, G., Gibbs, C. J., Mora, C. A., Rodgers-Johnson, P. E., Liberski, P. P., Gdula, W. J., and Zaninovic, V. (1989). Isolation and characterization of HTLV-I from symptomatic family members with tropical spastic paraparesis (HTLV encephalomyeloneuropathy). *J. Infect. Dis.* **160,** 371–379.

Miller, G., Pegram., S., Kirkwood, B., Beckles, G., Byam, N., Clayden, S., Kinlen, L., Chan, L., Carson, D., and Greaves, M. (1986). Ethnic composition, age, and sex, together with location and standard of housing as determinents of HTLV-I infection in an urban Trinidadian community. *Int. J. Cancer* **38,** 801–808.

Molgaard, C. A., Eisenman, P. A., Ryden, L. A., and Golbeck, A. L. (1989). Neuroepidemiology of human T-lymphotrophic virus type-I-associated tropical spastic paraparesis. *Neuroepidemiology* **8,** 109–123.

Montgomery, R. D., Cruickshank, E. K., Robertson, W. B., and McMenemey, W. H. (1964). Clinical and pathological observations on Jamaican neuropathy. *Brain* **87,** 425–462.

Morgan, D., Ruscetti, F., and Gallo, R. (1976). Selective in vitro growth of T-lymphocytes from normal human bone marrow. *Science* **193,** 1007–1010.

Morgan, O. (1990). Tropical spastic paraparesis clinical features. *In* "Human Retrovirology: HTLV" (W. A. Blattner, ed.), pp. 199–204. Raven Press, New York.

Morgan, O. C., Montgomery, R. D., and Rodgers-Johnson, P. (1988). The myeloneuropathies of Jamaica: An unfolding story. *Q. J. Med.* **67**(252), 273–281.

Murovska, M., Taguchi, H., Iwahara, Y., Sawada, T., Kukane, R., and Miyoshi, I., (1991). Antibodies to HTLV-I among blood donors in Latvia, USSR. *Int. J. Cancer* **47,** 158–159.

Murphy, E., Figueroa, J., Gibbs, W., Brathwaite, A., Holding-Cobham, M., Waters, D., Cranston, B., Hanchard, B., and Blattner, B. (1989). Sexual transmission of human T-lymphotropic virus type-I (HTLV-I). *Ann. Int. Med.* **111,** 555–560.

Murphy, E., Figueroa, J., Gibbs, W., Holding-Cobham, M., Cranston, B., Malley, K., Bodner, A., Alexander, S., and Blattner, W. (1991). Human T-lymphotropic virus type-I seroprevalence in Jamaica. I. Demographic determinants. *Am. J. Epidemiol.* **133,** 1114–1124.

Okochi, K., Sato, H., and Hinuma. Y. (1984). A retrospective study on transmission of adult T-cell leukemia virus by blood transfusion: Seroconversion in recipients. *Vox Sang* **46,** 245–253.

Osame, M., Usuku, K., Izumo, S., Ijichi, N., Amitani, H., Igata, A., Mastumoto, M., and Tara, M. (1986). HTLV-I associated myelopathy, a new clinical entity. *Lancet* **1,** 1031–1032.

Osame, M., Igata, A., Matsumoto, M., Kohka, M., Usuku, K., and Izumo, S. (1990a). HTLV-I-associated myelopathy (HAM) treatment trials, retrospective survey and clinical and laboratory findings. *Hematology* **3,** 271–284.

Osame, M., Janssen, R., Kubota, H., Nishitani, H., Igata, A., Nagataki, S., Mori, M., Goto, I., Shimabukuro, H., Khabbaz, R., and Kaplan, J. (1990b). Nationwide survey of HTLV-I-associated myelopathy in Japan: Association with blood transfusion. *Ann. Neurol.* **28,** 50–56.

Pan, I., Chung, C., Komoda, H., Imai, J., and Hinuma, Y. (1985). Seroepidemiology of adult T-cell leukemia virus in Taiwan. *Jap. J. Cancer Res. (Gann)* **76,** 9–11.

Paty, D. W. (1990). Multiple sclerosis clinical and MRI characteristics: Is there a link between HAM/TSP and MS? *In* "Human Retrovirology: HTLV" (W. A. Blattner, ed.), pp. 213–219. Raven Press, New York.

Poiesz, B. J., Ruscetti, F., Gazdar, A. F., Bunn, P. A., Minna, J. D., and Gallo, R. C. (1980).

Detection and isolation of type C retrovirus particles from fresh and cultured lymphocytes of a patient with cutaneous T-cell lymphoma. *Proc. Natl. Acad. Sci. USA* **77,** 7415–7419.

Popovic, M., Sarngadharan, M. G., Reed, E., and Gallo, R. C. (1984). Detection, isolation, and continuous production of cytopathic human T-lymphotropic retroviruses (HTLV-III) from patients with AIDS and pre-AIDS. *Science* **224,** 497–500.

Reeves, W., Saxinger, C., Brenes, M., Quiroz, E., Clark, J., Hoh, M., and Blattner, W. (1988). Human T-cell lymphotropic virus type-I (HTLV-I) seroepidemiology and risk factors in metropolitan Panama. *Am. J. Epidemiol.* **127,** 532–539.

Richardson, J., Newell, A., Newman, P., Mani, K., Rangan, G., and Dalgleish, A. (1989). HTLV-I and neurologic disease in South India. *Lancet* **1,** 1079.

Robert-Guroff, M., Clark, J., Lanier, A. P., Beekman, G., Melbye, M., Ebbesen, P., Blattner, W. A., and Gallo, R. C. (1985). Prevalence of HTLV-I in arctic regions. *Int. J. Cancer* **36,** 651–655.

Rodgers-Johnson, P., Gajdusek, D. C., Morgan, O. C., Zaninovic, V., Sarin, P. S., and Graham, D. S. (1985). HTLV-I and HTLV-III antibodies and tropical spastic paraparesis. *Lancet* **2,** 1247–1248.

Rodgers-Johnson, P., Morgan, O. C., Mora, C., Sarin, P., Ceroni, M., Piccardo, P., Garruto, R. M., Gibbs II, C. J., and Gajdusek, D. C. (1988). The role of HTLV-I in tropical spastic paraparesis in Jamaica. *Ann. Neurol.* **23**(suppl.), s121–s126.

Roman, G. C., (1987). Retrovirus-associated myelopathies. *Arch. Neurol.* **44,** 659–663.

Roman, G. C., (1988). The neuroepidemiology of tropical spastic paraparesis. *Ann. Neurol.* **23**(suppl.), s113–s120.

Roman, G. C., and Osame M. (1988). Identity of HTLV-I-associated tropical spastic paraparesis and HTLV-I-associated myelopathy. *Lancet* **1,** 651.

Roman, G. C., Spencer, P. S., and Schoenberg, B. S. (1985). Tropical myeloneuropathies: The hidden endemias. *Neurology* **35,** 1158–1170.

Roman, G. C., Spencer, P. S., Schoenberg, B. S., Madden, D., Sever, J., Hugon, J., and Ludolph, A. (1987). Tropical spastic paraparesis: HTLV-I antibodies in patients from the Seychelles. *N. Engl. J. Med.* **316,** 51.

Rosenblatt, J. D., Golde, D. W., Wachsman, W., *et al.* (1986). A second isolate of HTLV-II associated with atypical hairy-cell leukemia. *N. Eng. J. Med.* **315,** 372–377.

Rosenblatt, J. D., Chen, I., Wachsman, W., *et al.* (1988). Infection with HTLV-I and HTLV-II: Evolving concepts. *Sim. Hemato.* **25,** 230–246.

Rwandan HIV Seroprevalence Study Group. (1989). Nationwide community-based serological survey of HIV-1 and other human retrovirus infections in a central African country. *Lancet* **i,** 941–943.

Salker, R., Tosswill, J., Barabara, J., Runganga, J., Contreras, M., Tedder, R., Parra-Meija, N., and Mortimer, P. (1990). HTLV-I/II antibodies in UK blood donors. *Lancet* **336,** 317.

Scott, H. H. (1918). Investigation into an acute outbreak of central neurities. *Ann. Trop. Med Parasitol.* **12,** 109–116.

Strachan, H. (1888). Malarial multiple peripheral neuritis. *In* Sajou's "Annals of the Unversity of Medical Sciences," Vol. 1, pp. 139–141. Philadelphia.

Strachan, H. (1897). On a form of multiple sclerosis prevalent in the West Indies. *Practitioner* **59,** 477–484.

Temin, H. M., and Mizutani, S. (1970). RNA-dependent DNA polymerase in virions of rous sarcoma cells. *Nature (London)* **226,** 1211–1213.

Uchiyama, T., Yodoi, J., Sagawa, K., Takatsuki, K., and Uchino, H. (1977). Adult T-cell leukemia: Clinical and hematologic features of 16 cases. *Blood* **50,** 481–492.

Usuku, K., Sonoda, S., Osame, M., Yashiki, S., Takahashi, K., Matsumoto, M., Sawada, T., Tsuji, K., Tara, M., and Igata, A. (1988). HLA haplotype-linked high immune responsiveness against HTLV-I in HTLV-I-associated myelopathy: Comparison with adult T-cell leukemia/ lymphoma. *Ann. Neurol.* **23**(suppl.), s143–s150.

Verdier, M., Denis, F., Sangare, A., Barin, F., Gershy-Damet, G., Rey, J., Soro, B., Leonard, G., Mounier, M., and Hugon, J. (1989). Prevalence of antibody to human T-cell lymphotropic virus type I (HTLV-I) in populations of Ivory Coast, West Africa. *J. Infect. Dis.* **160**, 363–370.

Watanabe, T., Seiki, M., and Yoshida, M. (1984). HTLV type-I (U.S. Isolate) and ATLV (Japanese isolate) are the same species of human retrovirus. *Virology* **133**, 238–241.

Wiktor, S., Piot, P., Mann, J., Nzilambi, N., Francis, H., Vercauteren, G., Blattner, W., and Quinn, T. (1990). Human T-cell lymphotropic virus type-I (HTLV-I) among female prostitutes in Kinshasa, Zaire. *J. Infect. Dis.* **161**, 1073–1077.

Williams, A., Fang, C., Slamon, D., Poiez, B., Sandler, G., Darr, F., Shulman, G., McGowan, E., Douglas, D. Bowman, R., Peetoom, F., Kleinman, S., Lenes, B., and Dodd, R. (1988). Seroprevalence and epidemiological correlates of HTLV-I infection in U.S. blood donors. *Science* **240**, 643–646.

Yamanouchi, K., Kinoshita, K., Moriuchi, R., *et al.* (1985). Oral transmission of human T-cell leukemia virus type-I into a common marmoset (*Callithrix jacchus*) as an experimental model for milk-borne transmission. *Jap. J. Cancer Res.* **76**, 481–487.

Yodoi, J., Takatsuki, K., and Masuda, T. (1974). Two cases of T-cell chronic lymphocytic leukemia in Japan. *N. Eng. J. Med.* **290**, 572–573.

Zaninovic, V. (1986). Spastic paraparesis: A possible sexually transmitted viral myeloneuropathy. *Lancet* **2**, 697.

Zeng, Y., Lan, X., Fang, J., Wang, P., Wang, Y., Sui, Y., Wang, Z., Hu, R., and Hinuma, Y. (1984). HTLV antibody in China. *Lancet* **i**, 799–800.

II

Social and Behavioral Components of Neuroepidemiology

6

Patient-Based Assessments of Health Status and Outcome for Some Neurological Disorders

Ray Fitzpatrick • Ian Robinson
Graham Scambler

It is now widely accepted that states of health and illness cannot adequately be captured and described by means of biomedical parameters alone; these states are as much a reflection of the patient's perceptions and evaluations. Numerous developments might illustrate this expanded definition of health and illness, from the World Health Organization's broad vision of health as encompassing physical, social, and mental well-being to the growing emphasis now given in medicine to matters such as quality of life. For some observers, our new appreciation of the patient's perspective will provide the basis of a revolution in health care (Relman, 1988). At the core of this revolution are methods intended to assess the patient's views of his or her health needs and problems and perceptions of benefits obtained from health care (Tarlov *et al.*, 1989). Such methods are seen as making it possible, for the first time, to optimize the effectiveness and appropriateness of health services by providing evaluations from the patient's perspective (Ellwood, 1988). A number of instruments have been developed that use social science-type techniques to assess what has been variously termed subjective health status, functional status, and quality of life (Jette, 1980). These techniques have a range of important applications in, for example, planning individual patient care, clinical trials, and evaluation of health services (Steinwachs, 1989).

Neurological disorders impose a particularly wide range of personal, economic, and social costs upon the individual, the family, and the community. The primary purpose of health services for such chronic conditions should be to maximize the ability to function in everyday life and level of well-being or quality of life. It becomes evermore urgent therefore to define and assess patients' perceptions of neurological disorders—the ways in which disorders impact daily life—and also of the benefits obtained from medical care. This chapter examines patients' experiences with three contrasting neurological disorders: epilepsy, multiple sclerosis, and chronic headache. The chapter illustrates the use of medical sociological techniques to unravel the complex and diverse perspectives patients have of their illness and of the outcomes of medical care.

EPILEPSY

A Study of Sufferers' Perceptions

With very few exceptions, most evaluations of medical management of epilepsy have concentrated on strategies for antiepileptic drug prescribing and, to a lesser extent, surgery (e.g., Binnie, 1990; Shorvon, 1991). In such work, the patient's perspective has seldom been elicited. If references to the social and psychological sequelae of epilepsy are made at all, these typically take the form of ritualized addenda. Thus, Duncan (1991: 161) incorporates a short paragraph on "holistic issues," which begins "in addition to the pharmacological aspects, it is important to consider the implications and consequences of intractable epilepsy, *which are often more devastating than the seizures themselves* [our emphasis]." This is followed by a bland injunction to physicians to take "a personal interest" and proffer "advice on practical issues."

The study reported here was undertaken to make an exploratory assessment of the impact of epilepsy on the lives of adults living in the community. To qualify for inclusion in the study people had to (1) have experienced more than one nonfebrile seizure of any type and (2) either have experienced at least one nonfebrile seizure in the previous 2 years or be on antiepileptic drugs for more than one nonfebrile seizure in the past. Ninety-four people aged 16 or over, living in the London area, and meeting the medical criteria, were interviewed in their homes by a neurologist, to collect background medical data, and a sociologist. The latter used in-depth interviews to cover the onset of seizures; consulting behavior; diagnosis and patienthood; the impact and accommodation of epilepsy in friendships, families, and employment; and changing perceptions of self and self-worth. Interviews were recorded to facilitate quantitative and qualitative analysis (Scambler and Hopkins, 1990).

Epilepsy and Quality of Life

Evidence from the study determined that epilepsy had an important impact on at least four key dimensions of peoples' biographies (Scambler, 1989). The first and most important dimension was impact on *personal identity.* The physician's formal and authoritative diagnosis of epilepsy transformed "normal people" into "epileptics" (Scambler and Hopkins, 1986). This attribution of a new and unwanted status typically turned out to be more disruptive of people's lives than—actually or potentially—recurring epileptic seizures.

The source of people's underlying disquiet at the label "epileptic" was their perception of stigma. Many felt ashamed, and more feared rejection by "normal people," including erstwhile friends, solely because of their epilepsy. This fear of meeting with discrimination was termed *felt stigma* and is contrasted to actual episodes of discrimination, termed *enacted stigma.* Individuals with felt stigma reported a very strong fear of discrimination without ever having had an actual adverse comment or experience. Felt stigma predisposed people to conceal their condition whenever possible. Moreover, this first-choice strategy of secretiveness was frequently deployed within their own nuclear families as well as at work (Scambler and Hopkins, 1986). One consequence of this strategy was that the opportunities for others to discriminate against them were much reduced. In fact, overall, more distress was caused by felt stigma than by enacted stigma.

The second biographical dimension might be termed *family management.* People's epilepsy often started in childhood, and their understanding of what was happening to them was largely a function of their parents' theories and behavior. Schneider and Conrad (1980) have described some parents as "stigma coaches," training their offspring to feel ashamed and anxious about their epilepsy, prescribing secrecy by advice or example. This pattern was discerned in the London study and may be regarded as a form of overprotection. Parental overprotection was the most conspicuous source of anger and resentment among younger people with epilepsy. In adolescence and adulthood, felt stigma typically led to concealment. Not only were boyfriends and girlfriends rarely trusted: Two-thirds of formal engagements were characterized by a calculated concealment of seizures or diagnosis or both. Interestingly, there was little indication that open disclosure, or even exposure, was likely to lead to the termination of relationships, although this did occur occasionally.

Work opportunity was another predictable focus of concern. Felt stigma, together with some apprehension about meeting with discrimination in relation to driving or operating factory machinery, often prompted people to conceal their condition when the frequency of their seizures permitted it, a common finding in the United Kingdom and the United States (Scambler, 1987; Schneider and Conrad, 1983). Concealment reduced the prospects of encountering enacted stigma and other forms of discrimination. Felt stigma was itself, however, a negative factor in employment, causing people to avoid or withdraw from the labor market or decline opportunities for promotion or advancement. While the unemployment rate was not especially high for men, it was high for married women and was generally associated with low social class and a high frequency of seizures (Scambler and Hopkins, 1980). A recent study in northeast England, however, suggests that both men and women with epilepsy may be far more vulnerable than others to job losses in times and areas of high unemployment (Elwes *et al.*, 1991).

Fourth, *legal restrictions*, most obviously concerning driving, affected a number of people; many of these put a high premium on driving or were dependent on it for their jobs. Not infrequently, they drove illegally (one in five of those on the roads), taking advantage of the confusion among neurologists and family practitioners about the precise requirements of the law (Hopkins and Harvey, 1987).

The study therefore highlighted some of the major ways in which epilepsy can impede the quality of individuals' lives, and its findings are broadly congruent with a growing batch of studies in the United Kingdom and other Western societies. One such study appears to confirm the fundamental significance for quality of life of people's own perceptions of their epilepsy and of the effect of the diagnosis on their lives: "the discrepancy between current self perceptions and anticipated self without epilepsy was by far the most important correlate of well-being—those who believed that their lives would be little different if they did not have epilepsy tended to have high well-being and vice versa" (Collings, 1990: 169). Collings reports that seizure frequency and recent onset of seizures were also associated with low well-being, although much less so than was self-image discrepancy. Many studies, however, have found epilepsy to be associated with a depressed concept of self and life-style quite independently of any biomedical measure of severity, which suggests that physician commitment to an exclusively biomedical perspective on care may be inadequate.

Epileptic Label and Experiences of Health Care

The reaction of the majority of individuals to receiving their formal diagnosis of epilepsy was shock and considerable distress, largely because of its stigmatizing implications. Only 20% had considered the possibility before it was diagnosed by the doctor. After this initial phase of reaction to their diagnosis, people looked to physicians to counter their uncertainties by means of expert and comprehensible accounts of tests, etiology, therapy, and prognosis. However, lack of explanation was a common source of frustration:

> If I could understand the cause of it, then I could put everything together, but no one has told me what's the cause of it.

Another individual described her puzzlement at the significance of an electroencephalogram:

> He said: "There's something in your brain." God knows what he meant.

They also aspired to be treated effectively and with sensitivity to epilepsy's ramifications for quality of life. If not all their expectations were realistic given the current state of medical knowledge, it is interesting that dissatisfaction was most apparent in relation to physicians' apparent disinterest in the daily problems of coping with "being epileptic," a finding consistent with other studies in the United Kingdom (West, 1985) and the United States (Schneider and Conrad, 1983). The doctor was seen as being preoccupied with the diagnosis and drug therapies while ignoring the personal aspects of having epilepsy:

> I don't think doctors understand how you feel. I think they understand it medically to a certain extent, but I don't think they understand your problem mentally in trying to cope with the fact that you have seizures and to cope with life.

Or, as another individual succinctly complained,

> I think all they're interested in is finding the drug that will curtail it. . . . They didn't ask you how you managed your life around them.

The London study therefore threw light on specific sources of patient dissatisfaction with professional—largely biomedical—care. There was an expected overlap between the goals being pursued by physicians and their patients—cure whenever possible, but if not effective palliative therapy. But several patient-defined needs had clearly not been met: These were to do with broader aspects of care. Physicians have been perceived as lacking the motivation, time, or skills to elicit and address patients' own, lay perspectives on their epilepsy. Patients' concerns with regard to felt stigma, their needs to explain the meaning and sense of why they had epilepsy, and desires to develop active ways of coping with epilepsy and its sequelae were all generally neglected in medical consultations. Hospital-based specialists in particular were generally regarded as uninterested in matters beyond diagnosis and drug therapy.

MULTIPLE SCLEROSIS

Experiences Leading to Diagnosis

A similarly in-depth sociological study examined the personal and social consequences of MS (Robinson, 1988b). The study is based on a sample of 850 individuals obtained from a National Register of patients with MS held at Brunel, The University of West London. Data were gathered by a combination of mailed structured questionnaires and more detailed biographies obtained from a subsample.

Compared to many other chronic illnesses, a considerable period of time may elapse between the onset of first symptoms and the diagnosis of MS. In this sample, 57% of individuals reported a period of 5 or more years before formal diagnosis. Thus, compared to epilepsy, the personal experiences arising from MS have at least two significant and distinctive phases: before and after diagnosis. Initially, a diverse range of symptoms tend to be explained away as evidence of tiredness, overwork, aging, or, indeed, mental aberrations.

Eventually, such normal explanations prove unconvincing and the individual seeks medical help. This initial phase of contact with the medical profession is often satisfactory for the patient because the doctor, unable to find evidence of any serious lesion, provides support for a more normal and reassuring interpretation (Stewart and Sullivan, 1982). However, relationships with the doctor often begin to involve elements of doubt, mistrust, and conflict as patients become dissatisfied with their doctor's understanding of their condition. From a medical perspective, there may be considerable problems of differential diagnosis or, even if confirmed, the diagnosis may be withheld from the patient. From the patient's perspective, this is a frustrating period in which apparent discrepancies of judgment about the seriousness of the problem between the patient and the doctor often result in distressing and protracted uncertainty and a vigorous and active campaign to obtain more plausible explanations.

This study found, as have others (Scheinberg *et al.*, 1984; Elian and Dean, 1985), that, for as many as one-third of individuals, the discovery of the diagnosis of MS is made through means other than directly from the doctors (e.g., from overheard conversations or discussions with paramedical staff). Individuals may already have guessed something of the truth from their own understanding of the disorder. In one-quarter of cases, the neurologist may decide to tell the relatives first, and they may in turn, tell the patient.

The formal medical statement of the diagnosis in Scambler's study of epilepsy resulted in virtually universal shock and dismay among patients.

The reactions to the diagnosis of MS are more varied and complex (Robinson, 1988c). A majority of respondents described some degree of relief. This can be understood in terms of a number of factors. The diagnosis legitimized behavior that they feared would be considered malingering or neurotic. A long period of major uncertainty was at last resolved. Sometimes the diagnosis was viewed as less threatening than other possibilities such as a brain tumor. Equally common were reactions of anger, fear, and shock, especially when the transition from onset of symptoms to diagnosis was particularly rapid.

Coping with Problems of Multiple Sclerosis

The second and longer stage of MS follows the discovery of diagnosis. MS imposes a formidable array of challenges for the individual and his or her family (Robinson, 1988a). The individual increasingly comes to experience the body as unreliable, unpredictable, and indeed, in a sense, separate from the real person. One respondent described the development of MS as follows:

> I hated my body at the time, I felt it had let me down by being inadequate, too weak to withstand living. I felt and still do a year later that this "thing" which was taking over my body had nothing to do with "me" inside it.

At another level, uncertainty is a characteristic feature of this as of many other chronic illnesses. The individual is unsure of the future trajectory of MS and how he or she and relevant others such as the family will respond to the many unknown challenges to come. One major dimension of experience for many is some degree of reordering of relations with other people that may be summarized as dependence. The individual may be physically dependent on others to carry out basic day-to-day tasks, and this may be associated with a more fundamental sense of loss of reciprocity and mutual respect in relationships. Some experiences such as incontinence or the thought of dependence on a wheelchair may have such charged personal and social significance that they threaten to degrade or depress the individual.

As with the epilepsy study, one of the most striking results of the MS study is the absence of any linear relationship between severity of disease and the seriousness of personal or social consequences. Thus, no simple relationship existed between degree of physical disability, on the one hand, and levels of self-esteem or depression, problems within marriage, and difficulties with employment (Robinson, 1988b), on the other. Another study (LaRocca *et al.*, 1985) had also found that only a small amount of variance in employment status could be explained by means of measures of disease and disability in MS. Indeed, in this study, as in a similar investigation (Miles, 1979), there was very little relationship at all between level of physical disability and the individual's sense of ability to lead a normal life.

The study examined the concept of *managerial strategies* to account for this lack of relationship between disease severity and seriousness of personal problems. In other words, individuals' personal responses to their disorder played an important mediating role in relation to the disease. Sociologists have developed a number of concepts to examine the processes whereby individuals respond to the constraints of chronic illness. *Passing* (Goffman, 1968) refers to a social strategy of minimizing the public visibility of a disease and is similar to the concealment employed by individuals with epilepsy; however, the manifestations of MS may ultimately be more difficult to conceal than those of epilepsy, and another strategy—normalization (Davis, 1963)—is required. While accepting the social visibility of the individual's condition, every effort is made to lead as normal a life as possible. Above all, this involves a constant process of not allowing others to define the individual in terms of their condition and not allowing symptoms or limitations to intrude too much into interactions or relations. A third response, more commonly adopted by individuals with a strong sense of stigma associated with their disorder, was *social withdrawal.* Self-image was protected by reduced contact with others.

Most individuals did not adopt one managerial strategy to the exclusion of others; strategies fused into each other and varied according to context and over time. In nearly all instances, the adoption of any strategy involved the collaboration of important others such as the spouse.

At another level, the most common strategy adopted by individuals was a stance of "fighting" the disease. Individuals saw themselves as refusing to accept or be beaten by their disease. They regarded themselves as adopting a positive mental approach against their condition. One particular manifestation of this strategy was the active and experimental search for therapies. Individuals adopted a very wide range of treatments, particularly involving diet, "alternative" or unproven therapies such as evening primrose oil or hyperbaric oxygen, yoga, or planned approaches to rest or exercise. Generally individuals' expectations of such therapies were modest. Above all, they appreciated the sense of control that such therapies offered, combined with a sense of "feeling better." More generally, this active stance in relation to MS involved a constant search for relevant information. Information was seen as another vital component of gaining some degree of personal control. Rarely was hospital medicine cited as a potential source of the positive sense of control and hope that appeared to be the common goal of many strategies. While playing a crucial role at the diagnostic phase, consultations with the neurologist at later stages were commonly seen as ritualistic and a formality.

Yet, from the patient's perspective, what we may term the interpersonal aspects of their medical care were crucial. Patients hoped for frankness, a degree of caring concern, and preparedness to engage in a mutual exchange of information with the doctor. From respondents' comments, there was clearly dramatic variation in the extent to which such expectations were met. On the one hand, one woman commented,

> I requested an appointment with Dr. X. . . . I just feel a need to speak to him. More than anyone else in my life I get such a tremendous satisfaction from just speaking to him. Probably because I think he genuinely cares what happens to me.

By contrast, another woman explained,

> Everything I know and have found out about MS I have had to research for myself. I have never had a doctor who has sat down at any time with me and talked about my hopes and fears and how I feel. I think this is very bad. Doctors I have come across seem to say, "Well, you have MS, go home and live with it."

CHRONIC HEADACHE

Introduction to a Study of Patients Consulting for Chronic Headache

A study was carried out to examine neurological specialist management of chronic headache from the patient's perspective. Recently in the United Kingdom, a number of specialist clinics have been set up to provide more active advice and treatment for patients with migraine. Neurologists generally play a fairly limited role in the management of patients presenting with headache (Butler and Millac, 1980). They provide a differential diagnosis and, where appropriate, advise about drug therapy.

A sample of 95 patients was recruited, of whom the majority (69%) were women, with an average age of 37 years and a range of social backgrounds (Fitzpatrick and Hopkins, 1981b). None of the patients received diagnoses of a serious lesion; the majority of patients' symptoms were diagnosed as either "tension headache" or "migraine." The sample's headaches closely resembled in severity those reported for other clinic studies (Selby and Lance, 1960). As in other clinic surveys (Packard, 1979), the majority (67%) reported that their headaches had been a problem for more than 1 year.

Patients were first interviewed by researchers at the hospital clinic prior to their consultation with the neurologist. The focus of this interview was on the patient's perception of the problem and on expectations of clinic attendance. In a second and much longer research interview conducted in the patient's home, between 2 and 3 weeks after the hospital visit, a detailed account was obtained of the patient's perceptions and evaluations of the hospital visit. In-depth interviews were used to encourage respondents to describe events and perceptions in their own terms. This enabled the investigators to go beyond the basic assessment of satisfaction made in most patient satisfaction surveys. The data was tape-recorded, and tone and content of patients' accounts were taken into consideration when making ratings of the extent to which patients described their neurological clinic visits in positive, neutral, or negative terms.

Expectations and Concerns

Generally, patients had few expectations of the neurologist and did not expect extensive or dramatic benefits from clinic attendance, a common observation of this group of patients (Packard, 1979; Edmeads, 1984). If expectations were tentative, it was still possible to detect quite distinct concerns that patients had with regard to their symptoms. For some patients, the main concern was anxiety that their headaches might be symptoms of a more serious underlying disease. This concern arose either because patients' symptoms had persisted too long or had significantly changed pattern so that they could no longer be explained away as "normal headaches." For this group of patients, a concern for *reassurance* was a primary factor in seeking medical help.

A second and distinct group wanted an *explanation* for symptoms. Although not concerned about fears of brain tumors, they were puzzled by headaches that did not fit usual patterns. Different again were patients whose main concern was to obtain some *preventative intervention.* The common factor in this group was what they did not want—further symptomatic medical treatment. Many of this group had longstanding histories of migraine and had received a variety of symptomatic treatments from their general practitioner. Some of this group hoped that a specialist might recommend preventative medication; for others, prevention would require advice about life-style, diet, stress factors, etc. Many in this group had developed quite elaborate personal and experiential knowledge of their migraine in terms of provoking triggers, ameliorative actions, and advantages and disadvantages of alternative therapies.

A final group of patients were concerned primarily with obtaining *symptomatic relief.* As in other studies (Parnell and Cooperstock, 1979), few expected something miraculous from the specialist; instead, the view was that the neurologist was best for trying "something different" or "something new."

Satisfaction with the Clinic

Although patients were reluctant to express attitudes in terms of dissatisfaction, their accounts of their hospital visits were striking for the range of negative as well as positive responses (Fitzpatrick and Hopkins, 1983b). At one extreme, "I must say I was very impressed. I don't know whether I was very lucky. I felt at last something was getting done." This contrasted with "I was disappointed and annoyed—a waste of time." In many cases, it was as much the tone and manner of what was said as the content that revealed the patients' evaluations.

Those accounts rated as negative were examined. Those who were negative about the medical content of their consultations were variously disappointed with interpersonal aspects of the consultation (such as feeling that they had not been taken seriously), the limited history of their headaches taken by the doctor, lack or absence of investigations, and the appropriateness or lack of treatment. Those who were negative about the communication aspects of their consultations mainly focused on the lack of any explanation for the diagnosis offered to them (Fitpatrick and Hopkins, 1981a).

A number of variables were found to be related to dissatisfaction. First, patients with migraine, patients with longer histories of headache, and patients with a concern for preventative intervention were all significantly more likely than other patients to be dissatisfied with their consultations (Fitzpatrick and Hopkins, 1988). Closer inspection of these cases showed that a group of patients with longstanding histories of migraine had developed quite complex views of the nature and causes of migraine. This group was particularly dissatisfied with what appeared to be a very superficial and limited investigation of their personal circumstances, life-style, etc., by the neurologist. Many felt that they had not been taken seriously and felt disappointed that they had received no more attention than when they consulted their general practitioner. Their response arose from a mismatch between popular views that personalized advice about life-style could influence the course of headaches and the neurologist's more limited definition of his function.

A second source of disatisfaction could be traced to a different problem—the failure to reassure. The majority of patients with concerns about brain tumors or other such possibilities were impressed with the specialist's reassurance; however, a minority remained very concerned about their symptoms after the hospital visit. They were dissatisfied with the explanations they had received. Their dissatisfaction arose from problems of communication in the consultation. The neurologist often failed to identify the presence of such worries (Fitzpatrick and Hopkins, 1981a). Moreover, reassurance by assertion that nothing is wrong is not effective if unsupported by substantive information (Kessell, 1979).

A third factor that proved to be significantly related to dissatisfaction was the presence of psychiatric symptoms. In some cases, it appeared that dissatisfaction was part of a syndrome of unhappiness with the world in general (Barsky, 1981). For others, it was more likely that the patient had insight into the inappropriateness of referral to the neurologist given the limited psychosocial support role that he plays.

This brief explanation of the pattern of results has focused on the negative responses in the sample. It should be noted that many patients, particularly those wanting some alteration to their symptomatic treatment and also the majority of those in need of reassurance, expressed positive satisfaction with the hospital visit.

A curious form of construct validity for the measures of satisfaction was obtained. The sample of patients were followed up 1 year later, and a number of different assessments were made on the changes to patients' headaches. The severity of headaches as reported at the hospital visit was compared to severity at the 1-year follow-up, and patients also rated the degree of change in symptoms. By either method, improvement in headaches was significantly associated with positive satisfaction 1 year previously (Fitzpatrick and Hopkins, 1983a; Fitzpatrick *et al.*, 1983). Possible confounding effects such as severity of headache at consultation were ruled out. This result is very similar to that obtained in a Canadian study of patients presenting to their family doctors with headaches. The Headache Study Group (1986) found that the best outcomes after 1-year follow-up were in patients who felt they had been given sufficient opportunity to tell the doctor all they wanted to say at the initial visit.

The variance in satisfaction levels often is explained by patients' demographic characteristics alone and does not contribute to the evaluation of services received (Fitzpatrick, 1990). By examining in more detail patients' views, this study highlighted some important problems in neurological clinics. Patient satisfaction is least often measured with regard to outcomes (Hall and Dornan, 1988). This study would indicate that the contribution of patients to assessment of outcomes may be considerable.

DISCUSSION

All three studies set out to examine the experience of illness from the sufferer's perspective. They were based on a methodological approach to social research that emphasizes the respondent's viewpoint. This style of medical sociological research is particularly deserving of attention when health care systems and health professionals are widely criticized for their insensitivities and inabilities to recognize and respond to patients' main concerns, especially in the areas of chronic illness and disability (Calkins *et al.*, 1991).

In all three cases, conventional classifications of disease were unhelpful guides to experiential aspects of illness, and personal and social consequences of conditions were only moderately explained by medical measures of disease severity. Thus, individuals with well-advanced and disabling MS might establish a strong sense of normal life and a positive sense of control over their condition and, conversely, individuals presenting with what neurologists might regard as benign and, in medical terms, minor chronic headaches would experience their symptoms as severely handicapping.

Medical sociology has begun to develop a set of concepts to tease out the different sources of distress posed by chronic illness. The concept of stigma refers to a range of different ways in which the sufferer's sense of self is diminished or threatened (Goffman, 1968). For people with epilepsy, this might involve fear of rejection by others because of an epileptic identity; for individuals with MS, stigma might arise from failures of competence at everyday tasks or the particular fear of humiliation arising from incontinence. In a very different sense, uncertainty is also a pervasive and demanding dimension of illness experience: uncertainty about the next occurrence of an embarassing episode, uncertainty about the future trajectory of disease, and uncertainty about the extent to which life itself is threatened.

For many individuals with neurological problems, a sense of control and of the possibility of "doing something" is a crucial dimension of illness experience. In both MS and migraine, sufferers were found to look for changes in life-style or diet or to alternative treatments that might arrest or reduce symptoms or improve the individual's adjustment to his or her condition. Far from being gullible or expecting miracles, many sufferers have a realistic, modest, and essentially empirical awareness of the possibilities of such alternative strategies. In a culture that generally emphasizes the value of positive mastery over the environment, the search for active strategies may fulfill important needs to cope rather than to succumb (Robinson, 1988a). Access to information plays a pivotal role in acquiring a sense of control.

For other chronic illnesses, here illustrated by MS, physical limitations in the ability to perform daily tasks, often of symbolic or charged significance, may impose a more profound and demoralizing sense of dependence. Similarly, problems of mobility, in addition to physically limiting the ability to remain in contact with others, may also be associated with coping strategies of social withdrawal. These different dimensions of illness experience have been underlined not only because the conventional medical model fails to capture them but also to draw attention to limitations of many recent attempts to measure subjective health status and quality of life.

Considerable progress has been made in the development of instruments to assess the patient's perspective with regard to his or her illness. As well as achieving levels of reliability comparable to conventional medical measures (Feinstein, 1977), health status and quality of life instruments can show important differences between types of chronic illness (Stewart *et al.*, 1989) and, of particular importance, in some fields of chronic illness can be sensitive to important therapeutic benefits of treatments (Meenan *et al.*, 1984). However, despite the more comprehensive scope implied by their titles, many instruments in this field concentrate on a narrow range of dimensions of illness experience. Instruments most frequently assess areas such as ability to perform activities of daily life, physical function and mobility, pain, psychological well-being in the form of symptoms of depression or anxiety, and some aspects of "social function" such as degree of social contact with others. The neurological studies reported here suggest numerous dimensions of illness experience that may be missed by such instruments: stigma, sense of normality, dependence, sense of control, understanding regarding one's condition, etc. While these are apparently more fleeting and subjective dimensions of illness experience, systematic measures of such constructs are beginning to be developed in some areas of chronic illness (Nicassio *et al.*, 1985; Bradley *et al.*, 1990). Neurological disorders have received less attention in terms of such approaches, partly because medicine has traditionally focused more on diagnostic functions than on systematic approaches to a broader caring role. As neurological management widens its therapeutic goals, it will be essential to develop appropriate outcome measures, especially as evidence is found that styles of medical care may influence such outcomes (Kaplan *et al.*, 1989).

Similar arguments might be developed with regard to measures of patient satisfaction. To date, with a few exceptions, instruments to assess the patient's perceptions of health care have all too frequently produced unvarying and uninformatively positive results (Fitzpatrick, 1991) that are of little use in evaluation of services. They also tend to avoid those aspects of health care that are of particular significance to patients—in particular, perceptions of outcomes (Cleary and McNeil, 1988). At different stages of their illness and varying by condition, the patient groups discussed in this chapter have looked to medical care for information about their diagnosis, reassurance, support and encouragement to cope, and the opportunity to discuss the distress of chronic illness. The studies here underline the importance of such expectations and also the need to develop more sensitive measures of patients' assessments of treatment benefits that will be appropriate for the evaluation of treatment of neurological disorders.

References

Barsky, A. (1981). Hidden reasons some patients visit doctors. *Ann. Int. Med.* **94**, 492–498.

Binnie, C (1990). Progress in the treatment of epilepsy. *J. Neurol. Neurosurg. Psychiatry* **53**, 273–274.

Bradley, C., Lewis, K., Jennings, A., and Ward, J. (1990). Scales to measure perceived control developed specifically for people with tablet-treated diabetes. *Diabetic Med.* **7**, 685–694.

Butler, P., and Millac, P. (1980). The effect of a neurological clinic upon patients with tension headache. *Practitioner* **224**, 195–196.

Calkins, D., Rubenstain, L., and Cleary, P. (1991). Failure of physicians to recognize functional disability in ambulatory patients. *Ann Int. Med.* **114**, 351–353.

Cleary, P., and McNeil, B. (1988). Patient satisfaction as an indicator of quality care. *Inquiry* **25**, 25–36.

Collings, J. (1990). Epilepsy and well-being. *Soc. Sci. Med.* **31**, 165–170.

Davis, F. (1963). "Passage through Crisis." Bobbs-Merrill, Indianapolis, Indiana.

Duncan, S. (1991). Modern treatment strategies for patients with epilepsy: a review. *J. Roy. Soc. Med.* **84**, 159–162.

Edmeads, J. (1984). Placebos and the power of negative thinking. *Headache* **24**, 342–343.

Elian, M., and Dean, G. (1985). To tell or not to tell: The diagnosis of multiple sclerosis. *Lancet* **ii**, 27–28.

Ellwood, P. (1988). Outcomes management: A technology of patient experience. *N. Engl. J. Med.* **318**, 1549–1556.

Elwes, R., Marshall, J., Beattie, A., and Newman, P. (1991). Epilepsy and employment. A community based survey in an area of high unemployment. *J. Neurol. Neurosurg. Psychiatry* **54**, 200–203.

Feinstein, A. (1977). Clinical biostatistics, XLI. Hard science, soft data, and the challenges of choosing clinical variables in research. *Clin. Pharmacol. Ther.* **22**, 485–498.

Fitzpatrick, R. (1990). Measurement of patient satisfaction. *In* "Measuring the Outcomes of Medical Care" (A. Hopkins and D. Costain, eds.). pp. 19–26. Royal College of Physicians and King's Fund Centre, London.

Fitzpatrick, R. (1991). Surveys of patient satisfaction: I–Important general considerations. *Br. Med. J.* **302**, 887–889.

Fitzpatrick, R., and Hopkins, A. (1981a). Patients' satisfaction with communication in neurological outpatient clinics. *J. Psychosom. Res.* **25**, 329–334.

Fitzpatrick, R., and Hopkins, A. (1981b). Referrals to neurologists for headaches not due to structural disease. *J. Neurol. Neurosurg. Psychiatry* **44**, 1061–1067.

Fitzpatrick, R., and Hopkins, A. (1983a). Effects of referral to a specialist for headache. *J. R. Soc. Med.* **76**, 112–115.

Fitzpatrick, R., and Hopkins, A. (1983b). Problems in the conceptual framework of patient satisfaction research. *Soc. Health Illness* **5**, 297–311.

Fitzpatrick, R., and Hopkins, A. (1988). Illness behaviour and headache and the sociology of consultations for headache. *In* "Headache: Problems in Management" (A. Hopkins, ed.), pp. 351–385. W. Saunders, London.

Fitzpatrick, R., Hopkins, A., and Harvard-Watts, O. (1983). Social dimensions of healing: A longitudinal study of outcomes of medical management of headaches. *Soc. Sci. Med.* **17,** 501–510.

Goffman, E. (1968). "Stigma." Penguin, Harmondsworth, Middlesex.

Hall, J., and Dornan, M. (1988). Meta-analysis of satisfaction with medical care: Description of research domain and analysis of overall satisfaction levels. *Soc. Sci. Med.* **27,** 637–644.

Headache Study Group. (1986). Predictors of outcome in headache patients presenting to family physicians. *Headache J.* **26,** 285–294.

Hopkins, A., and Harvey, P. (1987). Epilepsy and driving. *In* "Epilepsy" (A. Hopkins, ed.). pp. 563–571. Chapman & Hill, London.

Jette, A. (1980). Health status indicators: Their utility in chronic disease evaluation research. *J. Chron. Dis.* **33,** 567–769.

Kaplan, S., Greenfield, S., and Ware, J. (1989). Assessing the effects of physician–patient interactions on the outcomes of chronic disease. *Med. Care* **27,** S110–217.

Kessell, N. (1979). Reassurance. *Lancet* **i,** 1128–1133.

LaRocca, N., Kalb, R., Schewinberg, L., and Kendall, P. (1985). Factors associated with unemployment of patients with multiple sclerosis. *J. Chron. Dis.* **38,** 203–210.

Meenan, R., Anderson, J., Kazis, L., Egger, M., Altz-Smith, M., Samuelson, C., Willkens, R., Solsky, M., Hayes, S., Blocka, K., Weinstein, A., Guttadauria, M., Laplan, S., and Klippel, J. (1984). Outcome assessment in clinical trials. *Arthritis Rheumatism* **27,** 1344–1352.

Miles, A. (1979). Some psycho-social consequences of multiple sclerosis: Problems of social interaction and group identity. *Br. J. Med. Psychol.* **52,** 321–331.

Nicassio, M., Wallston, K., Callahan, L., Herbert, M., and Pincus, T. (1985). The measurement of helplessness in rheumatoid arthritis: The development of the Arthritis Helplessness Index. *J. Rheumatol.* **12,** 462–467.

Packard, R. (1979). What does the headache patient want? *Headache* **19,** 370–374.

Parnell, P., and Cooperstock, R. (1979). Tranquillisers and mood elevators in the treatment of migraine. *Headache* **19,** 78–89.

Relman, A. (1988). Assessment and accountability: The third revolution in medical care. *N. Engl. J. Med.* **319,** 1220–1222.

Robinson, I. (1988a). Managing symptoms in chronic disease: Some dimensions of patients' experience. *Int. Dis. Stud.* **10,** 112–118.

Robinson, I. (1988b). "Multiple Sclerosis." Routledge, London.

Robinson, I. (1988c). Reconstructing lives: Living with multiple sclerosis. *In* "Living with Chronic Illness" (R. Anderson and M. Bury, eds.), pp. 43–56. Unwin Hyman, London.

Scambler, G. (1987). Sociological aspects of epilepsy. *In* "Epilepsy" (A. Hopkins, ed.). pp. 497–510. Chapman & Hall, London.

Scambler, G. (1989). "Epilepsy." Routledge & Kegan Paul, London.

Scambler, G., and Hopkins, A. (1980). Social class, epileptic activity and disadvantage at work. *J. Epidemiol. Community Health* **34,** 129–133.

Scambler, G., and Hopkins, A. (1986). "Being epileptic": Coming to terms with stigma. *Sociol. Health Illness* **8,** 26–43.

Scambler, G., and Hopkins, A. (1990). Generating a model of epileptic stigma: The role of qualitative analysis. *Social Sci. Med.* **30,** 1187–1194.

Scheinberg, L., Kalb, R., LaRocca, N., Geiseer, B., Slater, R., and Poser, C. (1984). The doctor patient relationship in multiple sclerosis. *In* "The Diagnosis of Multiple Sclerosis" (C. Poser, D. Paty, L. Schienberg, W. McDonald, and G. Ebers, eds.) Thieme-Stratton, New York.

Schneider, J., and Conrad, P. (1980). In the closet with illness: Epilepsy, stigma potential and information control. *Social Prob.* **28,** 32–44.

Schneider, J., and Conrad, P. (1983). "Having Epilepsy: The Experience and Control of Illness." Temple University Press, Philadelphia.

Selby, G., and Lance, J. (1960). Observations on 500 cases of migraine and allied vascular headache. *J. Neurol. Neurosurg. Psychiatry* **23,** 23–33.

Shorvon, S. (1991). Medical assessment and treatment of chronic epilepsy. *Brit. Med. J.* **302,** 363–366.

Steinwachs, D. (1989). Application of health status assessment measures in policy research. *Med. Care* **27,** S12–S26.

Stewart, A., Greenfield, S., Hays, R., Wells, K., Rogers, W., Berry, S., McGlynn, E., and Ware, J. (1989). Functional status and well-being of patients with chronic conditions. *J. Am. Med. Assoc.* **262,** 907–913.

Stewart, D., and Sullivan, T.(1982). Illness behaviour and the sick role; the case of multiple sclerosis. *Social Sci. Med.* **16,** 1397–1404.

Tarlov, A., Ware, J., Greenfield, S., Nelson, E., Perrin, E., and Zubkoff, M. (1989). The Medical Outcomes Study: An application of methods for monitoring the results of medical care. *J. Am. Med. Assoc.* **262,** 925–930.

West, P. (1985). Becoming disabled: Perspectives on the labelling approach. *In* "Stress and Stigma: Explanation and Evidence in the Sociology of Crime and Illness" (U. Gerhardt and M. Wadsworth, eds.). pp. 104–128. Macmillan, London.

7

The Epidemiology of Wernicke–Korsakoff Syndrome and Related Neurologic Disorders Due to Alcoholism

Heather Spencer Feigelson • Craig A. Molgaard

In 1881, Carl Wernicke first reported clinical and pathological findings of a previously unrecognized disease. His observations were made in three patients. The first was a young woman who had swallowed sulfuric acid in a suicide attempt; the other two were alcoholic men. The descriptions Wernicke gave have remained the classic diagnostic features for the syndrome that now bears his name, Wernicke's encephalopathy (WE) (Wernicke, 1881).

The characteristic pathology of WE is small punctate hemorrhages occurring symmetrically around the third and fourth ventricles of the brain. The "classic triad" of symptoms associated with WE are ataxia, often manifested as a staggering gait, ophthalmoplegia (i.e., paralysis of the eye muscles), and global confusion. The patient is typically disoriented with regard to place and time, cannot recognize familiar people, and is unable to maintain a coherent conversation. Polyneuropathy (pain, weakness, or loss of sensation) in the arms and legs is also common.

Without treatment, the symptoms of WE progress and the patient dies within about 2 weeks. If the patient is treated with large doses of parenteral thiamine (vitamin B_1) the symptoms improve, or even completely subside. However, very few patients will show a complete recovery from the mental changes (Butters, 1981).

Six years after Wernicke's first paper, S. S. Korsakoff described an amnestic syndrome based on a study of 20 patients. In later articles, Korsakoff described additional patients and provided a clinical description, which remains accurate today and characterizes the disorder that bears his name, Korsakoff's syndrome (KS) (Victor *et al.*, 1989).

The hallmark signs of KS include confusion, confabulation, and anterograde amnesia. This anterograde amnesia is the most striking feature of KS. The patient who suffers from KS is unable to learn new information from the time of onset of illness. Events that occurred hours or even minutes before cannot be recalled, nor can the names or faces of commonly encountered people, such as the patient's nurse or physician. Retrograde amnesia, the inability to recall past events, is also a consistent feature of KS. It appears to have a temporal gradient and is usually most pronounced for events occurring just prior to the onset of illness. Very remote events from childhood or young adulthood are often clear. The confabulation associated with KS is not necessarily a constant or permanent feature of this disorder. Generally, it is seen in the early stages of the disease and becomes less noticeable as the patient adjusts to the illness. Despite the severity of memory impairments, the intellectual function of KS patients as measured by IQ tests remains intact. This is an important difference between KS and dementia. Finally, the personality changes occurring in KS patients are interesting to note. With the onset of KS, impulsiveness, aggression, and severe alcohol abuse are replaced by apathy, passivity, and a virtual disinterest in alcohol (Butters, 1981). This is true even in patients who were known to be "barroom brawlers" or who had a history of domestic violence.

The relationship between WE and KS was not realized until long after Wernicke's and Korsakoff's classic works. In fact, even today controversy still exists, and the Wernicke–Korsakoff syndrome (WKS) is variably defined in the literature. Some authors refer to either WE or KS alone, others as if it is one syndrome. KS is referred to by many names, including Korsakoff's psychosis. The *Diagnostic and Statistics Manual,* 3rd ed., rev. (American Psychiatric Association, 1987), defines KS under Alcohol Amnestic Disorder. For the purpose of this review, we will refer to WKS as a single disorder that consists of two stages: WE, the acute phase that may be improved or even reversed with the administration of large doses of thiamine, and KS, the chronic, irreversible stage identified primarily by the amnestic disorder.

Although much work has been done to define the psychological and pathological features of this disease (Butters, 1981; Grant, 1987; Harper and Kril, 1990; Victor *et al.*, 1989), little is known about the epidemiology of WKS. The aims of this paper are to assess the amount and type of epidemiologic research on WKS to date, examine current research theories regarding the etiology of WKS, and to suggest areas for further epidemiologic research and potential public health interventions.

REVIEW OF DESCRIPTIVE STUDIES

This review includes seven studies that provide descriptive data about the distribution and occurrence of WKS. The first study to be discussed reports findings from both clinical and pathological data, five studies report incidence estimates of WE from necropsy data only, and the seventh study estimates the prevalence of KS from a survey of health care institutions. Because these methodologies are vastly different, the six studies with autopsy data will be reviewed and discussed first. The prevalence study will then be reviewed separately. The results of all seven studies are summarized in Table I.

Victor *et al.* (1989) have provided both a clinical description of WKS and an estimate of incidence from necropsic exam. Their work is the most frequently referenced descriptive study to date. Although epidemiologi-

Table I

Summary of Descriptive Studies

Study	Study design	Sample size	Rate	Sex ratio
Victor *et al.*, 1978 United States	Autopsy	3548	2.2%	1.3:1
Cravioto *et al.*, 1961 United States	Autopsy	1600	1.75%	1.8:1
Torvik *et al.*, 1982 Norway	Autopsy	8735	0.8%	4:1
Harper, 1983 Western Australia	Autopsy	4677	2.8%	3:1
Harper *et al.*, 1989 Sydney, Australia	Autopsy	285	2.1%	5:1
Lindboe and Loberg, 1989 Norway	Autopsy	6964	0.75%	2:1
Blansjaar *et al.*, 1987 The Netherlands	Prevalence (survey)	[a]	4.8/10,000	2:1

[a] Used the city population for the denominator.

cally imperfect, it is the only work reporting long-term follow-up for a large cohort of WKS patients.

The clinical description of WKS was derived from a heterogeneous group of 245 patients. Ninety of these patients were obtained from Boston City Hospital between 1950 and 1951, 129 cases from Massachusetts General Hospital were added between 1952 and 1961, and an additional 26 cases were studied at Cleveland Metropolitan General Hospital between 1963 and 1966. Some of these patients were followed for over 10 years; 82 of them had complete postmortem exams.

The sex ratio for these clinically diagnosed cases was 1.7 : 1 (154 males, 91 females) and was uniform across all three hospitals. The onset of signs and symptoms appears to be earlier in women and than in men. The highest frequency of cases occurred between the ages of 40 and 69 years for men and 30 and 59 years for women. The occurrence of WKS in the 20–29-year-old age group was approximately 2% ($n = 3$) in men and 12% ($n = 11$) in women. In the 70–79-year-old age group, 6.5% of the cases in men were reported, and no cases in women.

All but two of the cases were alcoholic, usually with a history of several years of alcoholism. No correlation was found between any particular type of alcoholic beverage and specific signs of WKS. Eighty-four percent of the cases were malnourished. In general, the dietary habits of WKS cases were different from those of "spree" or periodic drinkers. Nutritional deficiency among WKS patients occurred over a period of several months or even years. Spree drinkers can restore any nutritional deficiencies during their periods of sobriety.

Less than one-third of the cases presented with the classic triad of symptoms occurring together: ataxia, opthalmoplegia, and confusion. The most common presenting syptom was "mental confusion" (66%). "Staggering" was noted in 52% of cases, ocular signs in 40%, and polyneuropathy in 36%. Other common presenting signs were memory loss (20%), exhaustion or collapse (20%), and alcohol withdrawal syndrome (13%). In 25% of the cases, the patient was simply bedridden, perhaps as a result of ataxia or weakness.

The prospective nature of this study allowed some mortality data to be obtained. Excluding cases in whom the diagnosis of WKS was made postmortem, 216 were available for long-term follow-up. However, the period of clinical observation was highly variable (from less than 1 month up to 13 years) and incomplete. Of those with adequate follow-up to assess mortality, 93 (43%) died.

The mortality patterns were very different in patients who died in the acute stage (mean time of 8 days) compared to those who died several months or years after the initial onset of WKS. Death in chronic cases was not related to the original neurologic disease. Primary or secondary cause of death in 44 cases who died in the acute phase was infection in 77% and cirrhosis in 52%. In chronic cases, infection and cirrhosis were also common findings (41% and 35%, respectively), but carcinoma (27%) and pulmonary embolism (14%) were also common findings.

These researchers also reported incidence data from postmortem exams obtained at the Cleveland facility between 1963 and 1976 (Victor and Laureno, 1978). From 3548 autopsies of patients 18 years and older, 77 cases of WKS were identified, resulting in an incidence of 2.2%. The male:female ratio of WKS was similar to the overall ratio of autopsies, 1.3:1. This is the only series that has reported any specific information on the racial distribution of WKS. Cases of WKS were nearly twice as common in Whites than in Blacks (48 versus 29), but the frequency of black women was higher than white women (19 versus 12). An unexpected finding was the high frequency of oropharyngeal–esophageal carcinoma in WKS patients (8%).

An important observation by Victor *et al.* (1989) was the discrepancy between the sex ratio for alcoholism and that for WKS. They reported that the rate of alcoholism in 1966 was 4 times higher in men, whereas the rate of WKS observed in men was not even 2 times the rate in women. Although the prevalence of alcoholism was probably grossly underestimated in women, these results suggested that women may be more vulnerable to the development of WKS than men. Sex differences were also seen in the age of onset of symptoms. For women, the peak age at diagnosis was about 10 years younger than for men. Unfortunately, neither of these hypotheses have been adequately investigated.

One concern about the work by Victor *et al.* (1989) was the case definition used for the clinical portion of the study. A precise case definition was not specified, so it is unclear how these subjects were determined to have WKS, or what the potential rate of misclassification may be. The classic signs of WE were often absent, thus many cases may go undiagnosed. No information was given about confirming the diagnosis of WKS in the cases that had postmortem exams. It is assumed that all were found to indeed have WKS. A specific case definition would have helped future researchers replicate this study or improve upon the methodology employed.

In 1961, Cravioto *et al.* reported on 28 cases of WE diagnosed from histopathological findings at autopsy. Cases were identified from all patients (including children) who came to autopsy over a 3-year period at a single New York hospital, resulting in an incidence of 1.75%. Among the 28 cases, 18 were males and 10 were females (a ratio of 1.8:1) and they ranged in age from 32 to 82 years, with a mean age of 54.

A review of the clinical records revealed all but one of the cases were chronic alcoholics. The triad of ataxia, opthalmoplegia, and mental confusion was present in only 14% ($n = 4$) of the cases. However, at least one of these signs was present in the majority of cases. The most common finding, present in 26 of the 28 cases, was organic mental syndrome. Although some clinical signs of KS were reported, whether or not any of these cases could be classified as KS is unclear.

The duration of illness was impossible to estimate accurately based on the clinical and pathological information alone. Fifty percent of the cases died within 10 days of hospitalization for the acute episode; the remaining died within 3.5 months. Unfortunately, specific causes of death were not noted by the authors.

In 1982, Torvik *et al.* reported their findings from 8735 autopsies performed over a 5-year period (1975–1979) in Norway. Of those, 713 (8%) were cases of suspected or confirmed alcoholism. Seventy cases of WE were identified, resulting in an incidence of 0.8%. The incidence among known or suspected alcoholics was 12.5%. The sex ratio among cases was 4 : 1 (56 males, 14 females). The mean age of males was slightly older (64 versus 59 years). The 70 cases of WE were further classified as "active" ($n = 22$) or "inactive" ($n = 48$). The sex ratio for active WE was 1.4 : 1 (male : female) and 8.6 : 1 for inactive WE.

Clinical records were examined for 19 (86%) cases of active WE and 40 (83%) cases of "inactive" WE. Among the active cases, the correct diagnosis was made in only one case. Drowsiness and coma were the predominant symptoms in 18 cases. Of the inactive cases, the most common diagnoses were dementia and alcoholic psychosis.

The ratio of men to women among the known or suspected alcoholic subgroup was 4.2 : 1. This suggests that women are overrepresented among cases of active WE and underrepresented among cases of inactive WE. However, the overall ratio of WE is similar to that of alcoholics. This discrepancy may be explained by many factors independent of the disease state, including sex differences in admission or treatment, or by differences in severity of the disease in men and women.

Harper (1983) diagnosed 131 cases of WE prospectively from 4677 autopsies performed on patients over 20 years of age in Western Australia between 1973 and 1981. This is an overall incidence of 2.8%. Cases in this study were obtained from both a coroner's office (83 cases) and from a teaching hospital (48 cases). The incidence from the coroner's sample was 4.7% compared to 1.7% from the hospital sample. The ratio of WE cases occurring in males to females was 3 : 1, and the peak incidence occurred in the fifth decade (41%).

Good clinical documentation was available for 97 of the 131 cases of WE. Review of clinical records showed 97% of the cases were chronic alcoholics. Only 34% of the cases had a clinical diagnosis of WE or WKS. Sixteen percent had the classic triad of signs, 28% had two of the three signs, 37% had one, and 19% had none of the three.

The author notes that 12% of the total sample was of aboriginal decent. However, only 2.4% of the population of Western Australia is aboriginal; thus, this sample is substantially enriched. Unfortunately, possible explanations for this are not adequately discussed. This disproportion may result from many factors and may be real or artifactual. Aborigines are known to have a higher prevalence of alcoholism; however, differing patterns in hospitalization or autopsy may also contribute to the observed discrepancy.

The incidence rate in this study was higher than that in any other study. This increased rate may reflect different drinking patterns in this region of Australia compared to those of other study sites. However, twice as many cases were obtained from the coroner's office as compared to the hospital, which may also explain this higher rate. The high proportion of Aborigines, as discussed, was a likely contributor to this higher rate as well.

A later prospective necropsy study by Harper *et al.* (1989) refined the methodology from the previous study and estimated the incidence of WKS in Sydney, Australia. The sample included all hospitals and the morgue in a defined geographic area. Only subjects whose residential address was within the study area and who were over 15 years of age were included in the analysis. To adjust for potential seasonal variation, data were collected during two 3-month periods (March to May and September to November). The total sample size was 285. Approximately one-half of the subjects (n = 140) were from the coroner's office and the other half from hospitals (n = 145). The age and sex distributions between the forensic and hospital subgroups were identical. Men outnumbered women in the sample by more than two to one. The age range was 17–93 years, and the mean age for men and women was similar, 64 and 65, respectively. Six cases of WKS were identified from the sample, resulting in an incidence of 2.1%. Five cases were male and one was female. The age range was 44–61 years. Although the incidence reported from this sample is similar to that of other reports, the small number of cases makes it impossible to develop firm conclusions about these results.

A study by Lindboe and Loberg (1989) reported findings from 6964 autopsies performed during a 5-year period at a single hospital in Oslo. WE was classified as "active" or "inactive," and subjects as alcoholic or nonalcoholic. Based on medical records, 604 (8.7%) of all those autopsied were classified as alcoholic. A total of 52 cases of WE occurred, resulting in an incidence of 0.75%. Of these, 12 cases (23%) occurred in nonalcoholics. The ratio of males to females was about 2:1 overall, 4:1 in alcoholics and 1 : 1 in nonalcoholic cases. Medical records were reviewed for 18 cases (35%) classified as active WE. The correct diagnosis was made in only four cases, all of whom were alcoholic. The most common symptoms were disorientation and, in later stages, coma. No cases exhibited the classic triad of symptoms.

The classification of alcoholics versus nonalcoholics based on clinical records alone is likely to result in misclassification of a large percentage of subjects. However, the authors note that none of those classified as nonalcoholic had significant liver disease, pancreatitis, or cerebellar atrophy, whereas 61% of the alcoholic group had one or more of these conditions.

In reviewing these studies, the biases introduced by the use of autopsy data must be considered. Cases seen at autopsy tend to be a select group of hospitalized patients, who are themselves select (Kelsey *et al.*, 1986). Furthermore, the proportion of deaths that are autopsied has been decreasing in recent years. Interesting or undiagnosed cases are more likely to be seen at autopsy. Males are more likely to be autopsied than females, and younger people compared to old. Bias may result from the selection of cases for autopsy if a researcher has a particular disease of interest and requests autopsies on suspected cases.

The reported rates may be higher than the true rate of WKS in the general population if indeed the underlying cause of death in these cases is often undiagnosed, or if the researchers are searching harder for these cases and producing an enriched sample for autopsy. However, these rates also may be lower than the actual rate if mild cases are not brought to autopsy, and only a small proportion of all deaths are brought to autopsy. The fact that more men than women are autopsied, but the proportion of WKS cases found in women was consistently high in these studies, adds to the argument that women have an increased susceptibility to WKS.

Autopsy data are an excellent source of prevalence data for nonfatal diseases if the nonfatal disease is no more or less likely to be autopsied (Kelsey *et al.*, 1986). Whether or not this holds for WKS is unclear. Acute cases of WE often present in coma and are undiagnosed; therefore, they are likely candidates for autopsy. On the other hand, chronic cases of KS appear to die of apparently unrelated causes, such as cancer, and therefore may be no more likely to be autopsied than other chronic conditions.

Blansjaar *et al.* (1987) estimated the prevalence of KS in The Hague, The Netherlands, using data obtained from a survey of health care facilities. Representative workers from health care institutions and organizations in the municipal area were interviewed and information was obtained for each KS patient receiving treatment, housing, or care. The diagnosis of KS was accepted as valid whenever it was made during admission to a hospital or psychiatric nursing home, after detoxification.

A total of 215 cases of KS were identified, resulting in a prevalence of 4.8 per 10,000 city population. Sixty-eight percent of the cases were men and 32% were women, a ratio of just over 2 : 1. The mean age of the total case group was 62 years, although the mean age in men was slightly younger than in women (61 versus 65). The age distribution in men approximated a normal curve and peaked between the ages of 50 and 64. The age distribution in women suggested a bimodal curve, with peaks at 55–59 and 70–74 years of age.

The authors noted that this type of survey will not include mild cases of KS who have not been admitted to a hospital or nursing home. However, they do not consider the possibility of missed cases resulting from atypical presentation of symptoms, or those that may be masked by other illnesses such as dementia. A consistent finding in the necropsy studies was the lack of good clinical diagnosis; the majority of cases with WKS are probably never diagnosed. It is impossible to evaluate the reliability of this reported prevalence without a specified case definition. An exhaustive chart review of all cases seen in every facility in a specified period of time may have provided a better estimate of point prevalence. Minimally, all the hospital records for the cases identified in this sample should have been systematically reviewed by an unbiased reviewer for consistency. A random sample of medical records from these institutions of cases not diagnosed with KS would have also helped to assess the accuracy of KS diagnoses and the percentage of cases misclassified.

The results of these studies are summarized in Table I. In general, the incidence rates obtained from autopsy studies suggest that the rate of WKS in European countries is just under 1%, whereas the rates in the United States and Australia are around 2%. The studies consistently show a higher proportion of women than expected, suggesting that women may be at increased risk for WKS compared to men. WKS also appears to occur earlier or more severely in women.

CURRENT RESEARCH TOPICS

The Continuity Hypothesis

Ryback (1971) first proposed the continuity hypothesis, suggesting a continuum of cognitive impairment where the social drinker, the long-term alcoholic, and the WKS patient all represent separate points on the same scale. Since that time, many studies have investigated this theory, and Butters (1981) provides an excellent review. Recent reports (Alderdice and Davidson, 1990; Williams and Skinner, 1990) have refined the study designs of earlier work by controlling for potential confounding variables, including age, sex, socioeconomic status, IQ, and education level, and the findings have remained consistent. In general, these investigations have supported Ryback's hypothesis and demonstrated that some of the specific memory impairments that characterize WKS are also evident in detoxified long-term alcoholics in attenuated forms. Evidence for impairment in social drinkers, however, has been inconclusive (MacVane *et al.*, 1982; Parker and Noble, 1977; Grant, 1987).

The Relationship of Wernicke–Korsakoff Syndrome to Other Alcoholic Disorders

"Alcoholic dementia" is often referred to in the same context as WKS. The term dementia denotes a clinical syndrome composed of failing memory and loss of other intellectual functions due to progressive degenerative disease of the brain. There is no single alcoholic dementia syndrome; rather, this term is used to describe patients who have apparently irreversible cognitive changes, possibly from diverse causes, in the midst of chronic alcoholism (Braunwald *et al.*, 1987). The chronic alcohol population, as a group, has an intelligence that falls within normal range, even in patients with WKS. (Victor *et al.*, 1989). Research has consistently found IQ to remain intact in WKS cases, and the memory defects are specific. Thus, the classification of alcoholic dementia appears to be a misnomer, used to label demented patients with a history of alcohol use. It is not an interchangeable term with WKS, nor should it be considered as part of the clinical progression of WKS. A complete review and discussion of the relationship between WKS and alcoholic dementia is presented by Victor *et al.* (1989).

Some evidence does suggest that "alcoholic cerebellar degeneration" and WKS represent the same disease process (Victor *et al.*, 1989). Alcoholic cerebellar degeneration is characterized by ataxia, usually in the legs, and occasionally impairment of speech and ocular motility. Pathologic evidence supports the hypothesis of similar etiology (Victor *et al.*, 1989). The mental signs of WE, however, are absent in alcoholic cerebellar degeneration. Whether cerebellar degeneration is caused by nutritional deficiency, the toxic affects of alcohol, or the interaction between the two is unclear (Harper and Kril, 1990). Victor *et al.* (1989) found that 75% of patients with alcoholic cerebellar degeneration had a history of prolonged malnutrition but not necessarily heavy alcohol use. Torvik *et al.* (1982) found that 27% of alcoholics had cerebellar atrophy at autopsy. Although it seems reasonable to conclude that these two syndromes have similar etiology, the specific relationship between WKS and cerebellar degeneration remains unclear.

The Effects of Alcohol in Women

Alcoholism and alcohol-related diseases have become an increasing problem, or at least a more recognized problem, in women since it has become socially acceptable for women to drink (Corti and Ibrahim, 1990; Saunders *et al.*, 1981). The results of the descriptive studies previously described suggested that women may be more susceptible to WKS than men and may develop WKS earlier. Studies have shown that women develop other alcohol-related diseases earlier than men (Ashley *et al.*, 1977; Saunders *et al.*, 1981), that women are at greater risk for brain damage (Jacobson, 1986), and that alcohol is metabolized differently in women compared to men (Cole-Harding and Wilson, 1987; Frezza *et al.*, 1990; Saunders *et al.*, 1981).

A review by Saunders *et al.* (1981) addresses these issues. Studies have shown that the male:female ratio for alcoholic liver disease is 2:1, while 5–10 times as many men as women are problem drinkers. These results suggest that women may develop alcohol-induced liver damage from smaller amounts of alcohol and that dependence may not be necessary for damage to occur. Evidence also suggests that women develop liver disease after a shorter history of problem drinking, perhaps as much as 5–10 years earlier than men. Other studies have suggested that female alcoholics have more severe liver disease than their male counterparts. However, different patterns of detection, referral, and diagnosis of liver disease may account, in part, for these findings.

This apparent increased susceptibility in women may apply to other alcoholic-related conditions as well. One study evaluating morbidity in alcoholics (Ashley *et al.*, 1977) found that, although there were no pronounced differences in the prevalence of disease in women compared to men, the onset of disease was earlier in women. This was true for fatty liver, hypertension, obesity, anemia, malnutrition, gastrointestinal hemorrhage, and ulcer. One explanation for these observed sex differences is that more women than men seek treatment, therefore allowing alcohol-related diseases to be diagnosed. Women, more so then men, may underestimate the amount of alcohol they consume or the length of time they have been drinking.

In a study by Jacobson (1986), a series of 26 female alcoholics and 41 controls of similar age and socioeconomic status were interviewed and examined by computed tomographic brain scan. Results showed that alcoholics had significantly greater ventricular enlargement and widening of the sulci and cortical fissures compared to controls. These abnormalities occurred after a much shorter drinking history and at a lower peak alcohol consumption than in male alcoholics, suggesting that the brain, as well as the liver, is more susceptible to damage by alcohol in women compared to men.

Differences in body composition between men and women has been sited as one contributor to the observed sex differences in alcohol-related diseases (Saunders *et al.*, 1981). Alcohol has a smaller volume of distribution in women because women have more adipose tissue, on average, than men. Replacement of food with alcohol is higher in women than men, and female alcoholics have a lower mean body mass than nondrinking females (Hellerstedt *et al.*, 1990). Cole-Harding and Wilson (1987) showed that women metabolized alcohol faster than men, and they tried to correlate these findings with hormonal levels and menstrual phase, but no significant differences were observed.

A recent report from Frezza *et al.* (1990) has proposed that "first-pass metabolism" of alcohol may contribute to the enhanced vulnerability of women to alcohol-related disease. First-pass metabolism refers to the local metabolism of ethanol in the gastrointestinal tissue, which affects the blood alcohol concentration. By comparing the blood alcohol concentration after intravenous and oral administration of alcohol in 20 men and 23 women, Frezza *et al.* (1990) found that the bioavailability for ethanol is much greater in women than in men, because women have less gastric first-pass metabolism of ethanol. This was associated with less gastric alcohol dehydrogenase activity in women. Furthermore, in alcoholic women virtually no first-pass metabolism occurred.

SUGGESTIONS FOR FUTURE EPIDEMIOLOGIC RESEARCH

It is clear from reviewing the literature and examining current theories that many areas for future epidemiologic research exist. Although several descriptive studies have been reported over the past 30 years, the epidemiology of WKS remains an enigma.

Before epidemiologic research can advance, a concise case definition must be developed. As with many neurologic diseases, this is a complicated problem because a definitive diagnosis can only be obtained by pathologic study of the brain. Previous studies have reported that the classic triad of clinical symptoms is insufficient to classify cases of WE clinically, yet specific additional criteria have not been suggested. Psychological studies have furthered our knowledge of the characteristics of WKS; however, the complex battery of psychometric testing is not ideal for the epidemiologic approach to case definition and ascertainment. A straightforward case definition comprised of both clinical and psychological signs that correspond to known pathological features could promote future work in this area and is needed.

Despite past research, accurate estimates for the incidence and prevalence of WKS still do not exist. A well-designed, population-based study is needed to truly understand the scope of the problem and the public health importance of WKS. Again, the estimation of incidence and prevalence would be aided by a clear case definition.

Many interesting age, ethnic, and sex differences in the distribution of WKS have been suggested in previous studies, although none proven. International differences have been shown, but not explained, and no data exist on the occurrence of WKS in developing countries and non-Westernized cultures. Research in any of these areas would further our knowledge of WKS and may also help us understand other alcohol-related diseases and neurologic disorders.

Cigarette smoking is positively associated with alcohol use and is inversely associated with body weight (Hellerstedt *et al.*, 1990). In addition, smoking and drinking interact with body mass index, and the relationships are different in men and women. Because WKS is brought on by nutritional deficiency and chronic alcohol use, the potential relationships among WKS, gender, smoking, and body mass index need to be investigated and may explain, in part, the sex differential in WKS.

Only two factors have been identified as causative for WKS—thiamine deficiency and alcohol toxicity—yet much about WKS remains unexplained. Because not all alcoholics develop WKS, even those with many years of chronic abuse, it seems logical to assume that other conditions or risk factors exist to predispose one to WKS. Retrospective case-control studies are needed to help identify other such risk factors that may interact with thiamine and alcohol.

PUBLIC HEALTH INTERVENTION

Numerous interventions have been proposed to address the problem of WKS. Taxation and education are public health measures commonly implemented to help reduce alcohol-related morbidity and mortality. Although education is ideally the method of choice for public health intervention, it has experienced limited success in reducing the prevalence of alcoholism and alcohol-related disease. Taxation of alcoholic beverages has been shown to be inversely correlated to cirrhosis of the liver and to automobile fatalities (Richardson, 1990). In addition, taxation is an attractive option because it places the financial burden directly onto the consumer. Whether or not taxation has impacted the prevalence of WKS, however, remains unclear (Price *et al.*, 1987).

Several researchers (Centerwall and Criqui, 1978; Price and Theodoros, 1979; Price *et al.*, 1987; Wood and Breen, 1980; Yellowlees, 1986) have proposed the fortification of alcoholic beverages with thiamine to prevent the occurrence of WKS. These studies have shown that the addition of thiamine to alcoholic beverages is feasible, safe, and cost-effective. Unfortunately, this practice has not been implemented. In the United States today, milk, flour and fruit juices are just a few of the products that are routinely vitamin-fortified. The resulting reduction in diseases such as pellegra and scurvy from these measures has been phenomenal. Although the etiology of WKS is not fully understood, thiamine deficiency and chronic alcohol abuse have been well established as primary causes, and the implementation of thiamine fortification would likely produce a marked reduction in the occurrence of WKS.

It is clear from a review of the literature that much about WKS remains unknown. Ongoing research has, in part, explained the clinical features of the syndrome and helped to define the roles of alcohol and thiamine in the causation of WKS, but epidemiologic information is sparse. Many interesting aspects of this syndrome are yet to be adequately investigated. However, public health interventions can be implemented to reduce the prevalence of WKS by targeting both alcohol abuse and thiamine deficiency.

References

Alderdice, F. A., and Davidson, R. (1990). The effect of alcohol consumption on recency discrimination ability: An early screening test for alcohol-induced cognitive impairment. *Br. J. Addict.* **85,** 531–536.

American Psychiatric Association. (1987). "Diagnostic and Statistics Manual," 3rd ed., rev. American Psychiatric Association, Washington, D.C.

Ashley, M. J., Olin, J. S., le Riche, W. H., Kornaczewski, A., Schmidt, W., and Rankin, J. G. (1977). Morbidity in alcoholics. *Arch. Intern. Med.* **137,** 883–887.

Blansjaar, B. A., Horjus, M. C., and Nijhuis, H. G. J. (1987). Prevalence of the Korsakoff syndrome in The Hague, The Netherlands. *Acta Psychiatr. Scand.* **75,** 604–607.

Braunwald, E., Isselbacher, K. J., Petersdorf, R. G., Wilson, J. D., Martin, J. B., and Fauci, A. S. (eds.). (1987). "Harrison's Principles of Internal Medicine," 11th ed, pp. 133, 2002–2003, 2107. McGraw-Hill, New York.

Butters, N. (1981). The Wernicke–Korsakoff syndrome: A review of psychological, neuropathological and etiological factors. *In* "Currents in Alcoholism," Vol. 8 (M. Galanter, ed.), pp. 205–232. Grune & Stratton, New York.

Centerwall, B. S., and Criqui, M. H. (1978). Prevention of the Wernicke–Korsakoff syndrome. *N. Engl. J. Med.* **299,** 285–289.

Cole-Harding, S., and Wilson, J. R. (1987). Ethanol metabolism in men and women. *J. Stud. Alcohol* **48,** 380–387.

Corti, B., and Ibrahim, J. (1990). Women and alcohol—Trends in Australia. *Med. J. Aust.* **152,** 625–632.

Cravioto, H., Korein, J., and Silberman, J. (1961). Wernicke's encephalopathy. A clinical and pathological study of 28 autopsied cases. *Arch. Neurol.* **4,** 510–519.

Frezza, M., di Padova, C., Pozzato, G., Terpin, M., Baraona, E., and Lieber, C. (1990). High blood alcohol levels in women. *N. Engl. J. Med.* **322,** 95–99.

Grant, I. (1987). Alcohol and the brain: Neuropsychological correlates. *J. Consult. Clin. Psychol.* **55,** 310–324.

Harper, C. (1979). Wernicke's encephalopathy: A more common disease than realised. *J. Neurol. Neurosurg. Psychiatry* **42,** 226–231.

Harper, C. (1983). The incidence of Wernicke's encephalopathy in Australia—A neuropathological study of 131 cases. *J. Neurol. Neurosurg. Psychiatry* **46,** 593–598.

Harper, C. G., and Kril, J. J. (1990). Neuropathology of alcoholism. *Alcohol Alcoholism* **25,** 207–216.

Harper, C. G., Giles, M., and Finlay-Jones, R. (1986). Clinical signs in the Wernicke–Korsakoff complex: A retrospective analysis of 131 cases diagnosed at necropsy. *J. Neurol. Neurosurg. Psychiatry* **49,** 341–345.

Harper, C., Gold, J., Rodriguez, M., and Perdices, M. (1989). The prevalence of Wernicke–Korsakoff syndrome in Sydney, Australia: A prospective necropsy study. *J. Neurol. Neurosurg. Psychiatry* **52,** 282–285.

Hellerstedt, W. L., Jeffery, R. W., and Murray, D. M. (1990). The association between alcohol intake and adiposity in the general population. *Am. J. Epidemiol.* **132,** 594–611.

Jacobson, R. (1986). Female alcoholics: A controlled CT brain scan and clinical study. *Br. J. Addict.* **81,** 661–669.

Kelsey, J. L., Thompson, W. D., and Evans, A. S. (1986). "Methods in Observational Epidemiology," pp. 69–70. Oxford University Press, New York.

Lindboe, C. F., and Loberg, E. M. (1989). Wernicke's encephalopathy in non-alcoholics. *J. Neurol. Sci.* **90,** 125–129.

MacVane, J., Butters, N., Montgomery, K., and Farber, J. (1982). Cognitive functioning in men social drinkers. *Q. J. Stud. Alcohol* **43,** 81–95.

Parker, E. S., and Noble, E. P. (1977). Alcohol consumption and cognitive functioning in social drinkers. *Q. J. Stud. Alcohol.* **38,** 1224–1232.

Price, J., and Theodoros, M. T. (1979). The supplementation of alcoholic beverages with thiamine—A necessary preventive measure in Queensland? *Aust. N.Z. J. Psychiatry* **13,** 315–320.

Price, J., Kerr, R., Hicks, M., and Nixon, P. F. (1987). The Wernicke–Korsakoff syndrome: A reappraisal in Queensland with special reference to prevention. *Med. J. Aust.* **147,** 561–565.

Richardson, J. (1990). Alcohol taxes: The case for reform. *Med. J. Aust.* **152,** 619–620.

Ryback, R. S. (1971). The continuum and specificity of the effects of alcohol on memory. *Q. J. Stud. Alcohol* **32,** 995–1016.

Saunders, J. B., Davis, M., and Williams, R. (1981). Do women develop alcoholic liver disease more readily than men? *Br. Med. J.* **282,** 1140–1143.

Torvik, A., Lindboe, C. F., and Rogde, S. (1982). Brain lesions in alcoholics. *J. Neurol. Sci.* **56,** 233–248.

Victor, M., and Laureno, R. (1978). Neurologic complications of alcohol abuse: Epidemiologic aspects. *In* "Advances in Neurology," Vol. 19, (B. S. Schoenberg, ed.), pp. 603–617. Raven Press, New York.

Victor, M., Adams, R. D., and Collins, G. H. (1989). "The Wernicke–Korsakoff Syndrome and Related Neurologic Disorders Due to Alcoholism and Malnutrition," 2nd ed. F. A. Davis Company, Philadelphia.

Wernicke, C. (1881). "Lehrbuch der Gehirnkrankheiten fur Aerzte und Studirende," Vol. 2, pp. 229–242. Theodor Fischer, Kassel.

Williams, C. M., and Skinner, A. E. G. (1990). The cognitive effects of alcohol abuse: A controlled study. *Br. J. Addict.* **85,** 911–917.

Wood, B., and Breen, K. J. (1980). Clinical thiamine deficiency in Australia: The size of the problem and approaches to prevention. *Med. J. Aust.* **1,** 461–464.

Yellowlees, P. M. (1986). Thiamine deficiency and prevention of the Wernicke–Korsakoff syndrome. *Med. J. Aust.* **145,** 216–219.

8

Cerebrovascular Disease
and Smoking

Deborah M. Parra-Medina • Erin Kenney
John P. Elder

Stroke is a manifestation of cerebrovascular disease (CVD) that results in damage to the brain due to an alteration of the blood supply. The effects of stroke vary, depending on the extent and location of the damage to the nervous tissue. Several types of stroke include but are not limited to, the following: large artery thrombosis (the intravascular coagulation of the blood), embolism (material carried by the blood current and impacted in some part of the vascular system), subarachnoid hemorrhage (SAH; a discharge of blood from a ruptured blood vessel), and aneurysm (a permanent arterial dilation usually caused by weakening of the vessel wall).

Recently, prevention intervention efforts in this area have concentrated on minimizing the consequences of stroke, or tertiary prevention. Rehabilitation and the prevention of subsequent strokes are examples of interventions in this area. Due to advances in medical technology, such as through computerized tomography (CT scan), secondary prevention and early detection have become more widespread. Secondary prevention (when successful) precludes or minimizes morbidity by halting the progress from the preclinical to the clinical phase of stroke. Finally, primary prevention efforts emphasize the control or elimination of risk factors for CVD. Special primary prevention emphasis has been placed on high blood pressure control but includes smoking and other such risk factors common to coronary heart disease as well.

As it has for coronary heart disease, lung and other cancers, and other chronic diseases, smoking prevention and control has been advocated as a method for prevention of stroke or its recurrence (U. S. Department of Health and Human Services, 1991). This chapter reviews the epidemiologi-

Neuroepidemiology:
Theory and Method

· 165 ·

cal evidence relating smoking to stroke and smoking reduction to its prevention.

ANALYTICAL STUDIES

Introduction

There are two analytic methods for observational studies of etiology: one retrospective, the other prospective. The purpose of these methods is to produce a valid estimate of a hypothesized cause–effect relationship between a suspected risk factor and a disease. In a retrospective study, cases, people diagnosed as having a disease, are compared to a comparison or control group, persons who do not have the disease. Retrospective studies compare cases with regard to the presence of some risk factor in their past experience. Prospective studies begin with a cohort of individuals who have a negative history of stroke and are currently disease free. Individuals in the cohorts vary in use of cigarettes, which is hypothesized as causing the disease. The cohort is followed over time, which allows investigators to track the incidence and details of the disease in relation to exposure of the risk factor in question.

The studies reviewed in this chapter are organized and presented in order of methodological rigor. The first level or group of studies reviewed is retrospective. In general, these studies focus on the incident cases of stroke and search for smoking as a factor shared in the past experience of individuals. No comparison or control group is used in this group of studies. The second level or group discussed is retrospective case-control studies, differing from the previous group only in that they use a control group. The validity of these studies varies with respect to the criteria used to select the case and control groups and the extent to which these are matched to control for confounders such as gender, age, and medical history. The final group of studies reviewed is prospective. In these studies, individuals are classified in relation to degree of exposure to cigarette smoke and then followed forward in time for the development of stroke.

Retrospective Studies

Many years ago, stroke was regarded as a sudden or chance happening that afflicted older persons without warning. Stroke was regarded fatalistically. Little was known about prevention of disease, and an individual's health status in early life was not seen as related to onset of disease. In 1966, Locksley observed that the peak age incidence of ruptured aneurysm was between 40 and 60 years. A postmortem study of children's brains conducted by Uttley (1978) indicated that aneurysms rarely occurred in this group. The combination of these two observations led researchers Bell and Symon (1979) to surmise that stroke probably arises after birth and may be related to a person's health status in earlier life. Bell and Symon (1979) also observed that the incidence and etiology of coronary heart disease (CHD) resembled that of CVD. Although smoking had been identified as an important risk factor for CHD, its role in stroke was less certain. As a result of these observations, Bell and Symon (1979) believed an investigation of the relation between smoking and cerebrovascular disease was warranted.

Bell and Symon (1979) conducted a retrospective study of 208 male and female patients admitted and diagnosed with SAH during the period of 1965–1978. Information on smoking habits was gathered via medical records and validated by sending a questionnaire to all traceable patients. The researchers then compared the incidence of SAH in smokers and nonsmokers to the expected incidence in the general population. Results suggest that continued smoking increased the relative risk (the ratio of the incidence of stroke among those individuals who smoke to the incidence for nonsmokers) of suffering a SAH by a factor of 3.9 for men and 3.7 for women. Researchers also concluded that other risk factors besides smoking must affect SAH because 29 cases of SAH were observed in lifelong nonsmokers.

In a study of 178 patients discharged after suffering a SAH, Taha and Ball (1983) found results similar to the previously described study. The relative risk of SAH for smokers compared to nonsmokers was 4.7 for men and 2.6 for women; former smokers were not at increased risk. Both studies are limited in generalizability because a select population of patients who had suffered a SAH was used and both lacked adequate comparison groups. In addition, neither study controlled for confounding factors such as hypertension.

Candelise *et al.* (1984) conducted a clinical study in Italy to examine the influence of several risk factors, including smoking, on cerebral atherosclerosis. Four-hundred sixty-two patients, who were referred for examination from 1977 to 1987 for symptoms of reversible ischemic attacks and received a cerebral angiography, were admitted into the study. The degree of atherosclerosis was quantified by two neurologists. The results indicated that the atherogenic effect of smoking in patients with CVD was independent of other risk factors. In addition, a statistically significant positive relationship between the number of cigarettes smoked and the severity of atherosclerosis was present, indicating a possible dose–response effect. No relative risk was calculated. Candelise *et al.* (1984)

conclude that the method by which smoking enhances the risk of stroke is still unknown.

Retrospective Case-Control Studies

The previous studies show a consistent association between stroke and smoking. The relative risk related to smoking, however, has ranged from 2.6 to 4.7, possibly due to limitations in study design or methods of analysis. Although some of these studies showed an association between smoking and CVD, none used a control group or factored out the potential confounding role of hypertension, oral contraceptives, and other risk factors on stroke. The following studies improve upon the previous ones reviewed by utilizing a control group and/or factoring out potential confounding factors.

Rogers *et al.* (1983) conducted a comparative study to assess the effects of smoking on cerebral blood flow, while controlling for other risk factors. The subjects, all right-handed Caucasians of either gender, were classified into three groups according to tobacco exposure. The classifications were lifetime nonsmokers ($n = 117$), current <1 pack per day smokers ($n = 14$), and current >1 pack per day smokers ($n = 61$). No ex-smokers were included. Once classified on exposure, the subjects were then subclassified according to the absence or presence of risk factors into either a risk or no-risk group. The risk group had at least one of the following risk factors: hypertension, hyperlipidemia, heart disease, or diabetes mellitus. The no-risk group was free of all previously stated disorders. Each subject participated in general medical and neurological examinations, including a detailed medical history. A health questionnaire was used to assess the quantity of cigarettes smoked as well as duration of the habit. Cerebral blood flow was measured by having patients inhale Xenon 133, a tracer isotope, and checking the rate of clearance of the isotope from both sides of the head. Comparison of mean hemispheric gray matter blood flow values showed significant reductions in blood flow related to cigarette smoking and stroke risk factors. The presence of cigarette smoking with other risk factors reduced cerebral blood flow in an additive manner when compared to subjects who did not smoke.

Cerebral atherosclerosis is more common and severe in hypertensives because hypertension increases atherogenesis. In 1986, Molgaard *et al.* conducted a case-control study to determine whether or not an association between smoking and CVD existed when controlling for blood pressure and included a measure of the dose–response relationship observed in the Candelise *et al.* (1984) study. Cases were recruited from the University of California, San Diego Stroke program data bank and matched three to one to controls on the basis of age, sex, and hospital of origin. Twenty-eight males and 12 females served as cases. All cases included in the study had suffered a cerebrovascular event. Information on the cases was obtained by the examining physician and transmitted to the stroke data bank and by a supplemental telephone interview with the patient to obtain specific data on smoking such as years smoked, preferred brand, and passive smoking. Analyses revealed that the most significant predictor of a cerebrovascular event was blood pressure. To gather dose–response information, the researchers constructed several indices related to smoking. The indices used were average number of packs smoked per year and standardized estimations of nicotine and carbon monoxide consumption. Although all three indices that measured the dose–response relationship were found to be consistently and significantly associated with onset of a cerebrovascular event, the number of packs smoked per year was the most significant ($p < 0.01$). The categorical smoking variable (categories included smoker, ex-smoker, and nonsmoker) was not significantly associated with outcome. The authors suggest that the categorical smoking variable does not detect the cumulative lifetime exposure that is reflected in the indices because the dose–response relationship is masked.

Researchers in Auckland, New Zealand, also investigated the relationship between cigarette smoking, hypertension, stroke (Bonita *et al.*, 1986), and SAH (Bonita, 1986). Both studies found a minimum threefold increase risk of stroke or SAH in cigarette smokers compared to nonsmokers. The increased risk for smokers remained significant after adjusting for hypertension. Evidence of a dose–response relationship between the number of cigarettes smoked and the risk of stroke was also observed in both studies. In addition, the studies suggest a synergistic effect (15–20-fold increase) on risk in those who both smoked and were hypertensives compared to those who neither smoked nor were treated for hypertension. Overall, both studies found that more cases of stroke and SAH could be attributed to cigarette smoking (37 and 43%, respectively) than to hypertension (36 and 28%).

Two more recent case-control studies assessed the role of cigarette smoke as a risk factor for ischemic stroke. In a study by Gorelick *et al.* (1989), 205 acute ischemic stroke patients hospitalized in three urban medical centers in Illinois were examined. For each case, two controls were selected and matched on age, race, gender, and method of hospital payment. Results from both studies indicate that stroke cases were more likely to have a past history of hypertension, to be current smokers, and to have a significantly higher number or mean pack-years exposure. A significant dose–response effect between smoking and stroke was observed. No relative risk was calculated. The authors conclude that smoking is an independent risk factor for ischemic stroke.

Donnan *et al.* (1989) used CT scans and a questionnaire of patients with a first episode of ischemic stroke to identify groups at increased risk for stroke. Four-hundred forty-two case patients were matched individually to controls by age and gender. The study results strengthen the findings of Gorelick *et al.* (1989) in that they also identify smoking as an independent risk factor for stroke. Current smoking was a significant risk factor for transient ischemic attacks with a relative risk of 5.2. The adjusted relative risk of ischemic stroke, examined by multiple logistic regression, for current smokers was 3.7 compared to 2.0 for ex-smokers and 1.0 for lifetime nonsmokers. Donnan *et al.* (1989) also found a dose–response effect. The risk of stroke among current smokers increased with the amount smoked. The authors also found a significant increased risk of suffering a stroke for those exposed to second-hand smoke. Individuals whose spouses smoked were 1.7 times more likely to suffer a stroke compared to those whose spouses did not smoke. Additionally, if a parent smoked, the child exposed to parental tobacco smoke had a risk of stroke 1.2 times higher than those not so exposed, although the increased risk was not statistically significant.

Prospective Studies

In a prospective study, healthy or disease-free individuals are grouped and followed forward in time for the development of disease. The advantage of prospective studies is that individuals are classified in relation to exposure to risk factors (e.g., smoking, hypertension) before the stroke occurs. This reduces bias (e.g., lack of consistency of information based on memory) found in retrospective studies. However, even in prospective studies, the low incidence of stroke continues to be a limitation in the study of its etiology. A large number of subjects must be followed for decades in order to observe enough cases to conduct analyses. Despite the limitations of the prospective design, the following group of studies provides further evidence for the association between smoking and stroke.

Petitti *et al.* (1979) investigated the relation of various factors, including smoking, to risk of SAH and other strokes. The subjects were mostly white middle-class women who participated in the Walnut Creek Contraceptive Drug Study from 1969 to 1971. From a cohort of 16,759 women in the study, there were 34 incident cases of SAH and other strokes during this time period. Information obtained via follow-up examinations, annual mail questionnaire, and medical records was used to compile a month-by-month profile of illness, hospitalization, oral contraceptive use, and the like. Cases were identified through self-report (i.e., a member of the original cohort reports that they had experienced a stroke). The self-reports were then verified via clinical records. For primary analysis, cases were matched with several controls, average of 200 per case, by year of birth. In the Walnut Creek Study cohort, smoking was associated with a significant increase in both SAH (relative risk = 5.7) and other types of stroke (relative risk = 4.8). In addition to this, smoking and oral contraceptive use was found to synergistically multiply the risk of SAH by a factor of 21.9.

From 1954 to 1969, Rogot and Murray (1980) studied two cohorts of U.S. veterans prospectively in order to report on specific causes of death and their association with smoking behavior. The two cohorts were from the same population of U.S. veterans ages 31–84. The first wave of surveys resulted in a response rate of 68%; 198,820 responded. This group is referred to as the 1954 cohort. In 1957, the nonrespondents were sent another survey; 49,226 responded. This group is referred to as the 1957 cohort. Almost all subjects were white males from upper and middle socioeconomic classes. During the 16-year follow-up, there were 2728 observed stroke deaths, 2075 expected stroke deaths, and a resultant 1.32 mortality ratio for current cigarette smokers. For ex-cigarette smokers there were 1279 observed stroke deaths, 1254 expected stroke deaths, and a 1.02 mortality ratio. No relative risk was calculated. A dose–response association was observed. When the mortality ratios (observed deaths/ expected deaths) for the ex-smokers were compared to those for current smokers, the ex-smokers had a lower mortality ratio at each level of smoking (<10 cigarettes/day, 10–20 cigarettes/day, 21–39 cigarettes/day, or 40+ cigarettes/day).

Salonen *et al.* (1982) conducted a longitudinal study in Eastern Finland to assess the relation of smoking to the risk of cerebral stroke. The subjects or population at risk, adults between 35 and 59 years old, were recruited at random from national population registers. A total of 4034 men and 4334 women from North Karelia and Kuopio participated in a field examination between February and April 1972. The examination consisted of a general health survey, a measure of blood pressure, and a blood test. Incidence of stroke among baseline survey participants was gathered via medical records and death certificates. The study participants were followed-up for approximately 7 years, during which time 77 men and 65 women suffered a cerebral stroke. In this study, the best predictors of stroke were age, blood pressure, a history of diabetes, and a previous stroke. A positive association also existed between the risk of stroke and smoking (p <0.001). The adjusted relative risk was 4.2 for cerebral infarction and 2.2 for all

other strokes in men, both of which were statistically significant ($p < 0.01$).
For women, the adjusted relative risk was 1.4 for cerebral infarction and
0.8 for all other strokes; however, these were not significant.

The Heart Disease Epidemiology, or Framingham, Study consisted of a
sample of residents from Framingham, Massachusetts (Sacco *et al.*, 1984).
The Framingham Study began in 1949 with a cohort of 5209 men and
women, aged 30–62 years. Study participants submitted to biennial physical examinations, laboratory tests, and routine personal medical history
surveys. At the first examination, 5184 men and women who were free
from stroke and were selected and followed prospectively for 26 years. In
this time period, 198 men and 196 women suffered some type of stroke,
including atherothrombotic brain infarction, cerebral embolism, intracerebral hemorrhage, transient ischemic attacks, and SAH. Of the total stroke
cases, 36 subjects suffered a SAH. The average age of onset was 63 years.
SAH cases were categorized by age and gender and each matched with
four controls from the same study. Study results indicate that cigarette
smoking, particularly heavy smoking ($\geq$20 cigarettes/day), was more frequent among cases. In more recent analyses of data from this cohort
(Wolf *et al.*, 1988), smoking continued to make a significant independent
contribution to the risk of stroke. In addition, the risk of stroke increased
as the number of cigarettes smoked increased, and the relative risk of
stroke in those individuals who smoked >40 cigarettes per day was twice
that of those who smoked <10 cigarettes per day indicating a dose–response relationship. Wolf *et al.* (1988) also investigated the effect of cessation or abstention from cigarettes on the risk of stroke. Results indicate
that risk of stroke decreased significantly after 2 years of cessation and
was at the level of nonsmokers by 5 years.

Certain risk factors, including history of hypertension, age, and smoking, have consistently shown an association with stroke in many studies,
yet few studies have examined these relations in older populations. In
the Rancho Bernardo Study, Khaw *et al.* (1984) surveyed 2107 men and
women between the ages of 65 and 84 for heart disease risk factors
including smoking between 1972 and 1974. The vital status, which includes blood pressure, obesity index, cholesterol, and glucose tolerance
of the subjects, mainly upper–middle class Caucasians, was determined
annually for an average of 9 years follow-up. A total of 58 individuals
who had a previous history of stroke were excluded from the study.
Comparisons between those with a stroke-associated death and all others
indicate that self-reported smoking habits were not significantly different
between these groups. Nonsmokers had fewer stroke deaths than current
or former smokers, but the differences were not significant; however,
using the Cox proportional hazards model, the researchers identified

smoking as an independent significant predictor of stroke-related death (relative risk = 2.6 for smokers, $p < 0.001$). In a prospective study conducted in Denmark, Boysen *et al.* (1988) also used the Cox regression model (Rosner, 1990) to evaluate the causative effect of smoking and other risk factors on the incidence of stroke. As in the Khaw *et al.* (1984) study, Boysen *et al.* (1988) also found a significant effect for smoking habits on the risk of stroke.

Study results have been inconclusive with respect to whether or not quitting smoking would benefit health by lowering the risk of suffering a stroke. Studies by Candelise *et al.* (1984) and Rogers *et al.* (1983) have shown that smoking contributes to atherothrombotic CVD (reduces cerebral blood flow), yet little is shown on the reversibility of these effects by cessation. Rogers *et al.* (1985) conducted a two-part study to investigate the effect of level of smoking exposure on cerebral blood flow. The first part of the study was cross-sectional in design. A group of 268 neurologically normal volunteers were recruited and classified into three smoking categories: nonsmokers, current smokers, and former smokers. As in the aforementioned studies, Rogers *et al.* (1985) found that subjects who continued to smoke showed reductions in cerebral perfusion levels compared to nonsmokers and that the magnitude of reduction was related to the average amount of cigarettes consumed.

In the second part of the study, Rogers *et al.* (1985) continued the investigation on the benefits of cessation on the health of cerebral circulation by conducting a prospective study on the effect of abstention from cigarettes on cerebral perfusion. As in the study by Rogers *et al.* (1983), this study measured cerebral blood flow by way of the Xenon 133 inhalation method. A group of 11 chronic cigarette smokers who were able to quit through the course of the study served as cases. These cases were matched with 22 controls according to age, duration of smoking habit, and time between baseline and follow-up measures. The data collected for the prospective study indicates that subjects who quit smoking had significantly higher cerebral perfusion levels than subjects who continued to smoke. Correlational analysis between the magnitude of cerebral blood flow change and the duration of cessation resulted in a significant linear increase in cerebral blood flow. This result confirms evidence from other studies (Rogot *et al.*, 1980; Taha and Ball, 1983; Wolf *et al.*, 1988; Donnan *et al.*, 1989) that have shown that former smokers were not at increased risk of suffering a stroke than life-long nonsmokers. The results of this and other studies suggest that there may be substantial benefits to quitting smoking, even for older chronic smokers, and that improvements in cerebral circulation can occur in a relatively short amount of time.

From 1965 to 1968, the Honolulu Heart Program conducted a prospective cohort study of 8006 men of Japanese ancestry (Abbott *et al.*, 1986). There were 7872 subjects who reported being free of stroke and were current or lifelong nonsmokers. To examine differences between smokers and nonsmokers, subjects were followed for any first-stroke event. During the follow-up period, there were a total of 288 initial strokes: 189 thromboembolic, 75 hemorrhagic, and the rest of some other type. Information on cerebrovascular events was obtained via hospital discharge, autopsy, and death records and was validated by a neurologist. Incidence rates were then computed according to group and age. Among nonsmokers there were 117 initial stroke events, and among smokers 171 initial events. Estimates of relative risk indicate that the risk of cigarette smokers was 2–3 times that among nonsmokers. The association between stroke and smoking was significant ($p < 0.001$), even after controlling for other risk factors. In this study, researchers found that subjects at highest risk for stroke were those subjects who continued to smoke through the entire study period (relative risk = 3.0–6.1). By comparison, the subjects who quit smoking during the follow-up period reduced their risk of stroke by more than one-half (relative risk = 1.7–3.9). Although these quitters were still at a slight increase risk of stroke than nonsmokers, this difference was not statistically significant. These results, along with those of Rogers *et al.* (1985), indicate that stopping smoking has significant benefits. In other analyses of data from this cohort (Reed *et al.*, 1988) smoking was associated with cerebral atherosclerosis. A pathologic evaluation of the brain and Circle of Willis of 198 men who died as a result of stroke indicated that autopsy-verified cerebral infarction was strongly associated with increasing severity of atherosclerosis. Other data from this cohort also identify cigarette smoking as an independent risk factor for thromboembolic stroke and as associated with increased risk of intracranial hemorrhage (Kagan *et al.*, 1985).

The studies reviewed thus far relate cigarette smoking to several types of stroke among men (Salonen *et al.*, 1982; Kagan *et al.*, 1985; Abbott *et al.*, 1986; Reed *et al.*, 1988). Although such data have confirmed the risk of stroke among male smokers, cigarettes have not been established clearly as a risk factor for stroke in women (Petitti *et al.*, 1979). Some studies that have included both men and women have observed an elevated risk among smokers (Bonita, 1986; Bonita *et al.*, 1986; Wolf *et al.*, 1988). To clarify the risk of stroke associated with smoking among women, Colditz *et al.* (1988) conducted a prospective cohort study of 118,539 women between the ages of 30 and 55 years. Women included in the study were mostly Caucasian nurses (98%) and free of CHD, stroke, and cancer at baseline. General health information and a current and past smoking history were gathered via health information questionnaires mailed every 2 years. During 8 years of follow-up, there were 274 incident cases of stroke. Cohort members were categorized into three categories: current smokers, past smokers, and never smokers. Women who smoked had a significantly higher risk of stroke and the risk increased with the number of cigarettes smoked. The relative risk for ex-smokers was 1.6; for those who smoked 1–14 cigarettes per day, 2.2; for those who smoked 15–24 cigarettes per day, 2.7; and for those subjects who smoked >25 cigarettes per day, 3.7. The relative risk for fatal stroke was strongest and is consistent with the levels reported for men in other studies (relative risk = 4.0 for 15–24 cigarettes/day and 5.8 for >25 cigarettes/day). These prospective data support a strong association between cigarette smoking and the risk of stroke among women.

CAUSATION

All studies reviewed in this chapter have addressed the relationship between smoking and stroke. Some studies conclude that smoking is an independent risk factor for and predictor of stroke. Additionally, when combined with other risk factors such as hypertension and contraceptives, it can increase the risk of suffering a stroke as much as 21-fold. Few studies, however, conclude a causal link between smoking and stroke, because strokes also occur in nonsmokers, which indicates that other factors may be involved. Although an experimental approach provides a direct method for establishing whether an association between two factors is causal, in the absence of experimentation several lines of reasoning have been advocated for assessing causality (Schlesselman, 1982). Hill (1965, 1971) discusses six conditions that must be fulfilled before a cause–effect relationship can be accepted. This final section will review Hill's criteria and use the evidence presented in this chapter to establish the extent to which a cause–effect relationship can be accepted.

The first condition of Hill's criteria is *strength of association.* In this condition, the larger the relative risk of stroke for smokers compared to nonsmokers, the greater the likelihood that smoking is causally related to the outcome, stroke. The relative risk calculated in studies reviewed in this chapter range from 2.6 to 6.1 for current smokers. This indicates that smokers are up to 6 times more likely to suffer a stroke than nonsmokers. When combined with other risk factors such as hypertension or contraceptive use, the relative risk may increase 20-fold. (Bonita, 1986; Bonita *et al.*, 1986; Petitti *et al.*, 1979). All the data presented in these studies demonstrate a strong association and, doing so, satisfy the first condition of causality.

The second criterion is the presence of a *biological gradient* or *dose–response relationship.* If a dose–response relationship is demonstrated, the likelihood of a causal relationship is strengthened. Several studies reviewed in this chapter demonstrate that with increasing levels of exposure to tobacco via cigarette smoking, a corresponding rise in occurrence of stroke is found. In this review, two types of dose–response relationships were present. In the first type of relationship, the dose, the quantity of cigarettes smoked, increases the response, stroke. A number of studies indicated that the more cigarettes smoked per day, the higher the risk of stroke (Molgaard *et al.,* 1986; Bonita, 1986; Bonita *et al.,* 1986; Gorelick *et al.,* 1986; Donnan *et al.,* 1989; Wolf *et al.,* 1988; Colditz *et al.,* 1988). In the second type of relationship, the quantity of cigarettes smoked was related to a decrease in cerebral blood flow, which is a precursor of stroke (Rogers *et al.,* 1983; Candelise *et al.,* 1984; Rogers *et al.,* 1985). The research presented in this chapter indicates that the dose–response condition is satisfied.

Consistency of association is the third criterion. This criterion requires that the association uncovered in one study persist on testing under other circumstances, with other study populations. The association between stroke and smoking has been very consistent across several studies examining a number of different populations. Studies conducted with several age groups and with both genders have found strong associations between smoking and stroke. In addition, these findings are consistent for various ethnic and culturally diverse populations (e.g., Japanese, Scandanavian, European, American). The study types presented include retrospective, retrospective case-control, and prospective; however, the specific data sources and collection methods varied. The association between smoking and stroke remained consistent when medical records, population registers, health screenings, mail surveys, interviews, and/or autopsies were used. The more often the association appears under diverse circumstances, the more likely it is to be causal in nature. In the case of stroke and smoking, an association is found consistently regardless of study type.

When attempting to fulfill the fourth criterion, that of a *temporal sequence,* exposure to smoking must antedate stroke incidence and allow for a necessary period of induction and latency. A temporal sequence is more difficult to establish in many chronic conditions such as stroke. One type of temporal evidence is found in the study by Rogers *et al.* (1985). For both light and heavy smokers, the incidence of stroke decreases with increasing duration of time off cigarettes. Additionally, stroke tends to occur later in life, many years after smoking cigarettes is initiated (Sacco *et al.*, 1984). Thus, to some extent the association is temporally correct.

Because stroke may be multifactorial in nature, it is important to evaluate the *specificity of effect*. This criterion refers to the extent to which the occurrence of one variable, smoking, can be used to predict the occurrence of the other, stroke. There are two models of multifactorial causation. In one model, there are alternative causal factors; in the other, the causal factors act cumulatively and none of the factors alone can cause the disease. In the case of stroke, several researchers used the Cox proportional hazards model to evaluate the causative effect of several risk factors on stroke, including smoking. Khaw *et al.* (1984) and Boysen *et al.* (1988) used this model to identify smoking as an independent significant predictor of stroke. Thus, the specificity condition is satisfied.

Collateral evidence and biological plausibility provide additional support for the causal nature of an association if a causal interpretation is plausible in terms of current knowledge about the factor and disease. Several of the studies in this chapter conducted autopsies and used the Xenon 133 inhalation method to investigate the physiological effects of smoking tobacco on the cerebrovascular system. Evidence suggests that smoking tobacco decreases cerebral blood flow much in the same manner as it does to the heart. This evidence supports biological plausibility.

In summary, the association between smoking and occurrence of stroke essentially meets the criteria proposed for judging such relationships.

CONCLUSION

This chapter has reviewed the epidemiological evidence relating smoking to stroke and smoking reduction to its prevention. Retrospective and prospective studies were reviewed. Taken together, these studies demonstrate a consistent, strong, and independent association between smoking and stroke—an association that becomes even stronger with increasing levels of tobacco use. Additionally, among those who quit smoking, the incidence of stroke decreases with increasing time off cigarettes. The evidence presented here indicates that the association between smoking and stroke essentially meets well-established criteria for judging causal relationships. This implies that smoking prevention and control should continue to be advocated at the clinical and community level as a method for prevention of stroke or its recurrence.

References

Abbott, R. D., Yin, Y., Reed, D. M., and Yano, K. (1986). Risk of stroke in male cigarette smokers. *N. Engl. J. Med.* **315**(12), 717–720.

Bell, B. A., and Symon, L. (1979). Smoking and subarachnoid haemorrhage. *Br. Med. J.* **March, 1,** 577–578.

Bonita, R. (1986). Cigarette cmoking, hypertension and the risk of subarachnoid hemorrhage: A population-based case-control study. *Stroke* **17**(5), 831–835.

Bonita, R., Skragg, R., Stewert, A., Jackson, R., and Beaglehole, R. (1986). Cigarette smoking and risk of premature stroke in men and women. *Br. Med. J.* **293,** 6–8.

Boysen, G., Nyobe, J., Appleyard, M., Sorensen, P. S., Boas, J., Somnier, F., Jensen, G., and Schnohr, P. (1988). Stroke incidence and risk factors for stroke in Coppenhagen, Denmark. *Stroke* **19**(11), 1345–1353.

Candelise, L., Bianchi, F., Galligoni, F., Albanese, V., Bonelli, G., Bozzao, L., Inzitari, D., Mariani, F., Rasura, M., Rognoni, F., Sangiovanni, G., and Fieschi, C. (1984). Italian multicenter study on reversible cerebral ischemic attacks: III—influence of age and risk factors on cerebrovascular atherosclerosis. *Stroke* **15**(2), 379–382.

Colditz, G. A., Bonita, R., Stampfer, M. J., Willett, W. C., Rosner, B., Speizer, F. E., and Hennekems, C. H. (1988). Cigarette smoking and risk of stroke in middle-aged women. *N. Engl. J. Med.* **318**(15), 937–941.

Donnan, G. A., Adena, M. A., O'Malley, H. M., McNeil, J. J., Doyle, A. E., and Neill, G. C. (1989). Smoking as a risk factor for cerebral ischaemia. *Lancet* **9,** 643–647.

Gorelick, B., Rodin, M. B., Langenberg, P., Hier, D. B., and Costigan, J. (1989). Weekly alcohol consumption, cigarette smoking, and the risk of ischemic stroke: Results of a case-control study at three urban medical centers in Chicago, Illinois. *Neurology* **39,** 339–343.

Hill, A. B. (1965). The environment and disease: Association or causation? *Proc. R. Soc. Med.* **58,** 295–300.

Hill, A. B. (1971). "Principles in Medical Statistics," 9th ed. Oxford University Press, New York.

Kagan, A., Popper, J. S., Rhoads, G. G., and Yano, K. (1985). Dietary and other risk factors for stroke in Hawaiian Japanese men. *Stroke* **16,** 390–396.

Khaw, K. T., Barrett-Connor, E., Suarez, L., and Criqui, M. (1984). Predictors of stroke associated mortality in the elderly. *Stroke* **15,** 244–248.

Locksley, H. B. (1966). Report on the Cooperative Study of Intracranial Aneurysms and Subarachnoid Hemorrhage. Section V, Part I: Natural history of Subarachnoid Hemorrhage, intracranial aneurysms and arteriovenous malformations. *J. Neurosurg.* **25,** 219.

Molgaard, C. A., Bartok, A., Peddecord, K. M., and Rothrock, J. (1986). The association between cerebrovascular disease and smoking: A case-control study., *Neuroepidemiology* **5,** 88–94.

Petitti, D. B., Wingerd, J., Pellegrin, F., and Ramcharan, S. (1979). Risk of vascular disease in women: Smoking, oral contraceptives, noncontraceptive estrogens, and other factors. *J. Am. Med. Assoc.* **242,** 1150–1154.

Reed, D. M., Resch, J. A., Hayashi, T., MacLean, C., and Yano, K. (1988). A prospective study of cerebral artery atherosclerosis. *Stroke* **19,** 820–825.

Rogers, R. L., Meyer, J. S., Shaw, T. G., Mortel, K. F., Hardenberg, J. P., and Zaid, R. R. (1983). Cigarette smoking decreases cerebral blood flow suggesting increased risk for stroke. *J. Am. Med. Assoc.* **250,** 2796–2800.

Rogers, R. L., Meyer, J. S., Judd, B. W., and Mortel, K. F. (1985). Abstension from cigarette smoking improves cerebral perfusion among elderly chronic smokers. *J. Am. Med. Assoc.* **253,** 2970–2974.

Rogot, E., and Murray, J. L. (1980). Smoking and causes of death among U.S. veterans: 16 years of observation. *Public Health Rep.* **95**(3), 213–222.

Rosner, B. A. (1990). "Fundementals of Biostatistics." PWS-KENT Publishing, Boston, p. 438.

Sacco, R. L., Wolf, P. A., Bharucha, N. E., Meeks, S. L., Kannel, W. B., Charette, J. L., McNamara, P. M., Palmer, E. P., and D'Agostino, R. (1984). Subarachnoid and intracerebral hemorrhage: Natural history, prognosis, and precursive factors in the Framingham study. *Neurology* **34,** 847–854.

Salonen, J. T., Puska, P., Tuomilehto, J., and Homan, K. (1982). Relation of blood pressure, serum lipids, and smoking to the risk of cerebral stroke. *Stroke* **13,** 327–333.

Schlesselman, J. J. (1982). "Case-Control Studies: Design, Conduct Analysis." Oxford University Press, New York.

Taha, A., and Ball, K. (1983). Subarachnoid haemorrhage: Another smoking related disease. *East Afr. Med. J.* **60**(2), 85–87.

U.S. Department of Health and Human Services. (1991). Healthy people 2000—National health promotion and disease prevention objectives. DHHS Publication No. (PHS) 91-50213. Department of Health and Human Services, Public Health Service, Washington, D.C.

Uttley, D. (1978). Subarachnoid haemorrhage. *Br. J. Hosp. Med.* **19,** 138ff.

Wolf, P. A., D'Agostino, R. B., Kannel, W. B., Bonita, R., and Belanger, A. J. (1988). Cigarette smoking as a risk factor for stroke, the Framingham study. *J. Am. Med. Assoc.* **259**(7), 1025–1029.

9

Alien Hand

Rachelle Smith Doody

Epidemiologic studies are best accomplished for diseases with known etiologies, such as infectious illnesses, and diseases that are clinically well defined. Explanations for many noninfectious neurological diseases still rely on the traditional concept of a cause–effect relationship between some pathogen, insult, or inherent deficiency in the nervous system and the occurrence of a particular disease. This type of disease model has been called reductionistic (Engel, 1977), yet it is obvious to most medical practitioners that such models are only sketches for more complicated disease processes. Diseases that are relatively easy to diagnose and confirm by laboratory techniques, such as Duchenne's muscular dystrophy, where there is a typical clinical picture as well as a genetic marker, fit with traditional disease concepts. Conditions in which the etiology is unknown and diagnosis remains tentative at least until autopsy [e.g., Alzheimer's disease, corticobasal ganglionic degeneration (CBD)] pose special problems, particularly when clinical phenomenology for several different entities overlap.

It makes heuristic sense that diseases actually precede their description or "discovery." Practitioners had clearly encountered cases of progressive cognitive decline before Alzheimer described the neuropathology of Alzheimer's disease. Kety (1974) suggests that the medical model of illness progresses from the recognition and palliation of symptoms to the identification of specific diseases with specific etiologies and, ultimately, specific therapies. Often, the recognition of syndromes, or aggregations of signs and symptoms (with an associated causative and abnormal process), is a step toward identification of specific diseases. Alien hand is an interesting example of a neurologic syndrome or disease in the making and raises questions about the status of epidemiology with respect to such inchoate entitites.

PHENOMENOLOGY OF ALIEN HAND

Review of the neurologic literature suggests that the term alien hand has been used to describe a wide variety of sensory impressions and motor behaviors. It seems to have been used at first as a sign, rather than as an element of a syndrome (Brion and Jedynak, 1972). Some reports clearly described alien hand before it was so named and have only been invoked as examples of alien hand after the fact (e.g., the work of Goldstein; Feinberg *et al.*, 1992). As published reports increased, attempts to localize the alien hand sign to some region of the brain predominated, but the localization process has not been entirely satisfactory, in part because the behaviors that are being localized have been diverse and not always clearly described. Descriptions include allusions to a feeling of foreignness or lack of ownership of the affected hand and a spectrum of visible motor abnormalities (Doody and Jankovic, 1992). The alien feeling ranges from a perception that the limb simply does not belong to the patient to personification of the limb, ascribing it with autonomous motivation. The motor behaviors constitute a spectrum of involuntary activities including action-induced trembling, patterned and rhythmical activity such as spontaneous levitation or posturing, forced grasping and groping, and sometimes even malevolent-seeming actions directed against the patient him- or herself. Additionally, many, if not most, patients have difficulty with actions that require the cooperation of both hands. Although wideranging, the behaviors associated with alien hand can be grouped into clusters around major signs or symptoms for the purposes of discussion.

Grasp Reflex and Motor Perseveration

The grasp reflex refers to an involuntary and sustained grasp in response to stimulation of the palm: It is normal in infants but usually becomes inhibited in the course of normal development. Patients with an abnormal grasp reflex may be unable to release their grip after a handshake. Motor perseveration is a related phenomenon in which the affected individual has difficulty shifting from one motor activity to another. For example, if asked to alternate a clenched fist with an open hand, the patient may persistently make a fist, loosen it slightly, and then make a fist again repeatedly without opening the hand in a smooth set of alternations. Both the grasp reflex and motor perseveration are associated with contralateral frontal lobe pathology.

Grasp reflexes have frequently been associated with the alien hand sign. Motor perseveration or its absence is not as often reported, but it was probably not examined in all cases. Shahani *et al.* (1970) described a patient with a right alien hand due to occlusion of the left pericollosal artery. Their patient had a grasp reflex and perseveration, and their discussion blends a description of his case with prior descriptions of grasp reflex and perseveration dating back to Liepmann at the turn of the century. Overall, the grasp reflex is commonly associated with the alien hand sign, particularly when the patient has well-defined frontal lobe pathology. As we will discuss, underlying pathology may vary.

Apraxia

Apraxia, the inability to perform skilled movements that is not due to weakness, akinesia, deafferentation (sensory disturbance), abnormal tone or posture, intellectual disorders, or uncooperativeness, is usually associated with injury to the dominant hemisphere (Heilman and Rothi, 1985). Some forms of apraxia occur as a result of corpus callosum injury as well. Watson and Heilman (1983) reported a case of apraxia following infarction of the corpus callosum. Their patient had a left alien hand and severe problems with bimanual coordination. When she went to select a blouse from her closet, each hand selected a different blouse; the left hand then attempted to put on one blouse, while the right arm went into the sleeve of the other blouse. The patient also experienced mirror movements (the right hand tended to mirror the left). The authors focused their discussion on her motor apraxia, which shifted from an ideational apraxia to an ideomotor apraxia during the course of her illness. Apraxia is frequently mentioned in association with alien hand, although the fact that apraxia is a diagnosis of exclusion raises the question of whether or not it can be properly tested for and properly diagnosed in the setting of alien hand.

Ataxia

Ataxia refers to muscular incoordination. It is usually associated with diseases of the cerebellum, but terms such as sensory ataxia and optic ataxia have been used to describe particular causes of uncoordinated motor activity. Lesions to the central sensory pathways can result in contralateral sensory ataxia: Sensory feedback is inadequate to guide the movements of a limb and ataxic movements result. Similarly, optic ataxia occurs when a central visual pathway lesion impairs visual information from the opposite side of the world, and the limb (usually an arm) on the affected side loses the coordinating power of visual guidance during tasks that require visual input. Visual guidance usually improves sensory ataxia, so the ataxia is worse in the dark or with eyes closed, and sensory information helps to compensate for the loss of visual information in optic ataxia.

Levine and Rinn (1986) described a patient who developed a left alien hand due to an infarct that affected the right thalamus (producing a left sensory defect) and right medial occipital cortex and temperooccipital white matter (giving optic ataxia). The authors concluded that this unique case of alien hand was due to the combined effects of these two lesions and their corresponding syndromes. Clinically, their patient treated her left arm like an alien presence with hostile motivations, and they observed the arm sometimes striking her or trying to choke her. Similar involuntary and disturbing activities have been reported in alien hand due to classic frontal lesions.

Movement Disorders

Some reports of alien hand have emphasized motor behaviors rather than the sensation of alienness or the relationship of the alien hand to other disorders of cortical functions. Feinberg *et al.* (1992) recently defined alien hand sign as "unwilled and uncontrollable movements of an extremity not due to a movement disorder." Such a definition excludes many important phenomena, such as sensory complaints or the inability to recognize that the limb belongs to the patient. These excluded phenomena have been consistently associated with alien hand in previously reported cases. Japanese reports of alien hand also tend to emphasize the movement disorder aspect and to exclude subjective sensory complaints; For example, Tanaka *et al.* (1990) described a patient with several types of "dissociative motor disturbances" who, by most accounts, suffered from consequences of alien hand. The article included a set of photographs showing how the patient's left hand attempted to pull down his underwear while the patient tried to pull them up with his right hand. The left hand acted at cross-purposes to the right, mirrored the right hand, and carried out irrelevant tasks while the right hand was engaged. The patient had great difficulty with activities that required the cooperation of both hands.

The authors suggested that the term diagnostic dyspraxia should be used to describe problems such as these, in which movement of one hand triggers a range of abnormal movements in the other. They suggested that alien hand sign should refer to abnormal movements, such as the compulsive manipulation of tools (often referred to as utilization behavior in Western literature) and self-destructive behavior *not* elicited by volitional movements of the other hand. Prior reports of alien hand have included patients who clearly had problems similar to what these authors reported. Although prior studies were not rigorous in reporting whether the abnormal, autonomous movements were triggered by movement of the other hand or nontriggered, this author has certainly seen both triggered and nontriggered movements in the same patient. Insufficient evidence supports the separation of alien hand (nontriggered) from diagnostic dyspraxia (triggered).

Finally, several papers have discussed alien hand sign as a manifestation of the neurodegenerative condition CBD. This disorder is in some ways similar to Parkinson's disease, but certain distinctive features suggest that it is a separate clinical entity, and a distinctive pathology has been described at autopsy (Riley *et al.*, 1990; Gibb *et al.*, 1989). The initial symptoms are usually tremor, apraxia, limb dystonia, or cortical sensory disturbances. Several patients have also presented with or developed alien hand and similar disturbances involving the leg (Riley *et al.*, 1990). Patients with alien hand due to CBD are more likely to have spontaneous levitation and posturing of the limb described, although whether this results from different observers (with movement disorders practices) or some difference in the manifestation of the sign resulting from this particular etiology is not clear. Patients are often afflicted with more than one alien limb in the course of this progressive illness.

Psychomotor Disturbance

Several authors have emphasized the relationship between the patient's complaint that his or her arm feels foreign or like it does not belong to him or her, and the autonomous, complex nature of the arm's involuntary movements. Many credit Brion and Jedynak (1972) with the first description of alien hand (*la main etrangere*), by which they meant a feeling of unawareness or strangeness of one side of the body vis-à-vis the other, supported by the patient's inability to recognize the alien limb when held by the normal limb with visual stimuli removed, such as when the arms were placed behind the patient's back. They reported this sign in patients with tumors of the corpus callosum, in contrast to the hemiinattention syndromes of right parietal lesions, which were previously well known. Furthermore, they noted that many such patients had difficulty transferring sensory information between the hemispheres, such as the inability to name objects felt with the left hand while having no difficulty naming those felt with the right. These authors did not report dramatic autonomous movements, although one of the quotations from a patient included in their report indicates that certain movements, such as writing, seemed to be carried out autonomously.

Other authors have emphasized the psychomotor nature of the disturbance in alien hand. Goldberg *et al.* (1981) described two patients with what they called a dissociation of conscious intention from purposeful movement. They had forced grasping and groping, motor perseveration, and apparently purposeful, although involuntary, movements, which sometimes resulted in intermanual conflicts. These patients often restrained the alien hand with their normal hands. Drawing on the work of Bogen, these authors emphasized the presence of "autocriticism," in which the patients expressed frustration over the actions of the alien limb. Although he was describing elements of a callosal disconnection syndrome, rather than the kind of frontal injuries suffered by Goldberg's cases, Bogen (1985) is credited for using the term alien hand to describe the situation where a patient's *behavior* feels foreign, rather than just the limb, as defined by Brion and Jedynak (1972). McNabb and Leiguarda have retained the spirit of Brion and Jednyak as well as the motor side of the psychomotor definition provided by Bogen in their discussions of alien hand (McNabb *et al.*, 1988; Leiguarda *et al.*, 1989).

ANATOMY AND ETIOLOGY OF ALIEN HAND

Many of the cases mentioned thus far have resulted from injury to one or more of the frontal lobes. The frontal lesions in these patients usually involve the supplementary motor area and the anterior cingulate gyrus, areas believed to be involved in motor planning and coordination of limb movements. Those cases that have claimed unilateral lesions did not adequately rule out corpus callosum involvement (Goldberg *et al.*, 1981; McNabb *et al.*, 1988), so whether or not a unilateral frontal lesion can cause the problem in the absence of corpus callosum injury is not clear. Section or damage to the corpus callosum can also cause alien hand, although the condition is usually transitory when it follows surgical section used to treat intractable seizures (Bogen, 1985). Many cases with frontal pathology have also had extensive injury to the corpus callosum (Watson and Heilman, 1983; Starkstein *et al.*, 1988; Leiguarda *et al.*, 1989; Banks *et al.*, 1989). Most likely, persistent alien hand sign requires frontal and callosal injury. Etiologies of the frontal and callosal damage have included vascular infarcts of the frontal lobes and/or corpus callosum, tumors of the corpus callosum, hemorrhages of anterior communication arteries affecting the frontal regions and corpus callosum, and penetrating head injury.

In addition to frontally located lesions, a few patients have had more posterior pathology, including that discussed by Levine and Rinn (1986). This neuroanatomy seems to be rarely associated with alien hand, despite the fact that right parietal lesions are fairly common. Their suggestion that a lesion of the central sensory pathway must occur *in combination with* a lesion affection in the central visual pathway may account for the relative rarity of this type of alien hand.

Alien hand is now a well-recognized feature of the degenerative condition known as CBD. The few cases of CBD afflicted with alien hand that have come to autopsy have shown cell loss in the substantia nigra, locus ceruleus, and nucleus ambiguous with corticobasal inclusion bodies, with or without cortical involvement (Gibb *et al.*, 1989; Riley *et al.*, 1990). The neuropathology of CBD patients with alien hand has not been shown to be significantly different from those who did not manifest alien hand sign.

A few recent case reports have related alien hand to unique anatomical correlations or etiologies. One report suggested that paroxysmal alien hand could occur as a result of seizures affecting the frontal lobes; one of the reported patients also had a lymphoma involving the right supplementary motor area (Leiguarda *et al.*, 1991). Another report diagnosed alien hand in two individuals with longstanding movement disorders (Walker and Hunt, 1991). One had right hemidystonia and athetosis in addition to alien hand secondary to a congenital left thalamic lesion; the other had a right alien hand in the setting of torsion dystonia, which had been treated by bilateral thalamotomy to relieve the movement disorder, before the onset of alien hand.

The various anatomical lesions discussed so far have given rise to a number of classification systems (Bogen, 1985; Tanaka *et al.*, 1990; Feinberg *et al.*, in press). These theories and systems rely on correlations between the part of the corpus callosum involved, the extent of frontal damage and whether it is unilateral or bilateral, and the prominent motor features displayed by the patients. At present, no definitive classification system encompasses all cases. Etiologic theories all have in common some notion of disconnection (right from left, or sensory from motor) and some notion of released inhibition affecting activities of the alien hand.

SOCIOCULTURAL ASPECTS OF ALIEN HAND

Prehistory

Alien hand is probably not a new phenomenon nor increasing in incidence, but these are not directly testable hypotheses. The fact that Goldstein reported something similar in 1908 suggests that it occurred almost a century ago, if not before. Experience with other signs, syndromes, and diseases as well as certain "folk" aspects of the condition suggest that it has probably been with us for centuries and is only now being described more often. There are several possible approaches to discovering whether or not the entity was known, perhaps by another name, long ago. One can examine ancient Greek and biblical texts, looking for allusions to similar phenomenon. An example of this approach is found in O'Neill's (1980) work on speech disorders. One can study archeological remains looking for clues, such as devices to restrain a limb, although the yield would likely be low and causality would be difficult to establish. Or one can actively search out the incidence and prevalence of alien hand in contemporary populations and then infer, from demographic information, the likely occurrences of alien hand in earlier times. For example, if it turns out to be a disease predominantly affecting the age group over 60 years, then we could infer that it was less common when people died younger.

Reconstructing currently defined syndromes or diseases in earlier historical contexts is not always a straightforward process. Examination of early allusions to speechlessness, for example, suggest that our current definition of aphasia is highly conditioned by universal literacy (Doody, 1991). The actual behaviors observed in preliterate aphasics were probably substantially different from what we see today in literate aphasics, and even in nonliterate people with aphasia, whose cognitive functions are influenced by the literate settings in which they live. Even if the behaviors were identical, earlier observers might have emphasized different features that they believed were important to making a diagnosis or prescribing treatment. As Kuhn (1970) has pointed out, observations are related to prevailing scientific paradigms, and as paradigms change, so do the observations.

Certain medical anthropological studies also have bearing on the question of changing concepts of disease. When a "new" medical condition begins to occur in a population, it is not automatically recognized and accepted by those newly encountering it (Farmer, 1990). For example, when acquired immunodeficiency syndrome (AIDS) first affected populations in rural Haiti, there was no collective representation of the disorder among them. At first, people treated the disease as if it were tuberculosis, because patients who had AIDS also had tuberculosis. Over time, the people incorporated AIDS into local beliefs about diseases in general such as the ability of magic to bring them on. Ultimately, medical information about the cause of AIDS and its prevention and prognosis came to exist in parallel to their other beliefs: They believed that AIDS was sometimes a result of sexual transmission and sometimes a result of magic (Farmer, 1990). The point of this example is to indicate a certain give and take with respect to new or newly recognized phenomena and old interpretive frameworks. This occurs even among members of the medical community. It is not unlikely that more physicians will begin to recognize alien hand after more patients and their communities begin to do so. Experience with Alzheimer's disease and the increased numbers of cases being diagnosed would support this.

Alien Hand as a Folk Illness

Folk illness is difficult to define, but it has something to do with the popular imagination and unofficial concepts of disease. A recent abstract presented at the American Academy of Neurology sparked much public interest in alien hand (Doody and Jankovic, 1991). As a result of that abstract, at least 60 newspaper articles were printed, 6 magazine articles published, and 5 radio interviews aired on the topic over the next 3 months. Several articles turned on lines such as "the right hand doesn't know what the left hand is doing," "one hand washes the other," or "hands out of control." Writers and the public seem to have little difficulty relating to this, until recently, rather obscure neurological problem.

At least in Western society, there seems to be a longstanding and subtle personification of the two arms as "agents," with different and sometimes opposing purposes. Sinistrality obviously means left-handedness, yet the root gives rise to related terms, such as sinister, and the idea of "wickedness" or ominousness has sometimes been associated with the "left." Furthermore, the motifs of intermanual conflicts and autonomous hands have occured in several films: *Dr. Strangelove, The Hand, The Fiend with Five Fingers, and Evil Dead 2: Dead by Dawn.* I have been asked whether or not the movie writers or film directors of these productions modeled their characters after patients with alien hand sign: Someone will have to interview them to find out. But it is more likely that these characters and their autonomous, sinister hands grew out of the imagination, which is, already, mixed with the bizarre occurrences of real life. These films illustrate the fact that alien hand is not something entirely new, even though it is only now being reported with any frequency. In addition, chances are that the popular notions of alien hand will in some way influence which patients are seen, diagnosed, and ultimately treated for this malady.

Signs versus Syndromes

Throughout this discussion, I have sometimes referred to alien hand as a sign and sometimes as a syndrome or part of a syndrome. This usage is consistent with what is found in the neurological literature, although the differences between the sign and syndrome have not been explicitly addressed in any of these articles. Kety (1974) pointed out that, in the medical model of human illness, symptoms are recognized first, and when it is realized that they occur in fairly regu'.ır clusters, these are described as syndromes. The syndromes are ultimately related to one or more pathogenetic or etiologic entities. This process is apparently taking place currently with alien hand sign. Various authors are describing syndromes in which an underlying neuroanatomical lesion (e.g., frontal versus callosal) or an underlying etiology (e.g., CBD) are more or less related to a cluster of signs and symptoms that include alien hand. So far, no syndrome has clearly been created that includes all cases with a given neuroanatomical lesion or fully characterizes clinical phenomena so well that the underlying etiology (stroke versus CBD versus tumor, etc.) can be predicted. According to Kety, syndromes also evolve and sometimes break up into subtypes on the basis of clinical or laboratory information. They become "diseases" only when a common pathogenesis clearly matches the clinical picture.

If symptoms are ultimately organized into clusters, what then happens to signs? And is alien hand a sign, or a symptom? Symptoms are generally taken to mean what the patient experiences in the way of altered sensation, function, or appearance. Signs are somehow more "objective" indicators of disease. Alien hand is both subjective and objective. It is perhaps not surprising that several medical discussions of it have emphasized the observable motor side of the phenomenon rather than the subjective "alienness" reported by patients.

Foucault (1973) emphasizes the "ocular" nature of science in general and of medical science in particular. For him, symptoms are the first level by which the form of a disease is made visible. Signs offer a basis for recognition of what has taken place (anamnestic signs), what will take place (prognostic signs), or what is now taking place (diagnostic signs). In many ways, symptoms become the disease itself and are treated as such: They provide support to the interpretation of signs. Because observation has assumed major importance in the diagnosis and treatment of diseases during the last two centuries, the absolute distinction between signs and symptoms has been erased, and both serve to reveal diseases to the physician. Every symptom may be a sign, but every sign is not a symptom. It seems inevitable that our construction of alien hand syndrome or syndromes will weigh signs differently than symptoms.

Epidemiologic studies of alien hand, then, will be rather difficult until the process of delineating its signs and their supporting symptoms is comprehensive and complete. Only then will we reach consensus about whether there are one or more syndromes of alien hand and what the relationship is between each syndrome and an underlying neuropathological lesion or disease process.

Social Construction and Alien Hand

I hope to have suggested that the social construction of the alien hand entity is actively taking place. Longstanding and anonymous ideas about the hands as agents and potential rivals are part of the process of construction. Recent medical presentations, publications, and the publicity surrounding them are also part of the process. Different medical researchers emphasize different signs and etiologies and sometimes put forward rival classification systems that will ultimately be resolved in the peer-reviewed medical literature. This aspect of the social construction of scientific knowledge is well described by Latour and Woolgar (1979), including the political aspects of the process. Consequences of enhanced interest in alien hand may include more awareness on the part of the public, more standardized diagnoses, attempts to differentiate alien hand from similar phenomena, and probably more frequent diagnoses. Last, but not least, experimental therapies will likely arise after consensus is reached on the different syndromes and their relationships to different neuroanatomies (likely surgical interventions) or disease processes (likely pharmacologic interventions).

The social construction of alien hand in no way detracts from its scientific study. Most illnesses have probably gone through this process in some way at some time. However, because of what I have called the folk aspects of alien hand sign, and the recently increased interest in the condition, it lends itself to such an analysis and may be informative with respect to other disease phenomena.

UNANSWERED QUESTIONS

Many questions about alien hand remain unanswered, including those most necessary for epidemiologic purposes. We do not know the incidence or prevalence of the sign, or syndrome, or whether or not we are even dealing with unitary phenomenona. Only crude estimates can be made; for example, by tallying how many new cases we diagnosed in our tertiary care medical center last year, and multiplying by the number of tertiary care centers in the country, we would guess that the incidence of diagnosed new cases is several thousand per year. Several more cases may be recognized in community care settings without referral to tertiary care centers. Undiagnosed cases probably exceed those that are diagnosed.

We cannot judge the risk of developing alien hand for specific etiologies, although we know that it has been associated with several different etiologies. Most stroke patients do not develop alien hand, even those with frontal infarcts. Since hemorrhages and tumors affecting the corpus callosum and frontal lobes are relatively uncommon, alien hand due to these etiologies must be rare. In addition, although several patients in each series of CBD are afflicted with alien hand, the incidence and prevalence of this disease are unknown. We do not know if there are specific risk factors that predispose to alien hand, such as age, sex, handedness, or genetic factors. Finally, we do not even know whether we are dealing with a new or an ancient phenomenon. We can be reasonably certain that we are dealing with a changing process, the consequences of which will include specific syndromes, standardization of signs, and continued interest in the phenomena known as alien hand.

Acknowledgment

The authors thanks the Hershel and Hilda Rich Philanthropic Fund for their support of this work.

References

Banks, G., Short, P., Martinez, A. J., Latchaw, R., Ratcliff, G., and Boller, F. (1989). The alien hand syndrome. *Arch. Neurol.* **46,** 456–459.

Bogen, J. E. (1985). The callosal syndrome. *In* "Clinical Neuropsychology" (K. M. Heilman and E. Valenstein, eds.). pp. 295–338. Oxford University Press, New York.

Brion, S., and Jedynak, C. P. (1972). Troubles du transfert interhemispherique. *Rev. Neurol. (Paris)* **126**(4), 257–266.

Doody, R. S., and Jankovic, J. (1992). The Alien Hand and Related Signs. *J. Neurology, Neurosurgery and Psychiatry.* **55**(9) (in press).

Doody, R. S. (1991) Aphasia as postmodern (anthropological) discourse. *J. Anthropol. Res.* **47**(3), 285–303.

Doody, R. S., and Jankovic, J. (1991). The alien hand and related signs. *Neurology* **41**(suppl. 1), 122.

Engel, G. L. (1977). The need for a new medical model: A challenge for biomedicine. *Science* **196**(4286), 129–135.

Farmer, P. (1990). Sending sickness: Sorcery, politics, and changing concepts of AIDS in rural Haiti. *Med. Anthropol. Q.* **4**(1), 6–27.

Feinberg, T. E., Schindler, R. J., Flanagan, N. G., and Haber, L. D. (1992). Two alien hand syndromes. *Ann. Neurol. Neurology* **42**(1), 19–24.

Foucault, M. (1973). Signs and cases. *In* "The Birth of the Clinic," ch. 6. pp. 88–106. Vintage Books, New York.

Gibb, W. R. G., Luther, P. J., and Marsden, C. D. (1989). Corticobasal degeneration. *Brain* **112,** 1171–1192.

Goldberg, G., Mayer, N. H., and Toglia, J. U. (1981). Medial frontal cortex infarction and the alien hand sign. *Arch. Neurol.* **38,** 683–686.

Heilman, K. M., and Rothi, L. J. G. (1985). Apraxia. *In* "Clinical Neuropsychology." (K. M. Heilman and E. Valenstein, eds.). pp. 131–150. Oxford University Press, New York.

Kety, S. S. (1974). From rationalization to reason. *Am. J. Psychiatry* **131**(9), 957–963.

Kuhn, T. S. (1970). "The Structure of Scientific Revolutions," 2nd ed. University of Chicago Press, Chicago.

Latour, B., and Woolgar, S. (1979). "Laboratory Life." Sage Publications, Newbury Park, California.

Leiguarda, R., Starkstein, S., and Berthier, M. (1989). Anterior callosal syndrome. *Brain* **112**, 1019–1037.

Leiguarda, R. C., Nogues, M., Berthier, M., and Starkstein, S. (1991). Paroxysmal alien hand secondary to a medial frontal cortex lesion. *Neurology* **41**(suppl. 1), 302.

Levine D. N., and Rinn, W. E. (1986). Opticosensory ataxia and alien hand syndrome after posterior cerebral artery territory infarction. *Neurology* **36**, 1094–1097.

McNabb, A. W., Carroll, W. M., and Mastaglia, F. L. (1988). Alien hand and loss of bimanual coordination after dominant anterior cerebral artery territory infarction. *J. Neurol. Neurosurg. Psychiatry* **51**, 218–222.

O'Neill, Y. V. (1980). "Speech and Speech Disorders in Western Thought before 1600." Greenwood Press, Westport, Connecticut.

Riley, D. E., Lang, A. E., Lewis, A., Resch, L., Ashby, P., Hornykiewicz, O., and Black, S. (1990). Cortico-basal ganglionic degeneration. *Neurology* **40**, 1203–1212.

Shahani, B., Burrows, P., and Whitty, W. M. (1970). The grasp reflex and perseveration. *Brain* **93**, 181–192.

Starkstein, S. E., Berthier, M., and Leiguarda, R. (1988). Disconnection syndrome in a right-handed patient with right hemisphere speech dominance. *Eur. Neurol.* **28**, 187–190.

Tanaka, Y., Iswasa, H., and Yoshida, M. (1990). Diagnostic dyspraxia: Case report and movement-related potentials. *Neurology* **40**, 657–661.

Walker, F. O., and Hunt, V. P. (1991). Dystonic alien hand. *Neurology* **41**(suppl. 1), 344.

Watson, R. T., and Heilman, K. M. (1983). Callosal apraxia. *Brain* **106**, 391–403.

10

Alzheimer's Disease and Related Disorders Among African Americans

E. Percil Stanford • Barbara Du Bois

In the field of gerontology and geriatrics, there has been a tendency to focus more attention on the physical or medical aspects of aging than on the mental health status of older individuals. Recently, more emphasis has been placed on the importance of general functional status rather than simply chronological age. Thus, research interest in defining how functional status can be more accurately measured is now increasing. Assessments of functional status commonly include determining levels of impairment in physical, activities of daily living, and mental health areas; however, assessments are also conducted to determine impairment in social and economic resources as well (Morton *et al.*, 1992). The levels of impairment in functional ability may, therefore, be affected by one's cultural background and experience. Long-term economic deprivation may result in a clustering of functional impairments that are unique among the poor elderly as compared to the wealthy elderly. Therefore, functional ability may vary depending on unique lifetime experiences. Butler and Lewis (1977) point out that people are the dynamic actors within a social system that includes their family environment, personal history, personality characteristics, the larger world that surrounds them, value orientations that emphasize faith, family, and work, and other mechanisms that enable them to cope. In examining the psychological, social, and emotional dimensions of the individual, credence must be given to the effect that the total environment has had on the individual over their lifetime.

Mental health does not have the same meaning across cultures or even across economic classes. In fact, some cultures do not recognize mental health as a viable concept (Stanford, 1990). Healthy community and family relations may be far more important as a concept than the individual's mental health in those populations that value the group over the individual.

DEMENTIA AND CULTURE

Dementia has been a familiar concept for physicians since the first century. The term originally meant "out of one's mind"; however, the concept has evolved to signify an organic mental disorder that is accompanied by deterioration of previous intellectual abilities, social and occupational functioning, abstract thinking, judgment, and impulse control (Reisberg, 1983; Stone, 1988). Dementia has continued to emerge as a perplexing and devastating phenomenon of late life.

The dementia syndrome is a common disorder in the United States, affecting approximately 15% of individuals over the age of 65. Nearly one-half of all Americans reach age 75, with approximately one-quarter reaching age 85. With increasing longevity, the risks for dementia, stroke, and Parkinson's disease also increase. Although there are many different sources of dementia, Alzheimer's disease (AD) accounts for the highest rates of cognitive impairment among the aged. AD is estimated to account for between 50 and 75% of all dementia cases (Mortimer and Schuman, 1981). At least 2 million American adults are victims of AD (Mortimer and Schuman, 1981). Thus, not only does the prevalence of all types of cognitive impairment increase with longer life expectancy, but AD reaches its highest rate among aging individuals.

Dementing illnesses result from dysfunction in the brain and, as such, are classified as organic mental disorders. Organic mental disorders are caused by aging, intake of substances that cause brain dysfunction, or physical diseases that cause the condition. Organic mental disorders share clinical features (George *et al.*, 1991). All involve an impairment to cognitive functioning, while common signs of this impairment are memory loss, disorientation to time and place, clouding of consciousness, impaired abstract thinking, and impaired judgment. Not all of these signs and symptoms will occur for each patient. In fact, the heterogeneity of clinical signs are affected by etiological factors. These factors produce different characteristics of the organic mental disorder (e.g., mood disturbance, personality change), age of onset, chronicity, and clinical course of the condition.

AD has been classically defined in pathological terms as the formation of neurofibrillary tangles in the brain, the formation of neuritic or senile plaques, neuronal degeneration or loss, and neurodendritic spine loss.

A concomitant buildup of β-amyloid protein in the brain often accompanies AD.

Accurate diagnosis of AD has improved significantly in the last 10 years from reported error rates of 30% down to approximately 10% (Ron *et al.*, 1979; Welsh *et al.*, 1991). Better accuracy or differential diagnosis of delineating clinical signs and symptoms of AD from other organic mental disorders arises from a better understanding of the clinical presentation and course of disease. Accuracy of diagnosis is reduced when patients present with concomitant dementing disorders such as those related to vascular disease (multiinfarct dementia), reversible dementias, Parkinsons' disease, amnesia, and the alcoholic Wernicke–Korsakoff syndrome.

As Mortimer (1990) indicates, the problem of dementia is global. There is an increasing diversity of epidemiologic and analytic studies being conducted on AD from industrialized to third-world countries, the scope of which is to determine if factors related to culture may predispose to dementia. The challenge facing researchers is to understand how to best combine the results of previous and current studies and to coordinate efforts so that more can be learned about the etiologic factors responsible for dementing illnesses.

The bulk of research on the frequency of diseases related to dementia as well as the neurologic presentation of abnormalities comes from typically white, urban samples (Wragg and Jeste, 1989). Cognitive assessment batteries for ethnic minorities have not been developed as culture-free instruments. Performance on cognitive assessment instruments may be influenced by educational level, ethnic and cultural background, and language barriers. Items that relate to orientation of time and to serial subtraction are difficult for those with limited education. Some test items may have different meaning or no meaning cross-culturally. A report by the Office of Technology Assessment recommended that assessment procedures be adapted for ethnic minority groups to improve evaluation of cognitive abilities, to plan adequately for long-term care, to use in eligibility determination, and to apply to policy. According to Mortimer (1990: 27–33), there is tremendous need for prospective studies in which the dementia syndromes, including AD, would be diagnosed with uniform criteria in different populations; however, researchers recognize that detection of dementing illness cross-culturally may depend on factors that are not easily controllable. To minimize the confounding effects involved with cross-cultural research, a suggested approach is to study comparable occupational groups or socially defined groups in different cultures (Mortimer, 1988).

The Epidemiological Catchment Area (ECA) studies were designed to estimate the prevalence of mental disorders in both treated and untreated

populations in the United States. Not limiting the sample to institutionalized patients, the ECA studies allowed for estimating prevalence rates
for both severe mental disorders more commonly found in institutional
settings and the less severe disorders more commonly found in the community. Five primary sites were selected: Baltimore, Maryland; New Haven, Connecticut; Piedmont/Durham, North Carolina; St. Louis, Missouri;
and Los Angeles, California. With regard to the aged and minority groups,
the epidemiological surveys were conducted in settings where there was
ethnic and socioeconomic diversity. Rates for Hispanics come largely from
the Los Angeles catchment area, where as rates for blacks come primarily
from the two sites of St. Louis and North Carolina. Appropriate sampling
frames were conducted to obtain a representative selection of subjects
from each ECA site. Assessment of mental health status represented a
significant component to the ECA studies and the first attempt to determine prevalence rates of cognitive impairment in older age groups. The
ECA data continue to be the largest, most representative cross-sectional
data on cognitive impairment to date.

DEMENTIA IN THE AFRICAN
AMERICAN POPULATION

Major interpretive generalizations are made about the mental health status of blacks in the absence of data from population-based epidemiological surveys that sample all economic and social classes of blacks. Much
of the data on mental health and ethnicity is based on psychiatric epidemiological community surveys that compare blacks and whites and that
focus primarily on indicators of distress. The focus on *between-group*
differences or race-comparative studies de-emphasizes the importance
that should be assigned to *within-group* differences for those interested
in documenting mental health needs of special population groups. The
majority of studies aimed at determining the health status of blacks are
confined to small geographic locations (Dressler, 1985, 1986; Du Bois *et
al.*, unpublished results). Although these studies have demonstrated the
importance of small-scale evaluations of psychosocial epidemiology, more
researchers interested in the field of ethnicity and mental health should
now direct their focus to within-group evaluations. This will assure more
reliable and representative estimates of health status indicators across a
broad spectrum of subjects. This is especially important when previous
investigators have found substantial race differences in outcome measures (Neighbors, 1986).

AD has become a more familiar syndrome in the black community and causes major concern because of its significant impact on the community and support structures of the patient. African American individuals may now be considered at special risk for developing severe cognitive impairment and other organic mental disorders (Folstein *et al.*, 1985). Other than the ECA data, which compare and contrast prevalence rates among whites, blacks, and Hispanics, a specific literature on cognitive impairment among blacks is very limited.

Demographics

Since 1930, the black population over age 65 has grown substantially faster than the white population (Manuel, 1988). Between 1960 and 1980, the black older population increased by 83% compared to the white older population, which increased by 57%. The faster rate of growth is projected well into the next century. Using 1985 statistics, elderly blacks represented slightly over 8% of the total black population ($N = 2,343,000$). This contrasts with the 12.5% proportion found among older whites. By the year 2000, older blacks will constitute 8.5% and by the year 2040 12.5%. The largest increases in population are among the oldest-old, those over age 85. Between 1980 and 1985, the oldest-old black age group increased approximately 27%, compared to the oldest-old whites group, which increased 19%. For both groups, the population figures were largely due to increases in female longevity (U.S. Bureau of the Census, 1980).

Using 1985 statistics, life expectancy for black males is 65 years of age. In 1940, life expectancy was approximately 50 years of age. Black female life expectancy is now 73 years of age in contrast to 55 years in 1940. The principle causes of death among males over age 65 are cerebrovascular disease, cancer, and coronary heart disease. Causes of death for women are cerebrovascular disease, coronary heart disease, and cancer. Jackson (1988) indicated that from 1950 to 1976, death rates from heart disease were higher for blacks than for whites.

Manuel (1988) projects that the future African American aged population will conginue to increase at a rapid rate, causing the gap of the relative age status of African Americans and whites to narrow. This narrowing of the gap will not be exceptionally evident until after the post-World War II baby-boom cohort enters the ranks of the aged, after 2020. Between 1980 and 2000, the percentage of white females will increase from 13.9 to 16.5%, and the similar increase for older black women will be from approximately 8.9 to 10.2%. Furthermore, in 2040 percentages of these populations that will be old are 26.2% for whites and 19.5% for blacks.

Whether this convergence will represent or reflect a homogenizing effect of similar life styles or circumstances within the respective population groups remains to be seen.

Prevalence Rates of Dementia

Two types of data will be presented that show rates of cognitive impairment in the African American population. Results from the ECA studies will be supplemented with data from small-scale studies. As previously mentioned, the ECA data compare rates among ethnic groups and, as such, will not explain the within-group differences of cognitive impairment that may be a function of cultural or environmental factors.

The ECA data compared rates of cognitive impairment among blacks, Hispanics, and whites using a cross-sectional design (George *et al.*, 1991). Epidemiologists used current cognitive status as their assessment focus because of the cross-sectional nature of the study. For this purpose, both the Mini-Mental State Examination (MMSE) (Folstein *et al.*, 1975) and the Diagnostic Interview Schedule (Robins *et al.*, 1981) were included in the ECA community surveys. The MMSE measures orientation, memory, attention, ability to name, ability to follow verbal and written instructions, ability to write a sentence spontaneously, and ability to copy a figure. The MMSE does not measure other abnormal mental processes, thinking, or mood. Although not a diagnostic tool but, rather, a measure of current cognitive status, the MMSE correlates highly with other mental function measures if valid. The MMSE has high external reliability (between 0.85 and 0.98) when comparing tests to retests over time intervals ranging between 24 hr and 28 days and when compared to verbal and performance scores on other tests (Wechesler Adult Intelligence Scale, reliability coefficients of 0.78 and 0.66). The measurement of cognitive impairment was done in two separate ways: by counting the number of errors on the MMSE and by counting the number of MMSE errors and refusals together as errors. (The latter would increase the rate of cognitive impairment significantly for prevalence rates but not substantially alter the correlations between cognitive impairment and other factors.) For ECA purposes and comparability to other research results, the investigators chose the method of not counting refusals as errors on the MMSE. Cutpoints were used on the scoring of the MMSE. Thirteen or more errors were used to assign severe cognitive impairment, 7–12 errors for mild cognitive impairment, and 6 or fewer errors for no cognitive impairment.

The prevalence of severe cognitive impairment in the general population over age 18 (counting MMSE errors only) is 0.85% ($N = 19,597$, $SE = 0.09$), whereas mild cognitive impairment has a prevalence of 4.2%

(SE = 0.21) (George *et al.*, 1991: 299–300). Those over 55 years of age have significantly higher rates of impairment. Among the 55 and older cohort, severe cognitive impairment shows a prevalence rate of 2.3% (N = 8396, SE = 0.25) and mild cognitive impairment a rate of 9.58% (SE = 0.49).

Table I reports prevalence rates of cognitive impairment by age, sex, ethnicity, and education for those 18 and older. For the entire adult population, prevalence rates of severe cognitive impairment were highest among those 75 and older (4.95%, SE = 0.96), blacks (2.04%, SE = 0.45), and those having fewer than 9 years of education (3.57, SE = 0.49). Rates between males and females were not substantially different (males = 0.68%, SE = 0.12; females = 0.70%, SE = 0.12). Similar patterns were demonstrated for those showing mild impairment, but the prevalence rates for all demographic characteristics were significantly higher. Age (being 75 and older), being black, and less than 9 years of education showed rates of 19.1, 9.6, and 19.24%, respectively. Clearly, age and education play important roles in the presentation of cognitive impairment.

Table II reports prevalence rates of cognitive impairment by age, sex, ethnicity, and education among those 55 years and older. The rationale for limiting the age range to 55 and over is that younger people will have very different etiological factors accounting for cognitive impairment than older individuals; thus, presenting the data in such a way provides a more accurate picture of organic brain disorders related to aging. Similar trends in the data are demonstrated with the exception that highest rates of severe cognitive impairment occur in those 85 and older (10.1%, SE = 2.7), blacks (5.7%, SE = 1.34), and those having less than 9 years of education (4.3%, SE = 0.57). For those with mild cognitive impairment, the rates increase significantly among those 75–84 (17.8%, SE = 1.6), those 85 and older (25.5%, SE = 4.1), females (10.2%, SE = 0.67), Blacks (27.7%, SE = 2.7), Hispanics (12.9%, SE = 3.24), and those having less than 9 years of education (21.95%, SE = 1.19).

These data show that age, ethnicity, and education differences in the prevalence of cognitive impairment are significant. Age differences play important roles for each category of educational attainment, such that regardless of level of education, age is a significant correlate and risk factor for cognitive impairment. Level of education continues to play an important role as a correlate of impairment but only partially explains age and ethnic differences. African Americans have statistically higher rates of both severe and mild cognitive impairment than either Hispanics or whites for all levels of education. Thus, ethnicity is also a significant correlate and risk factor for impairment. Some justification of the ethnicity correlate is warranted. Within the broad range of the educational experience, older blacks may have had a significantly different educational

Table I
Prevalence of Cognitive Impairment by Age, Race/Ethnicity, and Education

| | N^a | Severe cognitive impairment | | | | Mild cognitive impairment in those without severe impairment | | | | | |
| | | Errors only | | Errors and refusals | | | Errors only | | Errors and refusals | | |
		%	(SE)	%	(SE)	N	%	(SE)	%	(SE)
Total	19,354	0.69	(0.09)	1.11	(0.11)	18,990	4.12	(0.21)	5.76	(0.24)
Age										
18–34	6,863	0.24	(0.08)	0.32	(0.09)	6,842	1.13	(0.17)	2.31	(0.24)
35–54	4,283	0.29	(0.10)	0.69	(0.16)	4,249	3.12	(0.33)	4.80	(0.41)
55–74	5,911	1.01	(0.22)	1.63	(0.28)	5,783	7.54	(0.58)	9.72	(0.65)
75 and older	2,297	4.95	(0.96)	7.30	(1.15)	2,116	19.09	(1.79)	22.15	(1.91)
Sex										
Male	8,258	0.68	(0.12)	1.09	(0.16)	8,104	3.90	(0.29)	5.56	(0.35)
Female	11,096	0.70	(0.12)	1.13	(0.15)	10,886	4.33	(0.29)	5.94	(0.34)
Race/ethnicity										
Black	4,682	2.04	(0.45)	2.99	(0.55)	4,530	9.62	(0.96)	12.32	(1.07)
Hispanic	1,598	0.60	(0.34)	1.31	(0.51)	1,582	7.94	(1.21)	14.43	(1.58)
White/other	13,074	0.52	(0.08)	0.86	(0.10)	12,878	3.21	(0.20)	4.41	(0.23)
Education										
<9 years	4,692	3.57	(0.49)	5.09	(0.58)	4,400	19.24	(1.07)	24.12	(1.17)
9–11 years	4,171	0.58	(0.18)	1.02	(0.24)	4,125	3.87	(0.47)	5.52	(0.56)
12 years	4,627	0.07	(0.05)	0.25	(0.10)	4,613	1.62	(0.25)	2.69	(0.32)
>12 years	5,864	0.04	(0.04)	0.20	(0.08)	5,852	0.26	(0.09)	1.16	(0.18)

^{a} N's reflect some missing date for demographic variables.

[From L. K. George, R. Landerman, D. G. Blazer, and J. C. Anthony, 1991, Cognitive impairment. *In* "Psychiatric Disorders in America: The Epidemiologic Catchment Area Study" (L. N. Robins and D. A. Regier, eds.), pp. 291–327, Free Press, New York.]

Table II

Prevalence of Cognitive Impairment by Age, Race/Ethnicity, and Education among Those Aged 55 and Older

| | | Severe cognitive impairment | | | | Mild cognitive impairment in those without severe impairment | | | | | |
| | | Errors only | | Errors and refusals | | | Errors only | | | Errors and refusals | |
	N^a	%	(SE)	%	(SE)	N	%	(SE)	N	%	(SE)
Total	8,208	1.77	(0.22)	2.73	(0.27)	7,899	9.70	(0.49)	7,735	12.01	(0.55)
Age											
55–64	2,381	0.81	(0.22)	1.32	(0.28)	2,337	4.98	(0.53)	2,316	7.23	(0.63)
65–74	3,530	1.29	(0.32)	2.06	(0.41)	3,446	11.16	(0.91)	3,395	13.28	(0.98)
75–84	1,832	3.83	(0.80)	5.84	(0.97)	1,710	17.82	(1.62)	1,641	20.43	(1.73)
85 and older	465	10.14	(2.70)	14.07	(3.11)	406	25.45	(4.11)	383	30.18	(4.46)
Sex											
Male	3,118	1.76	(0.33)	2.60	(0.40)	2,991	9.06	(0.73)	2,926	11.93	(0.83)
Female	5,090	1.77	(0.29)	2.83	(0.37)	4,908	10.19	(0.67)	4,090	12.08	(0.73)
Race/ethnicity											
Black	1,479	5.71	(1.34)	8.50	(1.60)	1,358	27.73	(2.65)	1,290	33.32	(2.84)
Hispanic	309	2.18	(1.40)	3.35	(1.72)	299	12.91	(3.24)	291	25.67	(4.24)
White/other	6,420	1.39	(0.21)	2.17	(0.26)	6,242	7.98	(0.48)	6,154	9.69	(0.53)
Education											
<9 years	3,545	4.33	(0.57)	6.14	(0.67)	3,285	21.95	(1.19)	3,172	26.32	(1.27)
9–11 years	1,642	0.74	(0.32)	1.29	(0.42)	1,613	6.08	(0.88)	1,591	8.04	(1.01)
12 years	1,508	0.20	(0.16)	0.79	(0.31)	1,499	3.16	(0.61)	1,478	4.53	(0.73)
>12 years	1,513	0.26	(0.18)	0.62	(0.28)	1,502	1.12	(0.37)	1,494	1.93	(0.48)

[a] N's reflect some missing data for demographic variables.

[From L. K. George, R. Landerman, D. G. Blazer, and J. C. Anthony, 1991 Cognitive impairment, *in* "Psychiatric Disorders in America: The Epidemiologic Catchment Area Study" (L. N. Robins and D. A. Regier, eds.), pp. 291–327, Free Press, New York.]

experience than older whites, which may predispose them to poorer performance on cognitive test instruments; thus, ethnicity and educational differences should be more closely examined. In studies of depression, when income effects were controlled, differences in depression rates between whites and blacks were not significant. Similar confounding effects may be operant in the higher prevalence rates for cognitive impairment for blacks than nonblacks.

The ECA data also suggested that geographic differences were due to the higher prevalence of cognitive impairment in the Durham, North Carolina site. This site also has the highest proportion of blacks. A likely explanation is that geographic differences reflect ethnic composition (the Durham site has an approximately 50% white and black composition) as well as possible urbanization differences. These differences in turn may influence educational quality, which is evident in performance differences in cognitive tests among older black respondents. Previous studies do not show geographic differences in the distribution of cognitive impairment (Mortimer and Schuman, 1981); therefore, the differences between the ECA sites are most likely a function of sociocultural differences in the subject population rather than true differences related to dementia.

The sociocultural differences apparent in the ECA sites provided rationale for exploring urban and rural residential correlates to cognitive impairment. Urban–rural differences in the St. Louis ECA site showed a higher prevalence of severe cognitive impairment among urban rather than rural residents. The opposite pattern was apparent in the Durham ECA site. Rural residents showed slightly higher prevalence rates of cognitive impairment than urban residents. Such differences could be indicative of the residential patterns of the study subjects. In the St. Louis site, more blacks live in the urban area whereas the rural area was inhabited predominantly by whites. For the Durham site, urban–rural differences were not significant; however, there were more rural black residents than urban. Generalizing across the five ECA sites, urban–rural residential patterns were not strongly correlated to cognitive status.

Other small-scale studies of dementia in the African American population are few. As with the ECA studies, rates of dementing illness have been established from multiracial samples. No studies have examined within-group variability of cognitive impairment as a function of social, cultural, economic, or education differences within the black community. Thus comparisons are made between whites and blacks, and whites and nonwhites.

Data from death certificates are used to provide information on dementia in the black community (Lilienfeld and Lilienfeld, 1980; Baker, 1988). Establishing accurate mortality rates for dementia may be unreliable. This may be due to the fact that dementia is a very difficult disease to establish as the cause of death. Accurately diagnosing organic brain disorders requires observing the course of illness over time. Making a diagnosis of AD requires that all other potential causative factors are ruled out. The question of causality concerns the possibility that dementia causes death directly or is an underlying condition that may indirectly predispose to death. As it applies to older ethnic minorities and specifically to Blacks, cause of death may be listed as something other than dementia if the attending physician does not have a medical history of the patient. Additionally, if a black patient is exhibiting other forms of dementia that may be due to cardiovascular function or alcohol use, the assignment of senility due to AD may overinflate prevalence rates for the disease. Examining mortality rates by race, Chandra *et al.* (1986) found that the average annual age-adjusted mortality rates for death due to senility were higher for nonwhites than for whites. Senility was listed more frequently as cause of death for nonwhites. This may be a reflection of the lack of diagnostic scrutiny into the cause of death where those who are non-white, are poor, or have no health insurance are concerned. Although whites who die with senility present may have another condition listed as cause of death, this by no means can be offered as proof that senility is more prevalent or malignant in nonwhite communities than in white communities (Chandra *et al.*, 1986). Alternatively, the reported higher prevalence of dementia in the black community may also be indicative of the significant increase in longevity underway in the black older population.

Schoenberg *et al.* (1985) conducted a study of severe dementia in Copiah County, Mississippi. The distribution of subjects over age 40 was 39% black and 60% white. Table III reports the prevalence rates for severe dementia by sex and black–white ethnicity. The prevalence rates overall were similar to other studies, which also showed that rates for cognitive impairment increase with age. The prevalence of severe cognitive impairment was higher for black and white females after age 70 (black = 2.6, white = 1.4) but increased dramatically after age 80 (black = 9.5, white = 7.3.). Although black males had slightly higher rates after age 70 than white males (black = 2.1, white = 1.3), the trend reversed after age 80 and white males had a higher prevalence than black males (white = 5.9, black = 3.2). Addressing the significantly higher prevalence of dementia in the black population, Baker (1988) suggested that the majority of black older persons were primarily poor, had differential access to health care, and had risks from environmental exposures that may predispose older Blacks to higher rates of impairment. Case-control studies are recommended to screen for potential risk factors in the black population and

Table III
Prevalence Rates of Clinically Diagnosed
Dementia by Age, Race, and Sex per 100
Inhabitants in Copiah County, Mississippi

	Age groupings		
	60–69	70–79	80+
White males	0.538	1.265	5.882
White females	0.266	1.401	7.246
Black males	0.718	2.069	3.158
Black females	0.000	2.549	9.449
Total	0.351	2.550	6.807

[From B. S. Schoenberg, D. W. Andersen, and A. F. Haerer, 1985, Severe dementia. Prevalence and clinical features in a biracial U.S. population, *Arch. Neurol.* 42, 740–743.]

to determine if differential survival rates between blacks and whites are significant factors in the prevalence of dementia.

CONCERNS FOR CONDUCTING DEMENTIA RESEARCH IN THE AFRICAN AMERICAN COMMUNITY

The Problem of Misdiagnosis

African Americans are commonly overrepresented in hospital psychiatric wards, clinics, and community agencies that care for mentally ill patients. Many of the health care providers involved in their treatment are non-black, which may result in a lack of understanding of the cultural basis for presenting symptoms. Differences in economics, professional outlook, educational status, and use of language between the patients and their therapists may result in psychiatric misdiagnosis and treatment. Blacks are most often misdiagnosed as schizophrenic while affective disorders are consistently underdiagnosed (Stanford and Du Bois, 1992). The problems of misdiagnosis are further compounded by the myth that Blacks rarely, if ever, suffer from affective disorders (Mathura and Bayer, 1990).

The literature on misdiagnoses shows that approximately 10% of dementia cases are actually a consequence of nutritional, infectious, metabolic, and other disorders that can be treated (Roca *et al.*, 1984). Early detection of the dementia syndrome would make possible the treatment of many of these cases; however, some evidence indicates that diagnosis is often either missed or inappropriately applied in a variety of settings (Roca *et al.*, 1984). In using cognitive assessment batteries to screen for AD and other dementias, Roca *et al.* (1984) found that errors in sensitivity and specificity could be easily related to definable characteristics of patients under examination. Some patients with clouded consciousness were designated as demented despite the fact that their disturbances in consciousness precluded a diagnosis of dementia. In addition, many of the diagnoses tended to be overlooked in younger patients and also inappropriately applied to the less educated.

Misdiagnosis of black psychiatric patients has gained considerable attention (Baker, 1988). Without an adequate medical evaluation or an effective doctor–patient relationship, historical and clinical data essential for differential diagnosis may not be available.

Caregiving Support

Given the rapid increase of the older African American population, a major concern is the degree to which the population will be cared for in the later stages of life given the higher rate of dementing illnesses. Elder blacks and their caregivers will require more information and technical assistance from a sensitized health care system to be more aware not only of mental health needs and symptoms of impending mental illness, but also of specific caregiving requirements of certain courses of dementing illnesses (Carter, 1972, 1978, 1981). The care of AD patients is considered one of the more difficult types of care to provide: thus, AD is commonly considered a "catastrophic disease" because of its impact on the well-being of the patient and the caregivers.

The belief that the elder American population is better off now than any other group of citizens does not bode well for the well-being of minority older people. Government policies and various institutions may take the position that there is no real urgency in providing public support for the mental health and physical health needs of minority older people or their caregivers. This type of institutional neglect forces black patients upon their own communities for support.

As their health begins to decline, African Americans often rely on informal networks for support. This is largely due to limited access to health care resources. Kobata *et al.* (1980) point out that the family, church, and community are primary focal points of support in the black community. The black family perhaps best exemplifies its stability by fostering involvement in both the central and extended family by both those who are blood relatives and those who are members of the family through kinship and social networks. The black community fully utilizes the church as one of its primary outlets for a variety of emotional, social, and material supports. Blacks have demonstrated that there is a high degree of flexibility in developing support mechanisms for meeting the needs of individuals in the community, particularly older persons. Very old blacks often have a greater variety of available helpers and are more versatile than younger individuals in substituting helpers for one another (Jackson, 1981; Gibson and Jackson, 1987). Gibson (1986) cautions, however, that the nature of the supports in the black family could be greatly altered if the economic well-being of the black family declines. The readily available and dependable help from family, friends, and church members could become unreliable under adverse conditions. A major disruption could seriously challenge the in-home care of older blacks and could possibly have a damaging effect on their long-term health care needs (Saldo and Manton, 1985).

CONCLUSION

Literature has shown that cognitive impairment is more likely to occur among those who come from poor socioeconomic backgrounds, have poor health status, and have low educational attainment. Population trends show that ethnic minority people will constitute a higher proportion of the population in the future than they currently do. Thus, it is imperative that serious research efforts are undertaken to understand the etiology and risk factors associated with the development of AD and other dementias in susceptible populations. The paucity of data regarding dementias in the African American population supports this notion. Current and future research efforts will be directed to specifying the susceptibility profiles of dementia patients and elaborating the specific risk factors due to ethnic group membership. Epidemiological analyses currently underway will go far in specifying these conditions.

The problems associated with AD and related disorders continue to affect the health of the African American community. Until there is a collaborative effort and commitment among researchers, policymakers, and health care providers, problems will continue to exacerbate.

References

Baker, F. M. (1988). Dementing illness and black americans. *In* "The Black American Elderly: Research on Physical and Psychosocial Health" (J. S. Jackson, ed.), pp. 225–233. Springer, New York.

Butler, R. N., and Lewis, M. (1977). "Aging and Mental Health: Positive Psychosocial Approaches," 2nd ed. C. V. Mosby, St. Louis.

Carter, J. H. (1972). Psychiatry and aging. *J. Am. Geriatr. Soc.* **20**, 343–345.

Carter, J. H. (1978). The black aged: A strategy for future mental health services. *J. Am. Geriatr. Soc.* **26**(12), 553–556.

Carter, J. H. (1981). Treating black patients: The risk of ignoring critical social issues. *Hosp. Comm. Psychiatry* **32**(4), 281–282.

Chandra, V., Bharucha, N. E., and Schoenburg, B. S. (1986). Patterns of mortality from types of dementia in the United States, 1971 and 1973 to 1978. *J. Neurol.* **36**, 204–208.

Dressler, W. (1985). Extended family relationships, social support, and mental health in a southern black community. *J. Health Soc. Behav.* **26**, 39–48.

Dressler, W. (1986). Unemployment and depressive symptoms in a southern black community. *J. Nerv. Ment. Dis.* **174**(11), 639–645.

Du Bois, B. C., Stanford, E. P., Goodman, J., Happersett, C., and Morton, D. (unpublished). Depression and social resources in older black Americans. *J. Cross Cultural Gerontol.*

Folstein, M. F., Folstein, S. E., and McHugh, P. R. (1975). Mini-Mental State: A practical method for grading the cognitive status of patients for the clinician. *J. Psychiatr. Res.* **12**, 189–198.

Folstein, M., Anthony, J. C., Parhad, I., Duffy, B., and Gruenberg, E. M. (1985). The meaning of cognitive impairment in the elderly. *J. Am. Geriatr. Soc.* **33**, 228–235.

George, L. K., Landerman, R., Blazer, D. G., and Anthony, J. C. (1991). Cognitive impairment. *In* "Psychiatric Disorders in America: The Epidemiologic Catchment Area Study" (L. N. Robins and D. A. Regier, eds.) pp. 291–327. Free Press, New York.

Gibson, R. C. (1986). "Blacks in an Aging Society." Carnegie Corp., New York.

Gibson, R. C., and Jackson, J. S. (1987). The health of the black elderly. *Milbank Q.* **65**(suppl. to 1987), 422.

Jackson, J. (1981). Urban black Americans. *In* "Ethnicity and Medical Care" (A. Harwood, ed.), pp. 37–129. Harvard University Press, Cambridge, Massachusetts.

Jackson, J. S. (1988). Growing old in black America: Research on aging black populations. *In* "Black American Elderly Research on Physical and Psycho-social Health" (J. Jackson, ed.), pp. 3–16. Springer, New York.

Kobata, F. S., Lockery, S. A., and Moriwaki, S. Y. (1980). Minority issues in mental health and aging. *In* "Handbook of Mental Health and Aging" (J. E. Birren and R. B. Sloan, eds.). pp. 448–466. Prentice-Hall, New York.

Lilienfeld, A. M., and Lilienfeld, D. E. (1980). Mortality statistics. *In* Foundations of Epidemiology," pp. 66–83. 2nd ed. Oxford University Press, New York.

Manuel, R. C. (1988). The demography of older Blacks. *In* "The Black American Elderly: Research on Physical and Psychosocial Health" (J. S. Jackson, ed.), pp. 25–49. Springer Publishing, New York.

Mathura, C. B., and Bayer, M. A. (1990). Social factors in diagnosis and treatment. *In* "Handbook of Mental Health and Mental Disorder among Black Americans" (D. S. Ruiz, ed.), pp. 167–179. Greenwood Press, Westport, Connecticut.

Mortimer, J. A. (1988). Epidemiology of dementia; International comparisons. *In* "Epidemiology and Aging: An International Perspective" (J. A. Brody and G. L. Maddox, eds.), pp. 150–164. Springer, New York.

Mortimer, J. A. (1990). Epidemiology of dementia: Cross-cultural comparisons. *J. Adv. Neurol.* **51**, 27–33. *In* "Alzheimer's Disease" edited by (R. J. Wortman *et al.*, eds). Raven Press, New York.

Mortimer, J. A., and Schuman, L. M. (eds.). (1981). "The Epidemiology of Dementia. (p. 187). Oxford University Press, New York, p. 187.

Morton D. J., Stanford, E. P., Happersett, C., and Molgaard, C. (1992). Acculturation and functional impairment among older Chinese and Vietnamese in San Diego County, California. *J. Cross Cultural Gerontol.* **7,** 151–176.

Neighbors, H. W. (1986). Socioeconomic status and psychologic distress in adult Blacks. *Am. J. Epidemiol.* **124**(5), 779–780.

Reisberg, B. (ed.) (1983). "Alzheimer's Disease." Free Press, New York, p. 475.

Robins, L. N., Helzer, J. E., Croughan, J., Williams, J. B. W., and Spitzer, R. L. (1981). "NIMH Diagnostic Interview Schedule: Version III," May 1981. National Institute of Mental Health, Rockville, Maryland.

Roca, R. P., Klein, L. E., Kirby, S. M., *et al.* (1984). Recognition of dementia among medical patients. *ARC Intern. Med.* **144**(Jan.), 77–75.

Ron, M. A., Toone, B. K., Garralda, M. E., and Lishman, W. A. (1979). Diagnostic accuracy in presenile dementia. *Br. J. Psychiatry* **134,** 161–168.

Saldo, B. J., and Manton, K. G. (1985). Changes in the health status and service needs of the oldest old: Current patterns and future trends. *Millbank Memorial Fund Q./Health Soc.* **63**(2), 286–319.

Schoenberg, B. S., Anderson, D. W., and Haerer, A. F. (1985). Severe dementia. Prevalence and clinical features in a biracial U.S. population. *Arch. Neurol.* **42,** 740–743.

Standord, E. P. (1990). Mental health issues of minority elderly—An overview. *In* "Ethnicity and Aging: Mental Health Issues" (E. P. Stanford, S. A. Lockery, and S. A. Schoenrock, eds.), pp. 1–3. University Center on Aging, San Diego State University, San Diego.

Stanford, E. P., and Du Bois, B. C. (1992). Gender and ethnicity patterns. *In* "Handbook of Mental Health and Aging" (J. E. Birrens, R. B. Sloane, and G. D. Cohen, eds.) pp. 99–117. University of California Press, Los Angeles.

Stone, E. M. (ed.). (1988). "American Psychiatric Glossary." American Psychiatric Association Press, Washington, D.C., pp. 406–407.

U.S. Bureau of the Census (1980). Demographic aspects of aging and older populations in the United States. *Curr. Popul. Rep., Sp. Stud.* U.S. Government Printing Office, Washington, D.C.

Welsh, K., Butters, N., Hughes, J., Mohs, R., and Heyman, A. (1991). Detection of abnormal memory decline in mild cases of Alzheimer's disease using CERAD neuropsychological measures. *Arch. Neurol.* **48,** 278–281.

Wragg, R., and Jeste, D. V. (1989). Overview of depression and psychosis in Alzheimer's disease. *Am. J. Psychiatry* **146,** 577–587.

III

Population Surveillance in Neuroepidemiology

11

Prevalence at Birth of Neural Tube Defects in California: A Population-Based Study

Margarita E. Villarino • Amanda L. Golbeck
Craig A. Molgaard

Anencephaly, spina bifida, and encephalocele are congenital defects of the central nervous system collectively known as neural tube defects (NTDs). NTDs result from a failure of the neural tube to close by the 6th week of fetal development and their severity varies according to the location and size of the defect.

The etiology of NTDs is unknown. Thus, descriptive epidemiologic data has been the basis for hypothesis formulation of etiologic factors of NTDs. Because of the marked geographical variation in the prevalence rates of NTDs, it is important that these data be collected and analyzed for specific populations. Population-specific data also make it possible to identify demographic trends in NTD occurrences, to obtain information for planning prenatal diagnostic services for NTDs and health care programs for children with NTDs, and to evaluate the effectiveness of the programs already in place.

In this chapter, we summarize the prevalence rates of NTDs reported for the United States population. We also review the national and international studies on the epidemiologic patterns of NTDs and those studies that focus primarily on potential etiologic factors of NTDs. Finally, we describe the prevalence rates and epidemiologic characteristics of NTDs in the State of California for 1978–1985, estimated from the California Birth Cohort Perinatal Files (CBCPF) for the corresponding years. Our study represents one of the largest population-based studies of NTD births in a large, heterogeneous population, with a reported low prevalence rate of NTDs.

FREQUENCY OF NEURAL TUBE DEFECT BIRTHS IN THE UNITED STATES

The frequency rate of NTDs is usually estimated as the number of births affected with a NTD and the total number of births. The total number of births is defined as livebirths or total births (livebirths and stillbirths) from a specified gestational age, usually 20 or 28 weeks. This rate is sometimes called the prevalence rate at birth (Elwood and Elwood, 1980). Because approximately 50% of conceptuses with a NTD are spontaneously aborted (Creasy and Alberman, 1976), they are not included in these estimates of disease frequency.

The rates reported in some of the largest prevalence studies of NTDs in the United States are summarized in Table I. Overall, the prevalence rate of NTDs for the United States population appears to center around 1 per 1000 livebirths, although consideration should be given to the time periods analyzed and the type of case ascertainment used by the different studies.

EPIDEMIOLOGIC CHARACTERISTICS OF NEURAL TUBE DEFECT BIRTHS

Several epidemiologic characteristics of NTDs are helpful in understanding the relative importance that environmental or genetic factors might have in their etiology (Sever, 1982). These environmental or nongenetic factors are the seasonal and geographic variations, the maternal and socioeconomic effects, and the reported associations with the use of fertility drugs and dietary intake. The genetic or nonenvironmental factors are the sex and race differences in the rates of NTDs.

Environmental or Nongenetic Factors

Population studies have provided little evidence to suggest the role of a single teratogen as the sole cause of a significant number of NTDs. They have, however, provided suggestive evidence for the contribution of environmental factors to an increased risk of NTDs.

Geographic Variation

Geographic variation is wide, both between and within countries. Among predominantly caucasoid populations, reported prevalence rates range from 0.32 per 1000 births for anencephaly and 0.38 per 1000 births for

Table I

Reported Prevalence Rates (PRs) of Neural Tube Defects in the United States

Reference	Data Source	Geographical area	Time period	PR per 1000 live births	Type of defect	
					Anencephaly	Spina bifida
Khoury et al., 1982	Birth Defects Monitoring Program	Nationwide	1970–1978	Not stated	0.50	0.60
Khoury et al., 1982	Metropolitan Atlanta Congenital Defects Program	Metropolitan Atlanta area	1968–1979	Not stated	0.70	0.90
Sever, 1982	Multiple sources	Los Angeles County	1966–1972	1.1	0.52	0.51
Myrianthopoulos and Melnick, 1987	Collaborative Perinatal Project	12 urban medical centers nationwide	1959–1966	1.33	0.68	0.71

spina bifida in Finland, to 4.45 per 1000 births for anencephaly and 4.50 per 1000 births for spina bifida in Belfast, Northern Ireland (Leck, 1984). Leck (1984) in an analysis of a series of over 10,000 individuals worldwide found Great Britain and Ireland occupying the upper part of the international prevalence rates range, whereas most of the rates reported for North America and mainland Europe clustered toward the center and the lower end of the range. Within the British Isles, NTDs are more common in Northern Ireland than in southeast England (Seller, 1987). For mainland Europe, limited data does not reveal any regular geographical pattern. However, for both anencephaly and spina bifida, Hungary has the highest reported figures (Czeizel and Karig, 1985), which are more than double those observed in the neighboring countries of Czechoslovakia and Yugoslavia.

Variability has also been noted within the United States, with prevalence rates higher in the northeast and lower in the west, respectively (Khoury *et al.*, 1982). This east-to-west gradient is supported by the available studies, which have found spina bifida rates ranging from 1.6 per 1000 births in New York State, to 1.0 per 1000 births in the State of Iowa, to 0.5 per 1000 births in Los Angeles County, California (Sever, 1982).

Among descendants of immigrants, the prevalence rates of NTDs tend to be intermediate between the country of origin and the new country of residence (Myrianthopoulos and Melnick, 1987). Prevalence rates of anecenphaly in reports published between 1961 and 1976 were 2.6–3.3 per 1000 births in Scotland, whereas the rate in Canadian Scots was 1.5 per 1000 births (Elwood and Elwood, 1980). During the same period, rates for Ireland were 2.1–4.7, whereas the rates for Irish in Canada were 1.8 and in Boston were 1.2 per 1000 births (Rhoads and Mills, 1986).

Seasonal Variation

It is generally accepted that there is seasonal variation in the birth of children with NTDs. In Great Britain, infants conceived in March, April, or May (Campbell *et al.*, 1986) appear to be at highest risk; in Canada, September and October conceptions appear to result in the highest rate (Dallaire *et al.*, 1984). There was an absence of a seasonal effect in the study conducted by Sever (1982) in Los Angeles County, California, and the majority of North American studies have failed to detect any significant seasonal variation for either anencephaly or spina bifida (Elwood and Elwood, 1980).

In addition to the variation with time of conception, there appears to be a wide fluctuation in the prevalence rate for different years and decades, suggesting an epidemic pattern. A review of secular trends during this century revealed that various peaks of NTDs have occurred in different locations. Elwood and Elwood (1980) reported an increase in the prevalence of anencephaly in Dublin from 1 per 1000 births in 1900 to 8 per 1000 births in the 1960s, with peaks during 1938–1941 and 1960–1961. MacMahon and Yen (1971) found that the rates in Boston rose from 2.08 per 1000 births in 1900–1904 to 4.69 per 1000 births in 1930–1934. Subsequently, the rates decreased to 1.43 per 1000 births (1960–1965). Haynes *et al.* (1974) described the prevalence at birth of NTDs in Olmsted County, Minnesota, from 1935 to 1971: There was a peak in spina bifida and anencephaly prevalence in 1944–1945 but no evidence of an earlier peak.

A worldwide secular decline in the prevalence of NTDs over the last decade, which cannot be entirely explained by prenatal screening, has been shown in some studies. In the United States, a study that analyzed three different sources of data—the Birth Defects Monitoring Program (BDMP), the Metropolitan Atlanta Congenital Defects Program (MACDP), and the National Center for Health Statistics Data (NCHS)—over a 10-year period (1970–1979) found a decreasing trend in NTD rates with average annual percentage decreases of 3.1% for the NCHS, 5.7% for the BDMP, and 7.7% for the MACDP (Windham and Edmonds, 1982). The decrease was noted in all variables examined: race, sex, and birth status (livebirth or fetal death) for both anencephaly and spina bifida.

In 1972, the prevalence of NTDs in England and Wales was 4.26 per 1000 births; in 1984 it was 1.26 per 1000 births (Seller, 1987). In Dublin, four maternity hospitals reported a prevalence of 6.6 per 1000 births from 1970 to 1973 compared to a prevalence of 3.98 per 1000 births from the same area 10 years later (O'Dowd *et al.*, 1987).

Maternal Age and Parity

Many studies have described a U-shaped distribution of the prevalence rates of anencephaly or spina bifida with either maternal age or parity considered alone, with high risks in mothers under 20 years old and in primiparae, and also in those over 35 years old and those of high parity. The lower rates are usually in mothers aged 20–24 years and of parity one. This type of age distribution has been shown in British and North American populations (Elwood and Elwood, 1980). However, some reports that show a linear increase with parity and no age effect have come from Finland, British Columbia, Hungary, Australia, and the United States (Elwood and Elwood, 1980; Sever, 1982; Naggan, 1971), all areas of relatively low prevalence. It has been suggested that this pattern may be typical of low-prevalence regions, with the excess risk in primiparae being due to a separate etiological factor found only in high-prevalence areas (Naggan, 1971). The relationship of the prevalence of anencephaly and spina bifida to each factor taking into account effects of the second factor has also been described. Elwood and Elwood (1980), in their study of anencephaly in 14 Canadian cities, found a U-type distribution for maternal age and parity. The differences in risk by maternal age were not large, and a stronger risk was related to the total parity of the mother.

Factors that may potentially alter the age and parity distributions of mothers of children with NTDs are (1) those that affect all mothers in the population simultaneously (i.e., an exposure to an epidemic of infectious disease during pregnancy) and (2) those that affect the mothers before the pregnancy in question. If these latter maternal factors operate at a certain age, a secular trend in the rates of NTDs will be related to the mother's year of birth rather than to the year in which the children are born.

Socioeconomic Status

An inverse relationship between NTDs and socioeconomic status (SES) has been considered one of the strongest indicators of an etiologic role for nongenetic factors (Sever, 1982; Leck, 1984). The evidence for the influence of SES on the prevalence rates of NTDs has been more apparent in Great Britain. Several studies have shown a progressive increase in the prevalence rate of NTDs from higher to lower socioeconomic class as determined by the father's occupation (Carter, 1974). Sever's (1982) data on occupational class failed to support an important role for SES-associated factors in the etiology of NTDs in the Los Angeles population, and some of the most recent studies in Britian have found that the differences between the highest and lowest socioeconomic classes are no longer as great as in the past (Leck, 1974). A link with dietary deficiencies seems probable, because women of lower SES are more likely than others to have a poorly balanced diet.

Dietary Intake Studies

Four recent studies (three case-control studies and one cohort study) have been conducted to test the hypothesis that vitamin-supplement vitamin use is related to NTDs; three of them reported a protective effect associated with multivitamin-supplement use or high levels of dietary folate intake, and one reported no association between multivitamin use and NTDs. In the study by Mulinare *et al.* (1988), women in Atlanta, Georgia, who used supplements periconceptionally were found to have a significantly lower risk for all types of NTDs than women who did not use supplements. In Australia, Bower and Stanley (1989) found a fivefold increase in the risk of women in the lowest level of free folate compared to those in the highest level. In this study, several dietary factors, including fiber and vitamins A and C, were also found to confer protection against NTD births. Mills *et al.* (1989) studied case-mothers from Illinois and California and reported that high intake of vitamin supplements prior to pregnancy does not alter a woman's risk of having an infant with a NTD. The study by Milunsky *et al.* (1989) prospectively examined the relation of multivitamin intake to the risk of NTDs in a cohort of women who underwent amniocentesis or had serum α-fetoprotein assay at about 16 weeks of pregnancy and reported that multivitamin folic acid intake was protective for NTDs. A clear association between vitamin-supplement use and NTDs was not documented by any of these studies. Methodological differences between them might explain some of the differences observed in the findings.

Fertility Drugs

Studies of the potential association between fertility drug exposure and increased risk of a NTD birth have found inconsistent results. Case reports and some studies using birth defects registry data suggest an association (Schardein, 1980; Elwood and Elwood, 1980). However, others have not found an increase in NTDs among infants of women who were treated with ovulation-inducing drugs while attending infertility clinics (Cuckle and Wald, 1989). A recent case-control study by Mills *et al.* (1990) compared ovulation-inducing drug exposure in NTD case-mothers, abnormal control mothers, and normal control mothers and found no difference. A meta-analysis by Vollset (1990) found a significant association between fertility drugs and NTDs by adding together data from a number of reports. Milunsky *et al.* (1990) offer additional support from this claim. They compared the risk for occurrence of NTDs among users of clomiphene during the 3 months prior to pregnancy (2 of 438, or 0.5%) to the risk of occurrence of NTDs in women who did not report the use of clomiphene (47 of 22,317, or 0.2%). The relative risk estimate in this study was 2.2 (95% CI 0.6–8.6). Although their results are not statistically significant, they postulate a potential association of clomiphene citrate and NTDs, in the absence of a known biological mechanism of action.

Genetic or Nonenvironmental Factors

Population studies have emphasized the increased prevalence rates of NTDs in certain races/ethnic groups and the greater number of affected females than males as evidence of the role of genetic factors in the etiology of NTDs.

Ethnic/Racial Differences

Two ethnic groups known to have a high prevalence of NTDs are the British and Sikhs (Carter, 1974), with prevalence rates of up to 8 per 1000 births. Although the rate is somewhat decreased, a higher prevalence rate persists after migration of these groups to regions of low prevalence. In the cities in England and the United States were data for more than one primary race have been collected, infants of predominately negroid or mongoloid ancestry tend to be at lower risk of both anencephaly and spina bifida than their caucasoid neighbors (Leck, 1984). The black population in Africa has a low prevalence of NTDs (i.e., 1 per 1000 births in Lagos), and this low rate persists even after migration to areas of high prevalence such as Great Britain (Carter, 1974).

A higher incidence of anencephaly in whites than in blacks has been documented. Sever's (1982) Los Angeles County study reported a white:black ratio for anencephaly of 1.8:1, whereas the ratio for spina bifida was 1.4:1. Khoury's Atlanta-based study (Khoury *et al.*, 1982) found a white:black ratio for anencephaly of 3.1:1 and for spina bifida of 2.5:1. In a large prospective study that included data from 12 medical centers throughout the United States, Myrianthopoulos and Melnick (1987) found a significantly higher prevalence in whites (1.6 per 1000 births) than in blacks (0.9 per 1000 births). In this study, the white:black ratio for anencephaly was 3.7:1, whereas for spina bifida it was only slightly higher for whites than for blacks (1.2:1).

Distribution by Sex

In most communities, anencephaly and spina bifida are seen more frequently in females than in males. Within caucasian groups,the male proportion ranges from 0.23 in Belfast, Northern Ireland, to 0.46 in Sydney, New South Wales (Elwood and Elwood, 1980). In British and European populations, the male proportion of anencephaly appears to be higher in communities having a low prevalence at birth. However, reports from the United States find that blacks, who comprise a low-prevalence group, have high male proportions of anencephaly (Sever, 1982; Khoury *et al.*, 1982). This may suggest a difference between caucasian and other racial groups.

As presently estimated, cases of anencephaly represent those fetuses that have survived to 20 weeks of gestation. Thus, a female excess at this time may represent either more females being affected or more males being lost before this gestational age. It appears that the postulated female excess is more pronounced in anencephaly than in spina bifida (Carter, 1974). Khoury *et al.* (1982) found a race-adjusted relative risk for white females of 1.8 for Atlanta and 1.5 nationwide for the occurrence of isolated NTDs. Myrianthopoulos and Melnick (1987) found a male : female ratio of 0.54 : 1 for anencephaly, spina bifida, and encephalocele combined, and a male : female ratio of 0.50 : 1 for anencephaly alone, based on their data from the National Institutes of Health Collaborative Perinatal Project. In Los Angeles County (Sever, 1982), the male : female sex ratio for anencephaly was 0.59 : 1, for spina bifida 0.95 : 1, and for encephalocele 0.89 : 1.

METHODS

Subjects and Setting

California contains a total population of more than 24 million, distributed among 58 counties and a total land area of 156,573 square miles. San Diego County alone has over 2 million inhabitants distributed over approximately 4000 square miles of land area and the city of San Diego is currently the eight largest in the United States, with a population of 1,022,400 (U.S. Census, 1980). The state as a whole is very heterogeneous in its composition, with a multicultural, multilevel SES population, and its proximity to the Mexican border and recent influx of Southeast Asian refugees has contributed to a great diversity of ethnic groups. At present, 38% of California's population is from racial/ethnic minorities (40% for San Diego County), and it has been estimated that 24% of California State residents are women of childbearing age (U.S. Census, 1980). From 1978 through 1985 (the time period of this study), there were approximately 400,000 livebirths and 3000 fetal deaths per year reported for the State of California, and more than 30,000 livebirths and 300 fetal deaths per year reported for San Diego County.

California Birth Cohort Perinatal Files

The CBCPF are compiled by the Maternal and Child Health Branch of the California Department of Health Services. Each record in the CBCPF is a composite of livebirth, linked infant death (if the child dies within the first year of life), and fetal death records filed in California for a given calendar year (Oreglia and Tashiro, 1986). Some edits and enhancements are included in the CBCPF that are not available in the state's annual vital statistics birth and fetal death files (e.g., ethnicity codes; reallocation of certificates of livebirths, infant deaths, and fetal deaths that occurred out of state back to the state of residence; congenital malformation codes) thus, the CBCPF data are more complete and accurate. By using files with linked infant death records, cases of infants who died with a NTD who were not shown to have a NTD on their birth certificate were counted as misclassifications and included in the analysis.

At the time of our analysis, the most current CBCPF available was the 1985 file, a "first-stage" file containing 1985 fetal deaths and livebirths with linked neonatal deaths (deaths occurring within the first 30 days after birth). The most recent "complete" CBCPF was the 1984 file, a "second-stage" file containing 1984 fetal deaths and livebirths with linked neonatal *and* postneonatal deaths (deaths occurring within the first year of life, but after the first 30 days after birth). The CBCPF from 1978 through 1985 were used as the database for determining the prevalence at birth rates of selected NTDs. We believe that the absence of postneonatal deaths for the year 1985 did not seriously compromise the ascertainment of NTDs for that year, because most of the liveborn children with anencephaly not reported on a livebirth certificate probably died within the neonatal period. Cases of spina bifida not reported on a livebirth certificate may have been nonsevere cases with a low probability of dying even within the first year of life; thus, it would not have been possible to identify them using the infant neonatal or postneonatal death certificate. CBCPF from years prior to 1978 were not included in the analysis because the coding used for congenital malformations in these files differed greatly from the one used for the years 1978–1985.

Study Design and Case Definition

The study design was a population-based analysis of the prevalence at birth rates of NTDs from January 1, 1975 to December 31, 1985, for the State of California and San Diego County. Because the CBCPF provide complete coverage for the geographic area and the time period studied, the only sampling involved was the identification of eligible cases within the dimension of time specified. CBCPF were analyzed as "residence" files—all livebirths, fetal deaths, and infant deaths occurring to California residents regardless of where the birth occurred—with the intent of homogenizing the environmental influences affecting the maternal at-risk population before and during the pregnancy in question.

Out of all possible central nervous system anomalies found under the CBCPF malformation code, only the following ICD-9-CM (NCHS, 1986) categories were included: category 740 (anencephaly and similar anomalies) with subcategories 740.0 (anencephaly), 740.1 (craniorachischisis), and 740.2 (iniencephaly), and category 741 (spina bifida, excluding spina bifida occulta) with subcategories 741.0 (spina bifida with hydrocephalus occurring in any region of the spinal cord) and 741.9 (0–3) (spina bifida without mention of hydrocephalus occurring in any region of the spinal cord).

The justifications for including only these categories of NTDs in our analysis are (1) the majority of NTDs are evenly divided between spina bifida and anencephaly, (2) anencephaly poses few diagnostic problems because the malformation is dramatic and readily recognizable at birth, (3) spina bifida occulta is apparent only after a roentgenographic examination, which is not routinely done at birth, and (4) the ICD-9 category 742.3 (congenital hydrocephalus) was not included because even if the hydrocephalus was due to a NTD (there is no consensus that hydrocephalus is part of the NTD spectrum), this condition is not always apparent at birth and might be obvious only in the latter neonatal or infancy period and, thus, not recorded in the certificates included in the CBCPF.

In the CBCPF from 1978 through 1981, the ICD-9 congenital malformation categories 740–741 (anencephaly/spina bifida) were undiscernibly combined to create a single malformation category used for those years. Thus, the breakdown analysis for anencephaly and spina bifida could be done only for the years from 1982 through 1985. The overall analysis of prevalence at birth rates was done for the 8-year period (1978–1985) for anencephaly and spina bifida combined.

Denominator data were obtained from published vital statistics for the State of California (California Department of Health Services, 1978–1985).

Statistical Analysis

The CBCPF were analyzed using the appropriate SPSS^x computer program and the San Diego State University Cyber mainframe computer. The statistical analyses were performed using the StatView II computer program.

For the purpose of evaluating a possible difference among the proportion of NTDs between San Diego County when compared to the rest of the State of California, confidence intervals were estimated around the two independent proportions using methods described in Fleiss (1980).

RESULTS

Table II presents types of NTDs for all of California during the study period in terms of prevalence at birth per 1000 events. It should be noted that the rates for anencephaly and spina bifida combined were stable throughout the study period as well as when examined separately. An examination of 95% confidence intervals confirms this trend. Also, the slightly higher point estimate for anencephaly alone (0.4040 per 1000) in 1982 produced confidence intervals that were significantly higher than those for 1983 and 1985, but not for 1984.

Table III contains total births with anencephaly and spina bifida during the study period for San Diego County alone and California minus San Diego County. A distribution is made between fetal death and livebirth outcomes. As can be seen, there is no difference by 95% confidence interval by total outcome between regions. This is also the case for livebirths analyzed separately and fetal deaths analyzed separately.

Rates and confidence intervals for anencephaly alone and spina bifida alone by region are presented in Tables IV and V, once again distin-

Table II

Types of Congenital Malformations in California (per 1000), 1978–1985

Anencephaly and Spina Bifida			Anencephaly			Spina Bifida		
Year	Rate	CI	Year	Rate	CI	Year	Rate	CI
1978	0.5984	0.5223–0.6853	1978	NA	NA	1978	NA	NA
1979	0.5697	0.4977–0.6519	1979	NA	NA	1979	NA	NA
1980	0.4946	0.4296–0.5691	1980	NA	NA	1980	NA	NA
1981	0.4599	0.3987–0.5304	1981	NA	NA	1981	NA	NA
1982	0.5888	0.5197–0.6668	1982	0.4040	0.3474–0.4697	1982	0.1755	0.1392–0.2209
1983	0.4557	0.3957–0.5246	1983	0.2825	0.2359–0.3381	1983	0.1618	0.1273–0.2053
1984	0.5194	0.4559–0.5915	1984	0.3396	0.2889–0.3990	1984	0.1709	0.1358–0.2148
1985	0.4092	0.3546–0.4721	1985	0.2784	0.2339–0.3313	1985	0.1287	0.0993–0.1664

Abbreviation: NA, not available.

Table III

Anencephaly and Spina Bifida by Outcome Type in San Diego County and California Minus San Diego County (per 1000), 1978–1985

Year	Fetal death Rate	Fetal death CI	Livebirth Rate	Livebirth CI	Total Rate	Total CI
San Diego						
1978	0.0000	NA	0.8114	0.5212–1.2504	0.8045	0.5168–1.2398
1979	19.1571	7.0714–46.6574	0.2725	0.1267–0.5601	0.4389	0.2441–0.7720
1980	22.9008	9.3405–51.5918	0.4850	0.2817–0.8201	0.6732	0.4277–1.0484
1981	32.7273	16.0519–63.3294	0.3085	0.1567–0.5877	0.5811	0.3601–0.9261
1982	34.8101	18.4050–63.2234	0.4439	0.2579–0.7507	0.7623	0.5084–1.1342
1983	11.0701	2.8612–34.7047	0.4040	0.2299–0.6960	0.4867	0.2929–0.7970
1984	21.1268	8.6145–47.6643	0.2521	0.1230–0.4973	0.4168	0.2421–0.7049
1985	17.4216	6.4291–42.5005	0.3763	0.2142–0.6484	0.5068	0.3141–0.8077
California						
1978	0.0000	NA	0.5864	0.5079–0.6768	0.5814	0.5036–0.6710
1979	22.4719	17.6828–28.4730	0.3858	0.3247–0.4581	0.5807	0.5051–0.6673
1980	15.0060	11.2712–19.8976	0.3496	0.2932–0.4165	0.4797	0.4134–0.5565
1981	15.5958	11.7149–20.6774	0.3247	0.2715–0.3879	0.4498	0.3869–0.5227
1982	27.4282	22.0916–33.9671	0.3637	0.3078–0.4295	0.5739	0.5031–0.6545
1983	21.4789	16.6030–27.6894	0.3041	0.2536–0.3645	0.4530	0.3908–0.5249
1984	25.7909	20.4718–32.3979	0.3498	0.2960–0.4131	0.5283	0.4617–0.6043
1985	18.8046	14.3630–24.5278	0.2744	0.2283–0.3296	0.4008	0.3446–0.4660

Table IV

Anencephaly by Outcome Type in San Diego County and California Minus San Diego County (per 1000), 1982–1985

	Fetal death			Livebirth			Total		
Year	Rate	CI	Year	Rate	CI	Year	Rate	CI
				San Diego					
1982	25.3165	11.8186–51.2004	1982	0.2663	0.1300–0.5255	1982	.4984	.3000–.8162
1983	11.0701	2.8633–34.7081	1983	0.2020	0.0885–0.4363	1983	.2863	.1455–.5455
1984	21.1268	8.6167–47.6674	1984	0.2241	0.1042–0.4607	1984	.3890	.2214–.6704
1985	17.4216	6.4312–42.5035	1985	0.1882	0.0825–0.4064	1985	.3201	.1735–.5764
				California					
1982	21.2972	16.6330–27.1841	1982	0.2324	0.1884–0.2863	1982	.3960	.3377–.4641
1983	17.9577	13.5323–23.7320	1983	0.1571	0.1217–0.2023	1983	.2822	.2338–.3403
1984	20.6327	15.9125–26.6595	1984	0.1919	0.1529–0.2405	1984	.3353	.2829–.3972
1985	16.4540	12.3236–21.8757	1985	0.1637	0.1288–0.2078	1985	.2749	.2288–.3299

Table V
Spina Bifida by Outcome Type in San Diego County and California Minus San Diego County (per 1000), 1982–1985

	Fetal death			Livebirth			Total	
Year	Rate	CI	Year	Rate	CI	Year	Rate	CI
				San Diego				
1982	6.3291	1.0953–25.1856	1982	0.1776	0.0722–0.4075	1982	0.2346	0.1090–0.4822
1983	0.0000	NA	1983	0.2020	0.0885–0.4362	1983	0.2004	0.0878–0.4329
1984	0.0000	NA	1984	0.0280	0.0014–0.1819	1984	0.0278	0.0014–0.1804
1985	0.0000	NA	1985	0.1882	0.0824–0.4064	1985	0.1867	0.0818–0.4033
				California				
1982	5.8083	3.5520–9.3597	1982	0.1263	0.0947–0.1679	1982	0.1704	0.1333–0.2174
1983	2.8169	1.3101–5.7810	1983	0.1396	0.1064–0.1827	1983	0.1584	0.1230–0.2037
1984	4.1265	2.2371–7.4168	1984	0.1555	0.1207–0.1999	1984	0.1833	0.1454–0.2308
1985	2.3506	1.0320–5.0689	1985	0.1084	0.0805–0.1454	1985	0.1237	0.0938–0.1627

guishing between fetal deaths and livebirths. For spina bifida, there were no significant differences. For anencephaly, there were also no differences when comparing the two regions by fetal death or livebirth or total births.

Rates and confidence intervals by sex and region for anencephaly alone and spina bifida alone during the years when they were recorded separately (1982–1985) are presented in Tables VI and VII. Except for male anencephalics in 1982 (when San Diego rates were significantly higher than California), no statistically significant differences are evident. Rates and confidence intervals by race (white versus black) for anencephaly and spina bifida for California during the years when they were recorded separately are presented in Table VIII. There was a significantly higher proportion of white NTD births for anencephaly during this time period.

DISCUSSION

This study utilized data from the CBCPF to examine prevalence at birth of NTDs. The data suggest that California has at present low and stable rates of NTDs. Ericson *et al.* (1988) note that NTDs have decreased in rate in many populations. Given that environmental exposures such as water pollution, air pollution, and background radiation are unevenly distributed and that the genetic constitution of the California population is also geographically uneven, it is also of interest that the rates comparing this particular form of adverse outcome between San Diego County and the rest of California are as similar as they are.

Table VI

Anencephaly by Sex in San Diego County and California Minus San Diego County (per 1000), 1982–1985

	Male			Female	
Year	Rate	CI	Year	Rate	CI
		San Diego			
1982	0.7457	0.4147–1.3117	1982	0.2399	0.0768–0.6595
1983	0.2235	0.0716–0.6144	1983	0.3523	0.1432–0.8085
1984	0.3784	0.1658–0.8171	1984	0.4003	0.1754–0.8644
1985	0.4684	0.2286–0.9241	1985	0.1642	0.0424–0.5230
		California			
1982	0.3035	0.2346–0.3917	1982	0.4930	0.4025–0.6048
1983	0.2611	0.1981–0.3434	1983	0.3043	0.2342–0.3945
1984	0.2971	0.2302–0.3827	1984	0.3753	0.2977–0.4724
1985	0.2192	0.1639–0.2924	1985	0.3332	0.2621–0.4228

Table VII

Spina Bifida by Sex in San Diego County and California Minus San Diego County (per 1000), 1982–1985

	Male			Female	
Year	Rate	CI	Year	Rate	CI
		San Diego			
1982	0.2868	0.1056–0.7112	1982	0.1799	0.0464–0.5732
1983	0.1676	0.0433–0.5340	1983	0.2349	0.0752–0.6457
1984	0.0000	NA	1984	0.0572	0.0030–0.3713
1985	0.2082	0.0667–0.5724	1985	0.1642	0.0424–0.5230
		California			
1982	0.1420	0.0968–0.2067	1982	0.2003	0.1444–0.2767
1983	0.1741	0.1237–0.2438	1983	0.1420	0.0962–0.2082
1984	0.1839	0.1326–0.2541	1984	0.1827	0.1305–0.2547
1985	0.1253	0.0849–0.1837	1985	0.1220	0.0814–0.1816

The prevalence at birth rates of NTDs for the years 1978–1985 were 0.51 and 0.49 per 1000 births for California and San Diego County, respectively. For anencephaly alone, fetal deaths compromised 42.53% of the total sample. Of our total sample size for NTD births, 32% was ascertained through fetal death certificates. This finding is consistent with published figures that report the proportion of stillborn anencephaly births (Baird and Sadovnick, 1984; Sever, 1982), and it reflects the importance of utilizing data sources that include cases of stillborn infants with congenital defects in the ascertainment of the prevalence rates of such defects.

In our study, the estimated rates were higher for anencephaly than for spina bifida. This finding is not consistent with most other studies conducted in the United States (Myrianthopoulos and Melnick, 1987; Khoury

Table VIII

Anencephaly and Spina Bifida by Race in California (per 1000), 1982–1985

Race category	Rate	CI
	Anencephaly	
White	0.3355	0.3063–0.3674
Black	0.1819	0.1265–0.2601
	Spina Bifida	
White	0.1670	0.1467–0.1901
Black	0.1478	0.0986–0.2200

et al., 1982); however, Sever's (1982) Los Angeles County study found a higher prevalence of anencephaly than of spina bifida.

The prevalence rates of NTDs estimated by out study are low in comparison to other published studies for the United States (see Table I). This could be due to (1) not all observed malformations necessarily get recorded on the corresponding certificate, even though NTDs are almost always clinically obvious at birth, (2) diagnostic variability and inadequacy, (3) underdetection of subtle birth defects, (4) differences in case ascertainment, and (5) differences in time periods studied.

Except for Sever's (1982) Los Angeles County study, other published studies have all utilized databases specifically created for surveillance of congenital defects, and the two studies (Myrianthopoulos and Malnick, 1987; Khoury *et al.*, 1982) that reported summary prevalence rates included cases of encephalocele in their estimation, which our study does not. Our study analyzed prevalence rates of NTDs from 1978 through 1985. The most recent year analyzed by any of the other studies was 1979 (Khoury *et al.*, 1982), going back as late as 1959 (Myrianthopoulos and Melnick, 1987). A change in the diagnostic criteria of NTDs, such as if during the period of the earlier studies a greater number of congenital defects of the central nervous system were classified as NTDs than during the period of our study, would account for higher prevalence rates in the earlier studies, or the rates of NTDs may have actually declined from one study period to another. To support the latter hypothesis, statistical testing for significance in the difference among the rates estimated by the different studies would have to be accomplished by adjusting for the differences in case ascertainment. If this is somehow possible, it would be of great importance for establishing the presence of a true decline in the rates of these congenital defects in the western United States.

As expected, the prevalence rates estimated by our study were significantly higher in white NTD births (for anencephaly) than in black NTD births. The number of white NTD births was also significantly higher than the "other races" category (data not shown), but the great racial diversity among this "other" group precludes us from doing meaningful inferences. Also not unexpectedly, our study found that in California there is a female preponderance of NTD births mainly attributable to a female excess of cases of anencephaly.

In conclusion, the prevalence at birth of NTDs is low in California. Rates of occurrence may even be as low as the rates reported for traditionally very low prevalence populations such as Finland and Czechoslovakia. The estimated prevalence rates were found to be relatively stable across the time period studied.

Population-based studies of the prevalence and distribution of NTDs such as ours provide direct experience that is useful in planning services and assessing the impact of proposals for population screening. Investigations that focus on the etiology(ies) of these defects will define some of the epidemiological complexities related to them and, thus, will aid in identifying methods to prevent their occurrence. Until then, surveillance efforts, methods of screening, and improved prenatal diagnostic techniques of NTDs, along with optimizing the care for the children born with these defects, should continue to be priorities in health care.

References

Baird, P. A., and Sadovnick, A. D. (1984). Survival in infants with anencephaly. *Clin. Pediatr.* **23,** 268–272.

Bower, C., and Stanley, F. J. (1989). Dietary folate as a risk factor for neural-tube defects; Evidence from a case-control study in Western Australia. *Med. J. Aust.* **150,** 613–619.

California Department of Health Services. (1978–1985). Vital statistics of California. State of California, Sacramento.

Campbell, L. R., Dayton, D. H., and Sohal, G. S. (1986). Neural tube defects: A review of human and animal studies on the etiology of neural tube defects. *Teratology* **34,** 171–187.

Carter, C. O. (1974). Clues to the aetiology of neural tube malformations. *Dev. Med. Child Neurol.* **32,** 3–15.

Creasy, M. R., and Alberman, E. D. (1976). Congenital malformations of the central nervous system in spontaneous abortions. *J. Med. Gen.* **13,** 8–11.

Cuckle, H., and Wald, N. (1989). Ovulation induction and neural tube defects. *Lancet* **2,** 1281 (letter).

Czeizel, A., and Karig, G. (1985). Analysis of the changing prevalence of neural tube defects in Hungary. *Acta Morphol. Hung.* **33**(1–2), 89–99.

Dallaire, L., Melancon, S. B., Potter, M., Mathieu, J. P., and Ducharme, G. (1984). Date of conception and prevention of neural tube defects. *Clin. Gen.* **26,** 304–307.

Elwood, J. M., and Elwood, J. H. (1980). "Epidemiology of Anencephalus and Spina Bifida." Oxford University Press, Oxford.

Ericson, A., Kallen B., and Lofkvist, E. (1988). Environmental factors in the etiology of neural tube defects: A negative study. *Environ. Res.* **45,** 38–47.

Fleiss, J. (1980). "Statistical Rates and Proportions." John Wiley and Sons, New York.

Haynes, S. G., Gibson, J. B., and Kurland, L. T. (1974). Epidemiology of neural tube defects and Down's syndrome in Rochester. Minnesota, 1935–1971. *Neurology* **24,** 691–700.

Khoury, M. J., Erickson, J. D., and James, L. M. (1982). Etiologic heterogeneity of neural tube defects: Clues from epidemiology. *Am. J. Epidemiol.* **115**(4), 538–548.

Leck, I. (1974). Causation of neural tube defects: Clues from epidemiology. *Bri. Med. Bull.* **30,** 158–163.

Leck, J. (1984). The geographical distribution of neural tube defects and oral clefts. *Bri. Med. Bull.* **40**(4), 390–395.

MacMahon, B., and Yen, S. (1971). Unrecognized epidemic of anencephaly and spina bifida. *Lancet* **1,** 31–33.

Mills, J. L., Rhoads, G. G., Simpson, J. L., Cunningham, G. C., Conley, M. R., Lassman, M. R., and Walden, M. E., Deep, O. R., Hoffman, H. J., and the National Institute of Child Health and Human Development Neural Tube Defects Study Group. (1989). The absence of a relation between the periconceptional use of vitamins and neural tube defects. *N. Engl. J. Med.* **321,** 430–435.

Mills, J. L., Simpson, J. L., Rhoads, G. G., Graubard, B. I., Hoffman, H., Conley, M. R., Lassman, M., and Cunningham, G. (1990). The risk of neural tube defects in relation to maternal fertility and fertility drug use. *Lancet* **336,** 103–104.

Milunsky, A., Jick, H., Jick, S. S., Bruell, C. L., MacLaughlin, D. S., Rothman, K. J., and Willett, W. (1989). Multivitamin/folic acid supplementation in early pregnancy reduces the prevalence of neural tube defects. *J. Am. Med. Assoc.* **262,** 2847–2852.

Milunsky, A., Derby, L. E., and Jick, H. (1990). Ovulation induction and neural tube defects. *Teratology* **42,** 467.

Mulinare, J., Cordero, J. F., Erickson, D., and Berry, R. J. (1988). Periconceptional use of multivitamins and the occurrence of neural tube defects. *J. Am. Med. Assoc.* **260,** 3141–3145.

Myrianthopoulos, N. C., and Melnick, M. (1987). Studies in neural tube defects I. Epidemiologic and etiologic aspects. *Am. J. Med. Gen.* **26,** 783–796.

Naggan, L. (1971). Anencephaly and spina bifida in Israel. *Pediatrics* **47,** 577–586.

O'Dowd, M. J., Connolly, Y. K., and Ryan, A. (1987). Neural tube defects in rural Ireland. *Archives of Diseases in Children* **62,** 297–298.

Oreglia, A., and Tashiro, M. (1986). What are California's birth cohort files?—Questions and answers. Report No. 26–10144). Health Data and Statistics Branch, Sacramento, California.

Rhoads, G. G., and Mills, J. L. (1986). Can vitamin supplements prevent neural tube defects? Current evidence and ongoing investigations. *Clin. Obstet. Gynecol.* **29**(3), 569–579.

Schardein, J. L. (1980). Congenital abnormalities and hormones during pregnancy: A clinical review. *Teratology* **22,** 251–270.

Seller, M. J. (1987). Unanswered questions on neural tube defects. *Br. Med. J.* **294**(6563), 1–2.

Sever, L. E. (1982). An epidemiologic study of neural tube defects in Los Angeles County 11. Etiologic factors in an area with low prevalence at birth. *Teratology* **25,** 323–334.

Sever, L. E., Lowell, E., Sanders, M., and Monsen, R. (1982). An epidemiologic study of neural tube defects in Los Angeles County I. Prevalence at birth based on multiple sources of case ascertainment. *Teratology* **25,** 315–321.

United States Census Bureau (1980). *General Social and Economic Characteristics/ California Section 1.* 1982. Government Printing Office, Washington, D.C.

United States National Center for Health Statistics (1986). "International Classification of Diseases. 9th Revision, Clinical Modification," Vol. 1. Library of Congress Number 77-94472. Edward Brothers, Ann Arbor, Michigan.

Vollset, S. E. (1990). Ovulation induction and neural tube defects. *Lancet.* **335,** 178 (letter).

Windham, G. C., and Edmonds, L. D. (1982). Current trends in the incidence of neural tube defects. *Pediatrics* **70**(3), 333–337.

12

Lapse of Consciousness: The Impact of Litigation on Surveillance in a Defined Population

Louise S. Gresham • *Michele M. Ginsberg*

Disease surveillance systems are elemental in defining patterns of disease and measures of control and in estimating the public health burden of morbidity and mortality on human populations. Most epidemiological surveillance relies on passive reporting of cases from a health professional to the local health department, that is, the physician as an adjunct of the health department (Terence *et al.*, 1989; Trask, 1915; Centers for Disease Control, 1988). Passive systems are particularly affected by external factors, such as publicity or enhanced medical interest based on a new clinical entity or disease severity, which may introduce artifactual changes in case finding (Marier, 1977; Voght *et al.*, 1983). The influence of publicity on surveillance and volume of reporting has been documented with toxic shock syndrome (David and Vergeront, 1982) and hepatitis A (Levy *et al.*, 1977). Whenever a change in the occurrence of a disease or condition is observed, surveillance methods need to be scrutinized.

California statute outlines the legal reporting requirements for infectious diseases and conditions that include lapse of consciousness (LOC) (California Code of Regulations, 1989). Article 7, Section 410, broadened the scope of what was previously the reporting of epilepsy in the California Health and Safety Code to include LOC. The intent of the law is that information on individuals experiencing a seizure or LOC be used by the State Department of Motor Vehicles (DMV) to enforce provisions of the Vehicle Code of California. The data are confidential and used solely to determine eligibility of a person to operate a motor vehicle. The local health department serves only as a conduit for reporting to the DMV; there is no follow-up at the local level other than for completeness of report.

Neuroepidemiology:
Theory and Method

An estimated threefold increase in the monthly LOC episodes reported to the San Diego County Department of Health Services (DHS) was observed over a 4-month period, September to December 1989. An external event taking place in the County Superior Court provided an explanation. Approximately 6 years prior, a head-on car collision occurred when an 18-year-old epileptic lost control of her car, resulting in one death and one severe injury to a passenger. The passenger, a paraplegic subsequent to her injuries, sued a local neurologist, alleging that he failed to report to the health officer or to the DMV a "change" in LOC status of the driver's epileptic condition. Coincident to the dramatic rise in LOC reporting beginning September 1989, the court case concluded and a judgment of 3.2 million dollars was made against the neurologist. The trial generated extensive television and print media coverage. This is considered a landmark case that held a physician liable for the driving of his epileptic patient and, perhaps, will support a new growth area of tort law.

METHODS

Case Definition

California Health and Safety Code mandates reporting to the local health officer the name, birthdate, and address of every person diagnosed as having a disorder characterized by LOC. The local DHS serves as a conduit of reporting to the DMV. A person can be reported more than once, so that the reported numbers reflect events or episodes, not individuals.

A case of LOC is anyone 14 years of age or older who has experienced an occurrence of a LOC or episodes of marked confusion, including Alzheimer's disease, in the preceding 3 years. The vast breadth of this differential diagnosis is reflected in the potential causes, which include neurologic, cardiovascular, metabolic, and psychiatric conditions. Also included are trauma, severe intoxication from drugs or alcohol, human immunodeficiency virus (HIV)–dementia, and Alzheimer's disease, which became reportable as a separate entity in 1989 (Cochrane, 1989; California Department of Health Services, 1990).

Data Collection and Analysis

San Diego County DHS maintains a password-protected database containing all notifiable diseases/conditions reported since 1987. Abstracted data from the confidential morbidity surveillance card include patient name, birthdate, sex, ethnic/racial group, age, date of diagnosis, report date, and reporting facility. Demographics on LOC cases received after October 1990 were not entered into the database because of economic constraints on staffing posed by the volume increase. Dbase IV was used for data entry and management; descriptive analyses were conducted using SPSS PC. Ninety-five percent confidence intervals were constructed for yearly incidence rates.

RESULTS

The incidence of reported episodes of LOC per 100,000 people increased over a 4-year period: 1987, 53.3; 1988, 55.7; 1989, 111.9; 1990, 252.3 (Table I). Based on incidence rates, which are calculated using the number of reported cases and estimated population in the year interval, the increase is decidedly not due to population increase.

An average of 105 LOC cases were reported each month to the local health officer in San Diego County during 1987 and 1988; yearly cases totaled 1220 and 1300, repectively. The monthly average doubled to 225 in 1989, largely because of the sharp rise in reporting beginning in September of that year. There were 2705 LOC reports in 1989 and cases continued to be reported at a high level throughout 1990 with a total of 6303 cases; the monthly average was 525 cases, with a peak of 740 LOCs in December (Fig. 1).

The Superior Court hearing began in September 1989, reporting week number 35, and ended in week 41. Media coverage in the local newspaper was extensive during weeks 34–42. The number of reports rose sharply in week 38 (Fig. 2) In week 42 (directly following the end of the trial), LOC reports doubled from the usual 50 expected cases and tripled by the end of the year. Of the 2705 LOCs in 1989, 58% were reported in the last 18 weeks. Figure 3 shows the San Diego case reporting level by week in comparison to the State of California for 1989. San Diego represented 12%

Table I

Lapse of Consciousness Reports, Incidence
per 100,000, San Diego County, 1987–1990

Year of report	Incidence per 100,000	95% CI
1987	53.3	50.4, 62.9
1988	55.7	52.7, 58.8
1989	111.9	107.7, 116.6
1990	252.3	245.8, 258.3

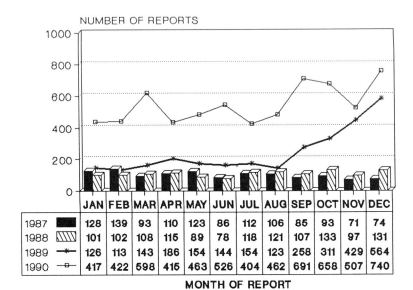

		JAN	FEB	MAR	APR	MAY	JUN	JUL	AUG	SEP	OCT	NOV	DEC
1987	■	128	139	93	110	123	86	112	106	85	93	71	74
1988	⧄	101	102	108	115	89	78	118	121	107	133	97	131
1989	—*—	126	113	143	186	154	144	154	123	258	311	429	564
1990	—□—	417	422	598	415	463	526	404	462	691	658	507	740

MONTH OF REPORT

Figure 1 Lapse of consciousness reports by month of report, San Diego County, 1987–1990.

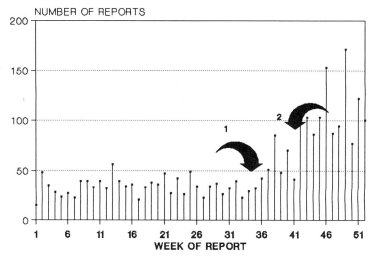

WEEK OF REPORT

Figure 2 Lapse of consciousness reports by week of report, San Diego County, 1989. 1, Superior Court case begins week 35; 2, Superior Court case ends week 41.

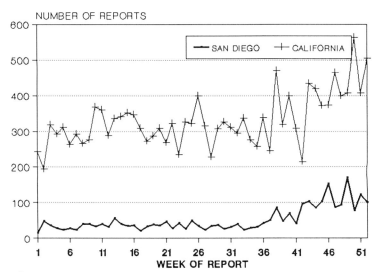

Figure 3 Lapse of consciousness reports by week of report, California and San Diego County, 1989.

of all reported California LOC cases in January 1989 and by December accounted for 25% of the cases.

The demographic profile of cases was consistent over a 3-year period, 1987–1989: 46% of the cases were female, 53% male; 78% white, followed by 8% Hispanic, 8% black, 2% Asian, and <1% American Indian. This underrepresents the proportion of Hispanics in San Diego County. The U.S. Census Bureau estimates the county's 1990 population as 20.4% of Hispanic origin and 79.6% non-Hispanic (74.9% white, 6.4% black, 7.9% Asian, and 0.8% American Indian). In 1988 and 1989, 2% of the case reports were missing some demographic data. This reflects much more complete recording than in 1987, when 27% of the cases lacked at least one demographic variable, usually ethnic/racial group.

Fifty-six percent of the cases were 40 years old or less at time of diagnosis. Table II shows a significantly higher percent of nonwhites in this age group when compared to whites. This phenomenon was consistent through 1989 and may suggest variation in health status or reason for the diagnosis to include alcoholism, trauma, or drug use.

The trend over time was for more private physicians and fewer hospitals to originate a LOC notification. In 1987, 54.7% of the confidential reports were from private physicians and 39.9% from hospitals. This is in contrast to 73.8% private physicians and 21.2% hospital-derived cases in 1989. The increase in private clinician notifications may reflect the level at which

Table II

Lapse of Consciousness Reports, Percentage
of Persons 40 Years of Age or Less at Diagnosis
by Ethnic/Racial Group

Year of report	% White	% Black	% Hispanic
1987	55.9	63.9	80.6
1988	56.5	76.8	83.6
1989	55.0	76.2	74.5

care was given or the type or severity of the condition reported. More
nonwhite patients were reported by hospitals, possibly attributable to
differences in the primary cause of the LOC or patterns of health care
facility utilization.

CONCLUSIONS

Clinicians reported more than 6300 LOC episodes in San Diego County
during 1990. That number is almost 5 times greater than the total for 1988.
The most plausible explanation for the significant increase in LOC reports
beginning in September 1989 is more complete reporting of cases diagnosed rather than an increase in actual disease of the magnitude reflected
in reporting. The addition of Alzheimer's disease reports, beginning in
April 1989, represents only 9% of cases and, alone, does not account
for the dramatic rise in reporting. The increase correlated closely with
extensive news media coverage of litigation. It is reasonable to attribute
this substantial change in reporting practice to increased awareness of
the requirement to report and sensitivity to the possible penalties and
monetary impact associated with the failure to do so. Future legislation
will likely focus on the legal responsibilities of physicians to report a
change in patient LOC status and restrict the definition of a reportable
LOC. The controversy remains over the equity between public safety and
the rights of those with seizure or memory disorders.

Nonwhite patients were more likely to be younger (40 years of age or
less) and to have received care at a hospital facility compared to white
patients. These observations may reflect possible differences in the risk
factors leading to the LOC diagnosis (i.e., alcohol and drugs), severity of
condition, or individual practices of health care utilization.

Four implications to clinicians and patients as a result of this litigation
in San Diego County are noteworthy. First, clinicians may be reporting

cases they would not have considered reporting before. Second, epileptics and alcoholics may be the target of discrimination regardless of their recovery or ability to control seizures (Krumholz *et al.*, 1991). Third, patients may choose to stay away from their physicians, viewing them as policemen, or withhold facts necessary for diagnosis and treatment in order to protect their driver's license. Last, because of the huge volume in cases, the DMV may not be able to process and review cases in a timely and thorough manner.

Physicians are not required to reveal the cause of the LOC when notifying the health department. It is unknown what potential contributions are made to the diagnosis by alcohol and drug use, neurologic sequelae, "spells," environmental exposures [i.e., cluster of patients with seizure attributable to Endrin poisoning (California Department of Health Services, 1988)] and HIV-related dementia. Memory loss and other forms of dementia can become severe in HIV/AIDS patients due to either encephalitis or direct destruction of frontal cortex neurons by the virus (Navia *et al.*, 1986). Reporting of HIV–dementia is particularly troublesome. Current California law does not permit a HIV–dementia report to be forwarded by DHS to the DMV. Physicians must mail two separate morbidity reports directly to the DMV: one report stating "AIDS" and the other stating "dementia" only.

Knowledge of risk factors is critical to assess accurately morbidity and define program planning toward intervention strategies and disease prevention. Also, there are severe economic and emotional implications for those people reported to the DMV and deemed ineligible to operate a motor vehicle. If young minorities are more likely to be reported related to drug and alcohol than Whites, they could experience the most severe economic impact through loss of driving privileges.

Completeness of reporting is not an attribute of passive surveillance systems (Eylenbosch and Noah, 1988). Many factors can lead to changes in surveillance and subsequent distortion of the incidence of a condition. Publicity surrounding litigation involving the reporting of LOC in San Diego greatly influenced the number and selectivity of reports of LOC. An indirect benefit of such publicity for compulsory notification systems may be the heightened awareness by health professionals of the value in reporting all legally notifiable diseases and conditions to the local health department. Further epidemiologic investigation is necessary to shed light on this disorder termed LOC and to test the feasibility of comprehensive and systematic data collection on cases. It is fundamental to understand the risk factors leading to a diagnosis of LOC and impaired fitness to drive and potential selective case reporting practices (Drachman, 1988; Gilley *et al.*, 1991). Only in this way can interventions be formulated to reduce associated health and economic burdens.

References

California Code of Regulations. (1989). Title 17, Sections 2500, 2572, Chapter 321. Health and Safety Code, Section 410.

California Department of Health Services. (1988). Seizure disorder from toxic taquitos (Endrin pesticide poisoning), Orange County. *Calif. Morbid.* 41, 1.

California Department of Health Services. (1990). Alzheimer's, other dementias now reportable to health departments. *Calif. Morbid.* **35/36,** 1.

Centers for Disease Control. (1988). Guidelines for evaluating surveillance systems. *MMWR* **37**(suppl. S-5), 1–18.

David, J. P., and Vergeront, J. M. (1982). The effect of publicity on the reporting of toxic-shock syndrome in Wisconsin. *J. Infect. Dis.* **145**(4), 449–457.

Drachman, D. A. (1988). Who may drive? Who may not? Who shall decide? *Ann. Neurol.* **24,** 787–788.

Eylenbosch, W. J., and Noah, N. D. (eds.). (1988). "Surveillance in Health and Disease." Oxford University Press, New York.

Gilley, E. W., Wilson, R. S., Bennett, D. A., *et al.* (1991). Cessation of driving and unsafe motor vehicle operation by dementia patients. *Arch. Intern. Med.* **151,** 941–946.

Krumholz, A., Fisher, R. S., Lesser, R. P., and Hauser, W. A. (1991). Driving and epilepsy, a review and reappraisal. *JAMA* **265,** 622–626.

Levy, B. S., Mature, J., and Washburn, J. W. (1977). Intensive hepatitis surveillance in Minnesota: Methods and results. *Am. J. Epidemiol.* **105,** 127–134.

Marier, R. (1977). The reporting of communicable diseases. *Am. J. Epidemiol.* **105,** 587–590.

Navia, B. A., Jordan, B. D., and Price, R. W. (1986). The AIDS dementia complex. I. Clinical features. *Ann. Neurol.* **19,** 517–524.

Cochrane, D. (1989). "Roche Handbook of Differential Diagnosis." Hoffmann-La Roche, New Jersey.

Terence, L. C., Berkelman, R. L., Safford, S. K., Gibbs, N. P., and Hull, H. F. (1989). Mandatory reporting of infectious diseases by clinicians. *JAMA* **262,** 3018–3026.

Trask, J. W. (1915). Vital statitics: A discussion of what they are and their uses in public administration. *Public Health Rep.* **30,** 1–51.

Voght, R. L., LaRue, D., Klaucke, D. N., and Jillson, D. A. (1983). Comparison of an active and passive surveillance system of primary care providers for hepatitis, measles, rubella and salmonellosis in Vermont. *Am. J. Public Health* **73,** 795–797.

13

Neuroepidemiology of Intrauterine Radiation Exposure

Lowell E. Sever

There has been evidence of the potentially devastating effects of *in utero* ionizing radiation exposure on neurological development since early in the history of radiology. From a group of 75 children identified as having been exposed to moderate levels of radiation *in utero*, 20 were described by Goldstein and Murphy (1929) as "microcephalic idiots." The authors directly attributed the microcephaly in at least 16 of the cases to embryonic exposure to radiation. The minimum estimated dose was >100 rad (Brent, 1979). While this is among the first recorded collections of adverse reproductive outcomes from embryonic exposures to therapeutic ionizing radiation, it unfortunately is not the last. For example, Dekeban (1968) reported on 26 infants who had been exposed to therapeutic radiation between 2 and 25 weeks of gestation. Twenty-two of these children, irradiated between 3 and 20 weeks of gestation, were microcephalic, mentally retarded, or both. In Dekeban's case series, the estimated protracted exposure was 250 rad and all of the malformed infants exhibited signs of generalized growth retardation (Brent, 1979).

Studies of the survivors of *in utero* radiation exposure at Hiroshima and Nagasaki provide much of our current knowledge of the effects of prenatal ionizing radiation exposure on neurological development and function. There are no accurate data on the true numbers of *in utero* exposures or survivors of *in utero* exposure from the bombings. When a national census was taken in 1960, a survey by the Atomic Bomb Casualty Commission (ABCC) revealed 2310 survivors who had been exposed *in utero* in Hiroshima and 1562 in Nagasaki [The Committee for the Compilation of Materials on Damage Caused by the Atomic Bombs in Hiroshima and Nagasaki (Committee), 1981]. The bulk of this review presents a summary and interpretation of what has been learned from the populations of these two cities.

The studies have been carried out for over 40 years, first by the ABCC and subsequently by the Radiation Effects Research Foundation. Initial reports came from studies of Hiroshima (Plummer, 1952) and Nagasaki (Yamazaki *et al.*, 1954). More recent reports have considered the two populations together, and there have been important improvements in the estimation of exposure and determination of risks by gestational age at time of exposure. In the discussion that follows, references to "weeks" refer to week of gestation or weeks after conception. Also, recent studies have included a variety of neurological outcomes in addition to microcephaly and severe mental retardation, the outcomes in the historical medical exposure studies.

EARLY STUDIES OF HEAD CIRCUMFERENCE AND MENTAL RETARDATION AMONG ATOMIC BOMB SURVIVORS, WITH RADIATION EXPOSURE BASED ON DISTANCE FROM THE HYPOCENTER

Plummer (1952) studied the health of 205 children from Hiroshima with *in utero* exposure during the first half of pregnancy. Eleven children were exposed within 1200 m of the hypocenter, the point directly under the center of the bomb when it exploded. Seven of these children were mentally retarded. These seven children had a mean head circumference of <45 cm in comparison to a mean head circumference of 48.6 ± 1.3 cm among 171 exposed children with normal mental function. Of the 194 children who were exposed beyond 1200 m, one child exposed between 2500 and 3000 m was mentally retarded.

The first extensive analysis of the outcomes of pregnancy in women exposed to the atomic bomb in Nagasaki was published in 1954. Yamazaki *et al.* (1954) examined pregnancy outcomes in women who were within 2000 m of the hypocenter at the time of the blast, comparing them to a control group of women who were 4000–5000 m from the hypocenter. The women within the 2000-m range were further categorized by the presence or absence of major radiation signs. Major radiation signs included epilation, oropharyngeal lesions, purpura, and petechiae. The authors considered an array of pregnancy outcomes; our discussion will focus on mental retardation and head circumference.

Sixteen mothers with major radiation signs had children surviving to the age of examination, 4.75–5.5 years old (Yamazaki *et al.*, 1954). Four of these children were mentally retarded; all their mothers had been within 850–1150 m of the hypocenter. One of these infants had microcephaly. The only information reported on gestational age at time of exposure was that three of the four retarded children were in the first half of pregnancy. The fourth was in the 36th week, and the child was reported to be "spastic" as well as mentally retarded. None of the 106 children in the 4000–5000-m control group were retarded.

Among the 16 children of mothers with major radiation signs, the mean head circumference was 47.18 cm, and the four children with mental retardation had the four smallest head circumferences in this exposure group. There was an observed difference of 1.85 cm between the mean head circumference for this exposure group and the 4000–5000-m control group, a difference that was statistically significant at $p < 0.01$. The authors do not provide any information on the sex of the children or whether or not there are differences between males and females in the negative association of head circumference with radiation exposure.

From the group of mothers within 2000 m who were without major radiation signs, 60 children were examined for intellectual function. The mean head circumference for this group was 49.5 cm, comparable to 49.03 cm for the control group. One of these children was mentally retarded and spastic. Information was not provided on gestational age at exposure.

Another early report dealing with reduced head circumference (microcephaly) and intellectual performance in the *in utero* exposure population is a paper published by Miller in 1956. This paper increases the number of cases of microcephaly reported earlier by Plummer (1952) and provides information on mental retardation. Miller (1956) presents head circumference data by gestational age at exposure and distance of the mother from the hypocenter. The gestational age groupings were 0–6 weeks, 7–15 weeks, 16–25 weeks, and 26–40 weeks. The distance data were grouped by 1200 m and under, 1201–1500 m, 1501–1800 m, and 1801–2200 m. Importantly, the members of the exposure groups are not evenly distributed across the gestational age groups; there is a deficit of cases in the 0–6 weeks gestational age group.

In this and ensuing ABCC reports, microcephaly or small head circumference was defined as a head circumference 2 or more standard deviations below the age–sex average. A total of 33 children with *in utero* exposures had microcephaly. Mental retardation was present in 15 of the 33 children, and the incidence of mental retardation was also related to distance from the hypocenter and gestational age. The incidence and severity of microcephaly increases as the distance from the hypocenter decreases. Twenty-four of the children with microcephaly were between the 7th and 15th week of gestational age at the time of the blast. All the subjects with mental retardation and head circumferences more than 3 standard deviations below the average (13 children) were between 7 and 15 weeks of gestation at exposure.

In a 1963 survey of children exposed *in utero* at Hiroshima, Tabuchi and Hirai and Tabuchi *et al.* as cited in Committee (1981) found 45 cases (8.3%) of microcephaly among 545 children whose mothers were within 3000 m of the hypocenter. This compares to 13 cases of microcephaly among 473 nonexposed controls.

With regard to the early findings from Nagasaki, Burrow *et al.* (1965) presented data based on 286 children with *in utero* exposure. Their major finding was a decreased head circumference among children whose mothers were within 1500 m of the bomb's hypocenter. Based on distance at the time of blast, the mean exposure for this group was estimated to be >50 rad. Reviewing their data by trimester and sex of the child, the authors observed that among females the head circumferences of children with first-trimester exposures were greater than those with second- and third-trimester exposures. Males with first-trimester exposure had slightly smaller head circumferences than those with second- and third-trimester exposures.

In one of the first reports to examine in detail mental retardation in the Japanese *in utero* survivors, Wood *et al.* (1967) evaluated a group of 1613 children with *in utero* exposure at Hiroshima and Nagasaki. They observed a total of 30 mentally retarded children, 22 from Hiroshima and 8 from Nagasaki. In Hiroshima, the incidence of retardation was significantly higher in children whose mothers were within 2000 m of the hypocenter than among the children in the control groups. In addition, the rates were significantly higher in the <1000-m group than among the 1500–1900-m exposure group. A marked dose–response relationship was noted, with effects diminishing in frequency and severity with increasing distance from the hypocenter. Among those cases from within 1500 m, most of the retarded children were 6–15 weeks gestational age at time of exposure.

There were 161 children examined whose mothers had been within 1800 m of the hypocenter. Of these, 29 had head circumferences 2 standard deviations or more below average. Among the offspring of women with exposure at <15 weeks gestation, 23 children had reduced head circumferences (9 with mental retardation) when 1.4 were expected. In the >15-weeks group, six cases of reduced head circumference (two with mental retardation) were observed when only two were expected.

STUDIES OF HEAD CIRCUMFERENCE AND MENTAL RETARDATION AMONG ATOMIC BOMB SURVIVORS, WITH RADIATION EXPOSURE BASED ON T65DR DOSIMETRY

The Plummer (1952) and Yamazaki *et al.* (1954) studies were based on opportunistic samples and made no systematic attempt to be complete. The first effort at the construction of an exhaustive clinical sample of the prenatally exposed survivors was in 1955 [International Commission on Radiological Protection (ICRP), 1986]. This led to the PE-86 sample. Multiple sources of ascertainment were utilized, but case identification was based primarily on birth registrations and interviews with women. No attempt was made to match the more distally exposed or the nonexposed by sex or prenatal age at the time of bombing with survivors exposed within 2000 m. In 1959, this sample was revised, and the latter group has been the basis of most subsequent analyses (Wood *et al.*, 1967; Miller and Blot, 1972); this is the revised PE-86 sample. Importantly, it included no survivors prenatally exposed between 2000 and 2999 m. Exposed individuals are limited to survivors prenatally exposed within 2000 m (the proximally exposed) or between 3000 and 5000 m (the distally exposed). Nonexposed persons include only those who were beyond 10,000 m and who were enumerated in ABCC First or Second Sample censuses. The survivors within the 3000–5000-m zone, as well as the nonexposed, were matched by sex and trimester of exposure with those exposed within 2000 m. Both examples include virtually all individuals with exposures (absorbed doses) of 0.5 Gy (50 rad) or more using the T65DR dosimetry.

The first major report to include dosimetric data in the analysis of the effect of *in utero* radiation on head circumference is a report by Miller and Blot (1972). This study is based on the ABCC fixed sample cohort PE-86 of Hiroshima and Nagasaki children who were *in utero* at the time of the blast. As already described, the sample consists of children of mothers within 2000 m of the hypocenter and a gestational age- and sex-matched control series based on children of mothers distally exposed or out of the city at the time of the blast. Individual radiation dose estimates were based on shielding and distance for almost all pregnant women in the study. These doses were based on the T65DR dosimetric system.

In this publication, Miller and Blot (1972) present data on small head circumference for each city by dose and gestational age at exposure. The data for Hiroshima showed that effects were the greatest when exposure occurred between 3 and 17 weeks of gestation. With regard to dose, the Hiroshima data showed a statistically significant excess of small head size in the group whose mothers received 10–19 rad. The frequency of small head size in the 0–9-rad group in the 0–17-week range was 7.6% compared to 4.8% in the controls, a difference that is not statistically significant. In the 10–19-rad group, 11.1% of the children had reduced head sizes, a statistically significant excess over the rate observed in controls. The frequency of small head size generally became greater as dose increased. In the highest dose group (150+ rad), 5 of 13 children exposed at <18 weeks had small head circumferences and mental retardation. In the 18+-week exposure group, 3 of 42 children had reduced head size. One of these children was in the 150+-rad exposure group and was also mentally retarded.

The head circumference and mental retardation findings from Nagasaki differ from those of Hiroshima (Miller and Blot, 1972). In the low-dose range at Nagasaki, two of four children in the 30–39-rad category, exposed at 0–17 weeks, had small head circumferences. Among nine children with exposures at 150+ rad before 18 weeks, eight had small head sizes, three of whom were mentally retarded. Among nine children with 150+-rad exposure at 18+ weeks, two children had small heads, and one of these two children was mentally retarded.

In a subsequent report, Blot and Miller (1973) analyzed the mental retardation data from both Hiroshima and Nagasaki using the T65DR dose estimation. In Hiroshima, the frequency of mental retardation was increased at doses as low as 50–99 rad and became more frequent with increasing dose. When the data were analyzed on the basis of gestational age at time of exposure, the risks of mental retardation were the greatest at <15 weeks. In the exposed group at Nagasaki, the mentally retarded cases came from the dose groups above 200 rad. It is only above this dose level that relative risk is elevated.

Miller and Blot (1972) discuss the differences in the findings between the two cities. In Hiroshima, progressive exposure effects begin in the low-dose group, whereas in Nagasaki effects occurred only among the heavily exposed. The interpretation of the intercity differences in effects of exposure on head circumference and mental retardation is uncertain. Initially these were attributed to differences in the types of radiation in the bombs at the two towns—specifically, to differences in the neutron component of the radiation exposure. Subsequently, it was found that the differences in neutron exposure were not as great as once believed (Yamazaki and Schull, 1990). Other explanations for the intercity differences have focused on adverse nutritional and economic conditions, with the devastation being more severe in Hiroshima (Yamazaki and Schull, 1990). The epidemiology of mental retardation is complex, and some evidence suggests that nutritional deprivation during gestation can lead to reduction in head circumference and intellectual function (Yamazaki and Schull, 1990). We will return to these issues in a later discussion.

STUDIES OF MENTAL RETARDATION AND IQ AMONG ATOMIC BOMB SURVIVORS, WITH RADIATION EXPOSURE BASED ON DS86 DOSIMETRY

Recent analyses of the data from Hiroshima and Nagasaki have been carried out using revised estimates of gestational age at time of exposure and of fetal dose. In addition, these studies have considered recent developments in understanding the sequence and timing of human brain development. Much of this work has been summarized by Schull and Otake (1986).

Otake and Schull (1984) determined the prevalence of mental retardation using revised organ dose measurements, the DS86 dose system. They found that the highest risk of forebrain damage occurred at 8–15 weeks of gestational age. Analyses of risk in this exposure age group were consistent with a no-threshold linear dose–response model. They estimated that the probability of increasing the incidence of mental retardation was 0.40% per rad. The data for exposures at later than 15 weeks did not show a similar dose–response effect. In the period 16–25 weeks, a linear relationship was not observed, suggesting a nonlinear association with a threshold during this period. In these analyses, Otake and Schull (1984) did not observe an increased risk of mental retardation with exposure prior to the 8th week or after the 25th week of gestation.

In a review of these data in ICRP49 (ICRP, 1986), it was reported that 30 of 1599 pregnancies in the revised clinical sample terminated in a child with severe mental retardation and 18 of these had head circumferences more than 2 standard deviations below the population mean. Of those pregnancies that terminated in a mentally retarded child, 19 were exposed in the 8th through 15th weeks of gestation. During the 8th through the 15th weeks of gestation, the risk of impaired neurological development was 5 times greater than the risk estimated for 16–25 weeks. As already noted, there is no evidence of a radiation-related increase in mental retardation in the interval from fertilization through the 7th week or after the 25th week.

With regard to severe mental retardation, the reanalysis of the data by Otake and Schull (1984) showed that the highest risk of mental retardation was during 8–15 weeks and that the severity of mental retardation appears to be linearly related to fetal dose. When the 0-dose group was removed, within the 8–15-week group the regression coefficient did not change much, and the predicted values do not differ significantly from the values observed, showing that the data are internally consistent.

The shape of the dose–response relationship for mental retardation appears to be linear, but there are exceptions regarding a threshold and its level. For example, the BEIR V report (Committee on the Biological Effects of Ionizing Radiations, 1990) states that "a threshold may exist at 0.2–0.4 Gy," whereas reference to the bar graph based on Otake and Schull (1984) shows little if any increase at exposures below 0.50–0.99 Gy (Miller and Brent, 1990).

In addition to severe mental retardation, the recent studies have considered data from intelligence tests conducted in 1955–1956. The IQ study population was established in Hiroshima in 1953 and Nagasaki in 1955 using a variety of sources (Otake *et al.*, 1989). The tests were conducted using the Japanese Koga and Tanaka-B intelligence tests, and the children were 10–11 years old at the time of testing. There are 1673 individuals with IQ scores and T65DR doses and 1202 individuals with IQ scores and DS86 doses.

There were two undesirable consequences of the sample redefinition (ICRP, 1986). First, by excluding individuals in the 2000–2999-m range, some individuals who may have had doses >0.01 Gy were removed. Second, it reduced the information available on IQ testing. The tests had been done in 1955 and not repeated later (at least by 1986). This was before the selection of nonexposed portion of the sample, and many persons in this group were never tested.

No evidence of a radiation effect on IQ test scores was observed among children prenatally exposed prior to the 8th week or at 26 or more weeks of gestational age. For the 8–15-week exposure group, the regression is possibly linear. The cumulative distributions of test scores suggest a progressive shift downward in scores with increasing exposure. Although there was no heterogeneity among the various dose groups in the variances of IQ scores, among children exposed at 8–15 weeks heterogeneity among the mean values under both dosimetry systems was significant. At midgestation, the mean test scores, but not the variances, are significantly heterogenous among individuals exposed at 8–15 weeks and, to a lesser degree, among those exposed at 16–25 weeks. In the 8–15-week group using a linear model, the estimate of the decline in IQ scores is 20–25 points per Gy with the DS86 doses compared to 17–21 points per Gy with the T65DR doses. Finally, when a linear quadratic model is applied to the individuals exposed at 8–15 weeks of gestational age, the reduction in intelligence test scores is 21–27 points per Gy of exposure using the DS86 doses. When controls receiving <1 rad are excluded, the effect is somewhat greater—33–41 points per Gy—but the two estimates are not statistically significantly different (Schull and Otake, 1986). The differences in mean scores of children exposed 16–25 weeks after fertilization was not as marked as at 8–15 weeks.

NEUROEPIDEMIOLOGIC ENDPOINTS, IN ADDITION TO HEAD CIRCUMFERENCE, MENTAL RETARDATION, AND IQ, STUDIED IN THE ATOMIC BOMB SURVIVORS

In addition to reduced head circumference, mental retardation, and reduced IQ, attention has been directed recently to other neurological effects of *in utero* exposure at Hiroshima and Nagasaki. Extensive data are available on the survivor's cohorts from both longitudinal and cross-sectional surveys. Although these data have not been analyzed or published as extensively as those on head circumference or mental retardation, they do add to our understanding of the neuroepidemiology of *in utero* radiation exposure.

Records of school performance have been analyzed for prenatally exposed survivors in Hiroshima and a comparison group (Otake *et al.*, 1989). The DS86 school performance study group consists of 929 of the 1090 individuals in Hiroshima with T65DR dose estimates. The mean dose estimates are very similar in the two samples, but there are 14 children in the 1.00-Gy group based on the DS86 dosimetry versus 4 using the T65DR doses. Comparisons of analyses using the two systems show that the dose–response trends are comparable, with a greater effect using the DS86 sample. Our discussion will focus on the DS86 analyses. Data were collected in 1956 when the children were 10–11 years old and most had completed the fourth grade. The school records included information on school attendance, performance in seven subjects, and the children's behavior and physical status.

In the first 4 years of school, which are included in the Hiroshima sample, students take seven subjects: language, civics, mathematics, science, music, drawing, and gymnastics (Schull and Otake, 1986). Their performance is evaluated on a percentile basis and scored on a 5-point scale. Schull and Otake (1986) examined scores for individual subjects using both linear and linear-quadratic dose–response models. For first-grade scores, they found that performance was significantly depressed in all school subjects in the 8–15- and 16–25-week exposure groups, but the nature of the relationship with dose was not clear. There was no evidence of a radiation-related effect in the 0–7- or 26+-week exposure groups.

Analyses that dealt with composite scores based on all subjects for each grade from first through fourth have also been published (Schull *et al.*, 1990). On the basis of average performance scores, damage to the 8–15-week fetal brain appears to be linearly related to absorbed dose. Damage to the fetus exposed at 16–25 weeks appears to be similarly linear, but the impact in terms of absolute average scores appears to be less (Schull *et al.*, 1989). Multivariate analyses using canonical and multiple correlations, which allow the simultaneous consideration of the effect of exposure on performances in the seven study subjects, also show a highly significant relationship of achievement in school to exposure at 8–15 and 16–25 weeks after fertilization. This trend is stronger in the earliest years of schooling.

The neuroepidemiologic endpoint of seizures has recently been studied in relation to *in utero* radiation exposure by Dunn *et al.* (1990). These researchers studied clinical histories of seizure disorders variously recorded as "seizure," "epilepsy," or "convulsion" among children of the PE-86 sample. The PE-86 sample consists of 2083 exposed and nonexposed children ascertained largely through birth certificates. These children were first examined in 1948 when they were about 2 years old, with follow-up examinations that included IQ tests in 1955–1956 and neuromuscular tests in 1961–1962. A history of seizures and relevant factors such as symptoms and duration was recorded but there was not enough information to permit clinical classification by seizure types. Thus, the investigators established three seizure categories on the basis of history: febrile, acute symptomatic, and unprovoked. The dosimetry used for this study was the DS86 dosimetry, which included calculated maternal uterine doses. Those doses were used to estimate fetal doses and are available for 1183 of the subjects who make up the sample in the Dunn *et al.* (1990) study. Most of the 900 exclusions had doses of <0.10 Gy in the T65DR dose system.

Dunn *et al.* (1990) looked at the occurrence of seizures by dose category in Gy and the gestational age groups 0–7, 8–15, 16–25, and 26+ weeks. They found no seizures reported among persons exposed at doses higher than 0.10 Gy prior to the 8th week of gestation. The highest frequency of seizures is seen in the highest dose groups exposed at 8–15 weeks of gestation. Importantly, this increase is accounted for by unprovoked seizures. When the mentally retarded individuals are included in the study sample, a consistent dose–response relationship for all seizures is observed between 8 and 15 weeks of gestation. Exposures during the

8–15-week gestation period led to an increased risk of seizures that was linearly related to dose with the highest seizure incidence in the >0.10-Gy exposure group. The risk ratios for unprovoked seizures in the 8–15-week exposure group are 4.35 (90% CI 0.45–40.9) for exposures in the range of 0.10–0.49 Gy and 24.9 (90% CI 4.09–192) following exposures of 0.50 Gy or more. When the 22 mentally retarded children are excluded from the analysis, a statistically significant risk is detected only at 8–15 weeks and then only in the group with unprovoked seizures.

Questions regarding the inclusion of persons with mental retardation are of mechanistic importance. Dunn *et al.* (1990) note that if seizures can arise following radiation exposure through two independent dose-related mechanisms, one that causes seizures and another that causes mental retardation in some persons who are then predisposed to develop seizures, then the mentally retarded must be excluded to explore the dose-response relation with the first mechanism. On the other hand, if mental retardation and seizures arise from a common brain defect manifesting itself in some instances as mental retardation and in others as seizures, then mentally retarded cases should not be excluded. Dunn *et al.* (1990) note that if mental retardation and unprovoked seizures are treated as different manifestations of a common pathway, the relative risks of either one occurring following exposure at 8–15 weeks is 12.2 (90% CI 4.4–33.4).

It is important to note that a better understanding of the associations among seizure disorders, mental retardation, and radiation exposure in this population requires a better understanding of neuropathology. Recommendations have been made regarding the use of noninvasive diagnostic techniques such as magnetic resonance imaging. In addition, it would be extremely informative if detailed microscopic studies could be carried out on the brains of these persons at death.

PROPOSED MECHANISMS FOR RADIATION EFFECTS ON CENTRAL NERVOUS SYSTEM DEVELOPMENT

Four gestational age categories at the time of the bombs have been established and the major events of brain development during each category described (Lione, 1987). The first period is 0–7 weeks; by the end of this period, the precursors of neurons and neuroglia, the two principal types of cells that give rise to the central nervous system, have emerged and are mitotically active. During the second period, 8–15 weeks, neurons increase in number, migrate to their final developmental sites, and lose their mitotic ability. During the period of 16–25 weeks, differentiation of the cells continues, the development of synapses continues, and the cellular architecture of the brain unfolds. The fourth period, 26 or more weeks of gestational age, is characterized by continued architectural and cellular differentiation and synaptogenesis.

On the basis of the timing of the gestational exposures discussed above, it is logical to focus on the period of 8–15 gestational weeks to examine possible mechanisms for central nervous system effects of *in utero* radiation exposure. During the 8th to 15th week of human development, there is a well-characterized period of neuronal proliferation and migration, when cells originating in the ventricular regions of the developing brain migrate into various layers of the emerging cerebral cortex. The progression of nerve cell migration has been monitored and the time of arrival of neurons at their destinations in the cerebrum calculated. The final mitotic division of neuronal cells is believed to occur before their migration into what will be the cerebral cortex. This mitotic activity is thought to be complete by the 16th gestational week. According to Lione (1987), evidence supports two waves of neuronal migration from the ventricular and pial surfaces of the developing brain, one wave from the 7th to the 10th week following conception and the second from the 13th to the 15th week. Neuronal differentiation, including the growth of axonal and dendritic processes leading to synaptic contacts with other neurons, occurs after the completion of migration.

Until 1984, researchers believed that ionizing radiation killed cells in the brain, causing small head size and, when severe enough, mental retardation. In 1984, Otake and Schull, reporting the preceding findings regarding gestational age-related differences in effects, suggested that exposure to ionizing radiation during weeks 8–15 impairs the process of cortical neurons proliferating or migrating to the cortex from areas near the ventricles. Cells killed before the 8th week of gestational age apparently can cause small head size without mental retardation because the neurons that will form the cerebrum are at a stage that is not susceptible to impairment by radiation. The glial cells, which provide structural support to the brain, are susceptible to depletion at this early stage (Miller, 1990).

The sensitivity of neuronal tissue during proliferation and migration suggests that either one or both of these processes can be adversely affected by radiation, leading to neurological impairment. Because there does not appear to be an effect during the first 8 weeks after conception, adequate replacement of lost cells has been suggested to occur (Lione, 1987). Effects of radiation on cell migration during weeks 8–15 may be the crucial histopathologic effect. The finding of small head size already discussed is related to reduction in cell number, but whether this has resulted from impairment of neuronal proliferation, massive cell killing, or a combination of these two processes is not clear (Otake and Schull, 1984). Because mental retardation has been found in the absence of small head size, this may result from a proliferation of glial cells in the brain after radiation exposure. The ability of glial cells to regenerate after radiation exposure has been demonstrated in animal studies (D'Amato and Hicks, 1965).

POSSIBLE CONFOUNDERS AND CONTRIBUTORS TO DIFFERENCES IN MENTAL RETARDATION BETWEEN HIROSHIMA AND NAGASAKI

Several potential confounders of the demonstrated relationship of radiation exposure to mental retardation may also partially explain the differences between Hiroshima and Nagasaki. For example, consanguineous marriages were common in both Hiroshima and Nagasaki, but especially in Nagasaki. This difference could, in principle, contribute to the intercity difference, not only in the frequency of severe mental retardation but also with the mean IQ score. Genetic differences are not likely to contribute to the shape of the dose–response curve in either city or the variation in risk by age groups (ICRP, 1986).

An aspect of the data of Otake and Schull (1984) that needs to be considered is the relatively high frequency of mental retardation in the control children, approximately 1%. The possible contribution of malnutrition in Hiroshima and Nagasaki following the bombings needs to be considered. Although there was terrible socioeconomic disruption in both cities, researchers generally agree that it was greater in Hiroshima (Yamazaki and Schull, 1990). In addition, the economic conditions prior to the bombing were worse in Hiroshima.

The extent of malnutrition in the pregnant women and its effects on mental development, separate from radiation, would be difficult to resolve and quantify. Effects of maternal malnutrition on mental retardation are controversial. The possible interactions between malnutrition and radiation damage have not been studied extensively. If the impairment comes from effects on neuronal number or migration, it seems unlikely that maternal malnutrition would restrict brain development as markedly in the second trimester as in the later, perhaps more sensitive, stages of gestation. It also appears that malnutrition would interfere more with the postnatal phases of brain development.

Another potentially contributing factor is an increased embryonic or fetal hypoxemia secondary to radiation damage to the hematopoietic system of the mother and/or her developing child. Anemia was demonstrated in the pregnant women who were exposed to relatively high radiation doses (ICRP, 1986). While low birth weight has been associated with reduced oxygen-carrying capacity of blood, mothers with congenital anemias are not known to have an abnormally high incidence of mentally retarded children (United Nations Scientific Committee on the Effects of Atomic Radiation, 1986).

The full impact of potential confounders will probably never be determined, but their possible importance has been recognized by several authors (Yamazaki and Schull, 1990). It must be stressed that the studies described herein were carried out following two of the most devastating events in human history. Thus, the knowledge gained from this research must be stressed, not the potential limitations identified retrospectively.

SUMMARY AND CONCLUSIONS

On the basis of the studies of the survivors in *in utero* radiation exposure, it is clear that prenatal exposure to ionizing radiation has important neurological effects. These effects include reduced head circumference, increased rates of mental retardation, reduced IQ, and increased risks of seizure disorders. While questions have been raised about differences between Hiroshima and Nagasaki in the impact of radiation on neurological development, the data discussed earlier point to major contributions to exposure timing and dose to subsequent neurological outcomes. The period of 8–15 weeks of gestational age appears to be the most sensitive time window for neurological insult. During this time, neuronal proliferation, migration, and differentiation are taking place. Thus, it appears that the developing brain during this period can be affected by an exogenous insult, such as ionizing radiation, in a way that leads to a variety of abnormal neurological outcomes.

While the question of exposure timing can be answered relatively well with the data from Hiroshima and Nagasaki, dose–response relationships are not quite so clear-cut. Apparently, there is an increasing frequency of neurological endpoints (i.e., microcephaly, mental retardation, and seizure disorders) at 0.50 Gy. Below that level, the findings are more ambiguous, although some of the studies apparently show an effect at 0.10–0.19 Gy. The question of whether or not there is a threshold remains unanswered.

One of the central areas of continuing interest is the mechanisms through which *in utero* ionizing radiation exposure affects the developing brain. Although, as has been pointed out, the effects seem to be on neuronal proliferation, migration, and differentiation, the specific mechanisms through which this occurs are a topic of considerable investigation (Schull *et al.*, 1990). Because much of what we know about brain development has been learned only recently, our understanding of the neuroepidemiology of *in utero* radiation exposure will probably increase as additional insight is gained into the relationships among exposure, mechanisms, pathogenesis, and health and behavioral endpoints.

Acknowledgment

This work was supported by the U.S. Department of Energy under contract DE-ACO6-76RLO 1830.

References

Blot, W. J., and Miller, R. W. (1973). Mental retardation following in utero exposure to the atomic bombs of Hiroshima and Nagasaki. *Radiology* **106**, 617–619.

Brent, R. L. (1979). Effects of ionizing radiation on growth and development. *In* "Contributions to Epidemiology and Biostatistics," Vol. 1 (M. A. Klingberg, ed.), pp. 147–183. S. Karger, Basel.

Burrow, G., Hamilton, H., and Hrubec, Z. (1965). Study of adolescents exposed in utero to the atomic bomb, Nagasaki, Japan, *JAMA* **192**, 357–364.

Committee on the Biological Effects of Ionizing Radiations. (1990). "Health Effects of Exposure to Low Levels of Ionizing Radiation. BEIR V." National Academy Press, Washington, D.C.

The Committee for the Compilation of Materials on Damage Caused by the Atomic Bombs in Hiroshima and Nagasaki. (1981). "Hiroshima and Nagasaki: The Physical, Medical, and Social Effects of the Atomic Bombings." Basic Books, New York.

D'Amato, C. J., and Hicks, S. P. (1965). Effects of low levels of ionizing radiation on the developing cerebral cortex of the rat. *Neurology* **15**, 1104–1116.

Dekaban, A. (1968). Abnormalities in children exposed to x-radiation injury to the human fetus: Part I. *J. Nucl. Med.* **9**, 471–477.

Dunn, K., Yoshimaru, H., Otake, M., Annegers, J. F., and Schull, W. J. (1990). Prenatal exposure to ionizing radiation and subsequent development of seizures. *Am. J. Epidemiol.* **131**, 114–123.

Goldstein, L., and Murphy, D. P. (1929). Microcephalic idiocy following radium therapy for uterine cancer during pregnancy. *Am. J. Obstet. Gynecol.* **18**, 189–195, 281–283.

International Commission on Radiological Protection. (1986). "Developmental Effects of Irradiation on the Brain of the Embryo and Fetus: A Report of a Task Group of Committee 1 of the International Commission on Radiological Protection." ICRP Publication 49, Pergamon Press, Oxford.

Lione, A. (1987). Ionizing radiation and human reproduction. *Reprod. Toxicol.* **1**, 3–16.

Miller, R. W. (1956). Delayed effects occurring within the first decade after exposure of young individuals to the Hiroshima atomic bomb. *Pediatrics* **18**, 1–18.

Miller, R. W. (1990). Effects of prenatal exposure to ionizing radiation. *Health Phys.* **59**, 57–61.

Miller, R. W., and Blot, W. J. (1972). Small head size after in-utero exposure to atomic radiation. *Lancet* **2**, 784–787.

Miller, R. W., and Brent, R. L. (1990). Low dose radiation exposure. *Science* **247**, 1166–1167.

Otake, M., and Schull, W. J. (1984). In utero exposure to A-bomb radiation and mental retardation; a reassessment. *Br. J. Radiol.* **57**, 409–414.

Otake, M., Yoshimaru, H., and Schull, W. J. (1989). Prenatal exposure to atomic radiation and brain damage. *Congential Anomalies* **29**, 309–320.

Plummer, G. (1952). Anomalies occurring in children exposed in utero to the atomic bomb in Hiroshima. *Pediatrics* **10**, 687–692.

Schull, W. J., and Otake, M. (1986). Neurological deficit among the survivors exposed in utero to the atomic bombing of Hiroshima and Nagasaki: A reassessment and new directions. *In* "Radiation Risks to the Developing Nervous System" (H. Kriegel, W. Schmahl, G. B. Gerber, and F. E. Stieve, eds.), pp. 399–419. Gustav Fischer Verlag, Stuttgart and New York.

Schull, W. J., Otake, M., and Yoshimaru, H. (1989). Radiation-related damage to the developing human brain. *In* "Low Dose Radiation: Biological Basis of Risk Assessment" (K. F. Baverstock and J. W. Stather, eds.), pp. 28–41. Taylor & Francis, London.

Schull, W. J., Norton, S., and Jensh, R. P. (1990). Ionizing radiation and the developing brain. *Neurotoxicol. Teratol.* **12**, 249–260.

United Nations Scientific Committee on the Effects of Atomic Radiation. (1986). "Genetic and Somatic Effects of Ionizing Radiation." United Nations, New York.

Wood, J. W., Johnson, K. G., Omori, Y., Kawamoto, S., and Keehn, R. J. (1967). Mental retardation in children exposed in utero to the atomic bomb in Hiroshima and Nagasaki. *Am. J. Public Health* **57**, 1381–1390.

Yamazaki, J. N., and Schull, W. J. (1990). Perinatal loss and neurological abnormalities among children of the atomic bomb. *JAMA* **264**, 605–609.

Yamazaki, J. N., Wright, S. W., and Wright, P. M. (1954). Outcome of pregnancy in women exposed to the atomic bomb in Nagasaki. *Am. J. Dis. Child.* **87**, 448–463.

14

Childhood Convulsions Associated with Cerebral Malaria in Ghana: An Example of Shoe-Leather Neuroepidemiology

Kathryn Bartmann • *Laura K. Wyman* • *Paul Dagbui*

This study examined the occurrence of childhood convulsions at St. Anthony's Hospital, Dzodze, Ghana. St. Anthony's is a 150-bed District Hospital in the southern part of Ghana's Volta Region. It is operated by the Catholic church and admits acutely ill patients of all ages regardless of socioeconomic status, 24 hours a day. The maternity ward has 30 beds, the adult ward (including the tuberculosis isolation ward) has 40 beds, and the children's ward has 80 beds. The activities of the hospital are both curative and preventive. The motivation for initiating this study arose from primary interest in convulsions associated with cerebral malaria in children; however, pediatric convulsions with a range of etiologies were also considered. Data regarding outcome of treatment is also presented. The study occurred from October to November 1989, when the first author was serving as a medical missionary associated with the Catholic diocese.

BACKGROUND

St. Anthony's Hospital is the only hospital in the Kefu District. The district encompasses a population of 250,000, with 32,000 residing in the town of Dzodze itself. The illiteracy rate in this community is high, which has a negative result on health education.

The major occupation is farming on a subsistence basis. The most important crops in the area are maize, cassava, and palm fruits. Ground-

Neuroepidemiology:
Theory and Method

nuts, tomatoes, bananas, onions, okra, and tobacco are also cultivated. The yield is limited by periods of drought, lack of fertilizers, farming equipment, and technical skills. There is no industry in the area. A few people are self-employed artisans such as carpenters, masons, blacksmiths, and fitters. Fishing is the main occupation along the coast. Domestic activities such as distillation of alcohol from sugar or palmwine is common. Many women are engaged in small-scale trading.

Malaria is identified as the highest prevalent common disease in the community. Others are worm infestation and diarrheal diseases. The age group most seriously affected is children under 5 years.

The incidence of malnutrition is very low in this community. The obvious acceptable reasons are that traditionally it is a rich farming area in food crops and fish. Obesity is replacing marasmus as the predominant nutrition problem in the middle-aged female group. Alcoholism and drug abuse are emerging as manifestations of social stresses and tension.

Other factors influencing health in this community are poor sanitation, illiteracy, poverty, and lack of transport. Progress in education and active community participation are effectively breaking the chains of disease causation. Notifiable diseases (cholera, yellow fever, etc.) are reported to the World Health Organization by the national health authority. Measures taken at the hospital level are completing notification forms, education, and feedback.

Although the exact rate of falciparum malaria in this district has not been estimated by epidemiologic studies, clinical experience suggests that it is a problem of hyperendemic proportion. Falciparum malaria (also known as malignant malaria) is frequently attended by the complication of cerebral malaria, which has a mortality rate of 20% even with good medical care. Presenting an unarousable coma in patients without focal neurologic findings, cerebral malaria is a symmetric encephalopathy usually associated with convulsions in children. Symptoms are thought to be initiated by masses of parasitized red blood corpuscles creating blockage of capillaries and precapillaries in the brain. Appropriate treatment is almost invariably successful, effecting complete recovery. However, the importance of prompt treatment in infantile cerebral malaria is paramount, because infants appearing well in the morning may be in coma by nightfall. While permanent sequelae malaria are rare in treated cases, they are of concern due to their severity: hemiplegia, cerebellar ataxia, and deafness (Benenson, 1990).

Acquired immunodeficiency syndrome has not yet been identified in this area, although several human immunodeficiency virus-positive cases have been recorded in Battor Hospital in the south of the Volta Region.

METHODS

The study population was defined as all patients discharged from the pediatric ward at St. Anthony's Hospital with a diagnosis of convulsion, cerebral malaria, or meningitis during the 3 year period 1986–1988. Patients who met these criteria were identified via examination of logs maintained by the nursing staff. The logs provided relevant demographic information, hospitalization dates, and brief summaries of diagnosis and disposition on discharge. Review of these patients' actual medical records was then employed as a means of case verification. The initial search for cases in the log review procedure revealed 301 patients with the discharge diagnoses of interest; however, 71 of these were excluded from further analysis because their status as cases could not be verified.

The figures presented in the results of this paper reflect only those cases that were found to have a corroborating diagnosis of convulsion ($n = 230$). Cerebral malaria and meningitis patients who did not have an accompanying diagnosis of convulsion were dropped from the study.

RESULTS

Age and sex-specific frequency of pediatric convulsions at St. Anthony's hospital during 1986–1988 is shown in Table I. Two hundred thirty cases of pediatric convulsion were identified, with the age at diagnosis ranging from 1 month to 13 years. Sixty-one percent of the cases occurred in children less than 3 years old. The incidence in males and females across all age groups was approximately equal.

Table II illustrates the distribution of cases across etiologic categories. The causes are listed as they were discovered during examination of the data, rather than being predetermined diagnostic groups created by the investigators. The majority of convulsions (57%) were revealed to be associated with a diagnosis of malaria (associated febrile convulsions and cerebral malaria convulsions). There were 43 convulsions (19%) of unknown etiology, and 24 (10%) were noted to have been nonmalarial febrile convulsions. Five cases were attributed to meningitis, one to epilepsy, and five to encephalities. One case was presumed to be related to brain damage status postmalaria, with no active infection.

Overall, outcome of treatment was positive, as reflected in Table III. In the records, 78% of the males and 71% of the females were listed in a condition that was "good" or needed "some improvement" upon release

Table I

Age- and Sex-Specific Frequency of Pediatric Convulsions, 1986–1988,
St. Anthony's Hospital, Dzodze, Ghana

Age (years)	Number of cases			% Total cases (male and female)
	Male	Female	Total	
0	19	19	38	16.5
1	28	24	52	22.6
2	28	22	50	21.7
3	13	15	28	12.2
4	9	10	19	8.3
5–9	16	20	36	15.7
10–15	3	2	5	2.2
Unknown	2	0	2	0.9
Total	118	112	230	100.0

Table II

Etiology of Pediatric Convulsions, 1986–1988, St. Anthony's
Hospital, Dzodze, Ghana

Causes of convulsion	Cases	% Total cases
Malaria other than cerebral malaria (febrile convulsion)	89	38.7
Cerebral malaria	66	28.7
Convulsion of unknown etiology[a]	43	18.7
Febrile convulsion[b]	24	10.4
Meningitis	5	2.2
Encephalitis	1	0.4
Epilepsy	1	0.4
Postmalaria brain damage—no active infection	1	0.4
All causes	230	100.0

[a] No cause listed in record.

[b] Febrile = nonmalaria (1 measles, 1 skin infection, 22 fever with no
specific origin noted or of unknown origin).

Table III

Outcome of Treatment in 230 Pediatric Convulsion Patients, 1986–1988,
St. Anthony's Hospital, Dzodze, Ghana

Age (years)	Cases	Good	Some Improvement	Satisfactory	Died	Discharge	Unknown
Male							
0	19	7	8	3	1	0	0
1	28	9	7	2	4	1	5
2	28	13	12	1	2	0	0
3	13	3	8	0	1	1	0
4	9	3	6	0	0	0	0
5–9	16	6	8	1	0	0	1
10–15	3	0	2	0	1	0	0
Unknown	2	0	0	0	2	0	0
Total	118	41	51	7	11	2	6
Female							
0	19	5	6	2	5	0	1
1	24	8	10	5	1	0	0
2	22	5	9	7	0	0	1
3	15	7	4	2	2	0	0
4	10	2	4	3	0	1	0
5–9	20	9	10	0	1	0	0
10–15	2	0	1	0	1	0	0
Unknown	0	0	0		0	0	0
Total	112	36	44	19	10	1	2

from the hospital. Mortality in this population for all age groups combined was approximately 9% in both males and females.

DISCUSSION

In light of resource constraints, the scope of this study was confined to providing a cross-sectional description of convulsion frequency in the pediatric population at St. Anthony's hospital. Unfortunately, information regarding the local population was not available for definition of denominators in calculating rates or performance age-adjustment of the case distribution. Comparisons between age groups and etiologic categories were restricted by lack of statistical reference materials.

Several sources of potential bias in the results presented are recognized. First, it is possible that incident cases of convulsion during the study period were overlooked in the initial case selection process. Because it was not feasible to review the medical records of every patient in the pediatric log book, cases of convulsion with a documented discharge diagnosis other than convulsion, cerebral malaria, or meningitis possibly may have been overlooked. Additionally, a substantial number of cases that were ascertained lacked specific etiologic notation (see Table II).

At St. Anthony's hospital, diagnoses based on clinical evaluation often could not be definitively secondary due to lack of laboratory, radiologic electroencephalogram, and other diagnostic support. Although treatment decisions based on clinical evidence alone are admirably successful at this hospital, for epidemiologic analyses, the situation was less than ideal. The laboratory did not have the capability to perform microbiology cultures, enzyme-linked immunoassay analyses, immunofluorescence assays, or chemical analyses necessary for discriminating many diseases. Malaria parasite smears were available; however, a diagnostic dilemma was posed by the fact that a positive blood film does not necessarily prove that a patient has malaria, and, at the same time, failure to locate malaria parasites in the blood does not exclude malaria.

Another potential source of bias existed in this study with regard to reliability of age reporting. In the society from which the study population was derived, birthdates were often neither recorded nor remembered. The hospital staff did attempt to assess patients' ages by estimation relative to the occurrence of local events, but the accuracy and precision of reporting remained questionable.

Preparation of this report was handicapped by inaccessibility of reference materials and time limitations. It is our hope that despite the shortcomings inherent in this study, it may provide support for forthcoming investigations or that the raw data collected will be useful to the hospital for other purposes.

References

Benenson, A. S. (ed.) (1990). Control of Communicable Diseases in Man. American Public Health Association, Washington.

15

The Epidemiology of Childhood Lead Poisoning

Omar Shafey

Lead poisoning, even at very low doses, can cause neuropsychological impairment. Lead toxicity in children can result in poor cognitive perception, behavioral disturbance, learning disability, and retarded intellectual development. In the United States, an estimated 4.8 million children aged 0.5–5 years old are currently lead-poisoned. Ten million more children in 44 million contaminated homes are at direct risk of lead poisoning by ingestion of lead-based paint chips. Lead-poisoned children are disproportionately African American, poor, and urban. Public health measures to combat the lead threat include remediation and cleanup of lead-contaminated buildings, intensive national urban screening programs, case-finding efforts, medical case treatment and follow-up activities, and extra-environmental action. Social costs arising from mass childhood lead poisoning exceed the estimated $100 billion needed for public health measures to prevent lead poisoning. Measures taken to date have been inadequate to control the persisting danger of mass childhood lead poisoning.

BACKGROUND

Lead was one of the earliest metals manipulated by humans. It is a natural constituent of the earth's crust with a low melting point, good malleability, high density, and an ability to form alloys. The metal was first smelted about 4000 years ago and Hippocrates first described the deleterious effects of lead in 370 B.C. (Nadakavukaren, 1986). Nikander, the Greek poet and physician of the second century B.C., noted lead toxemia among those who worked with cerussa (lead carbonate). In the following stanza,

Nikander describes neurologic symptoms of acute toxicity: hallucinations, colic, paralysis, and death suffered by lead workers 2000 years ago:

> The harmful cerussa, that most noxious thing
> Which foams like the milk in the earliest spring
> With rough force it falls and the pail beneath fills
> This fluid astringes and causes grave ills.
> The mouth it inflames and makes cold from within
> The gums dry and wrinkled, are parch'd like the skin
> The rough tongue feels harsher, the neck muscles grip
> He soon cannot swallow, foam runs from his lip
> A feeble cough tries, it in vain to expel
> He belches so much, and his body does swell
> His sluggish eyes sway, then he totters to bed
> Phantastic forms flit now in front of his eyes
> While deep from his breast there soon issue sad cries
> Meanwhile there comes a stuporous chill
> His feeble limbs droop and all motion is still
> His strength is now spent and unless one soon aids
> The sick man descends to the Stygian shades.
>
> (Landrigan, 1990) p. 61

Lead poisoning has been implicated in the decline of the ancient Greek and Roman empires (Trotter, 1990). The early Greek and Roman societies are known to have stored, cured, and fermented beverages in lead-lined containers. These practices insidiously poisoned the people, especially members of the higher social classes, who consumed processed food-stuffs. Presumed lead exposure among the children of nobility resulted in reduced intellectual capacity and socially disadvantageous alterations in behavior. Widespread neuropsychological impairment of an important leadership class may have been a factor relevant to the overall collapse of ancient Greek and Roman societal institutions.

The retarding effects of lead poisoning also may have hastened the decline of the British upper class in the 18th and 19th centuries (Landrigan, 1990). High rates of Port wine consumption resulted in elevated blood lead concentrations among the ruling classes of England in that period. Lead-contaminated drinking water was also a problem. As an aristocracy drawing its leadership from a small, closed population, British society was especially vulnerable to the effects of mass poisoning among the nobility.

A member of the British upper class, Sir Thomas Legge was appointed Medical Inspector of Factories for Great Britain in 1897 (Landrigan, 1990). He recognized the effects of lead poisoning among occupationally exposed plumbers and other metal workers. In 1899, lead poisoning became a reportable disease in England. As surveillance and workplace controls were instituted, reported cases of acute lead toxicity and deaths declined during the following decades, although total lead consumption and chronic low-level exposure in the general population continued to rise.

Lead uses in the industrializing United States accelerated rapidly throughout the 20th century (Cohen, 1970). Lead became disseminated commercially to the public in the form of leaded gasoline fuels, lead-based paints, pottery, toys, cookware, and lead acid batteries among other articles. These sources constitute major exposure routes and sources of residual contamination dangerous to children's health even today.

Aside from the acute toxicity usually seen in association with occupational settings, lead poisoning in children was first documented by the Australian J. L. Gibson in 1904 (Gibson, 1904). Literature specific to the childhood lead poisoning problem in the United States was first published in 1917 by K. D. Blackfan (1917). The neurologic implications of lead poisoning in children were recognized for about 50 years preceding 1960. In 1960, the U.S. government finally established a maximum acceptable level of blood lead concentration: 60 μg/dl of blood (Roberts, 1987). Today, a blood level of 60 μg lead/dl is considered a medical emergency.

The first federal legislation attempting to control lead poisoning in children was promulgated in 1971 (Mushak and Crocetti, 1990). The Lead Based Paint Poisoning Prevention Act provided states with funding to administer screening programs for lead exposure. This act also directed the U.S. Department of Housing and Urban Development (HUD) to prohibit the use of leaded paint in federal or federally assisted housing construction.

In 1975, a lower level of 30 μg/dl was designated by the Centers for Disease Control (CDC) as the new minimum level requiring treatment. In 1981, the recently elected conservative government dismantled the 1971 federal act funding states' lead poisoning screening programs and passed administrative responsibility to individual states as an element of the Maternal and Child Health Block Grant. As financial responsibility for child health was passed to the states by the federal government, research showed lead to be more toxic than previously believed. The minimum acceptable blood lead level for children (according to the CDC) was reduced yet again in 1985 to 25 μg/dl.

In 1989, the federal government required all states participating in the Medicaid program to test poor children for trace blood lead levels as a condition for receiving federal Medicaid funds. The required testing program in California alone would have cost approximately $15–20 million annually (Hilts, 1991a). California and almost all other states failed to conduct the required testing of poor children. Five children's advocacy groups filed a lawsuit against the State of California on this issue in 1990. In October 1991, Governor Pete Wilson settled the suit by signing a bill authorizing funding to test 500,000 children for lead poisoning.

While federal agencies espouse screening for ever-expanding populations of children at risk for lead toxicity, federal funding for this urgent public health need is minimal. Only $8 million was spent nationally for lead screening in 1991 and only $14.9 million was requested by Health and Human Services (HHS) for fiscal year 1992. These amounts would be insufficient for California alone.

Most recently, in October 1991, the acceptable level for blood lead levels was reset even lower to 10 μg/dl (Hilts, 1991b). Acceptable limits on blood lead concentrations may continue to come down in response to the mounting evidence that even very low levels of lead are associated with subtle adverse neurologic and other health effects.

Paint manufacturers recognized early the negative health effects of disseminated lead but chose, with government acquiescence, to self-regulate their industry. Between the 1950s and 1977, paint manufacturers voluntarily agreed to limit lead concentrations to no more than 1% of paint by weight (Mushak and Crocetti, 1990). This level amounts to approximately 10,000 ppm, well above the level necessary to result in acute systemic toxicity. Finally, in 1977, Congress mandated the Consumer Product Safety Commission to require reductions in paint lead levels to <0.06%.

The Environmental Protection Agency (EPA) has had regulatory control over the use of lead in gasoline since 1973 (Hammond and Dietrich, 1990). In 1975, lead was declared a criteria pollutant basing its control requirement on ambient air standards. Since the mid-1970s, lead content in auto fuel has declined because the newly required automobile emissions control equipment (catalytic converters) were damaged by lead. In 1982, the EPA set limits of 1.1 g lead/gal of gasoline. These limits were lowered to 0.1 g/gal in 1986.

The current EPA criterion demands that air lead levels be no more than 1.5 μg lead/m^3 ambient air (Mushak and Crocetti, 1990). Many lead smelters and waste incinerators were forced to close due to their inability to meet air quality standards. Local airborne lead fallout from these point source polluters continues to expose children via residual soil and dust contamination.

Lead contamination of drinking water supplies is exacerbated by the prevalent use of lead pipes and soldering in household plumbing. In 1986, the EPA banned the use of lead solder and lead piping in household plumbing, but no provision was made for remediating the millions of homes already built. The current drinking water maximum contaminant level is 5 μg/liter of water, down from 50 μg/liter level effective as recently as 1988. About 20% of the U.S. population is exposed to water lead levels 4 times in excess of current maximum safe standards.

Lead contamination of the food supply is regulated by the Food and Drug Administration (FDA). In 1979, the FDA set a goal of limiting food lead levels to a maximum of 100 μg/day/child (Mushak and Crocetti, 1990). Through voluntary industry actions, the percentage of lead-soldered cans used in manufactured food products has declined from 90% in 1979 to 6% in 1988. Pesticide and engine exhaust contamination of food supplies contribute to the foodborne lead threat.

Lead poisoning has been a problem for many societies over the course of human history and contemporary societies are no exception. Net lead consumption has not decreased, but many countries have taken steps to reduce the amount of dispersed and directly available lead in the environment. The mounting negative health consequences of environmental lead pollution forced the U.S. government to reduce the allowable concentration of lead in paint, automotive fuels, canning, and printing materials. The control of dispersive lead contamination has been associated with subsequent reductions in median blood lead levels throughout the United States; however, due to continuing refinement in knowledge about low-level lead toxicity and an inability to remediate some known sources of contamination, the overall prevalence of lead toxicity has persisted and not fallen in tandem with the drop in median blood lead levels.

Sources of Lead Poisoning

Lead can be found in air, food, and drinking water. Higher lead concentrations can be found in dust and soil contaminated by automotive exhaust, lead smelter and waste incinerator discharge, and/or lead-based paint chips. The most frequent significant exposure to lead for children comes from peeling lead-based paint on residential interior and exterior walls.

Paint

Peeling lead-based paint in old urban, low-income housing units poses the greatest preventable environmental public health threat to the health of urban low-income children (Landrigan *et al.*, 1987). At least one-half of all HUD facilities, 900,000 housing units, require lead abatement of painted surfaces. A housing unit requires abatement under a standard with a ceiling of 1 mg lead/cm painted surface area. The projected costs for a 5-year remediation program of HUD housing exceeds $2 billion.

These estimates do not include privately held contaminated properties not administered by government housing programs. In total, an estimated 44 million structures in the United States are contaminated with lead-based paint. Thirteen million children live in these housing units. A 1-g lead paint chip containing 5% lead will deliver a potential dose of 50 mg (50,000 μg) of lead. The amount of lead absorbed by the body varies with the size of the chip and the child's nutritional state, but clearly the toxic risks are great. The cost of adequate remediation for these buildings approaches $90 billion.

Unremediated buildings painted with lead-based paint prior to the 1977 paint regulations are now peeling and flaking toxic chips. Ironically and tragically, sloppy remediation of residential leaded paint by sanding, sandblasting, or other paint-stripping techniques serves to increase environmentally available lead in the form of inhalable paint chips and dust (Schwartz and Levin, 1991). Lead-based paint is still available for maritime use, farm and outdoor equipment, and road stripe painting and in old paint still available in discount stores. Dilapidated low-income housing and the continued availability of lead-based paint implicate paint as the major source of childhood lead poisoning.

Soil

Lead in dust and soil is the second major source of environmental lead contamination (Mushak and Crocetti, 1990; Thornton *et al.*, 1990). In rural areas, concentrations rarely exceed 200 ppm. In urban areas exposed to both a high density of automotive gasoline combustion and lead-based paint flakes, soil lead levels can exceed 3000 ppm. In industrial areas surrounding smelters and waste incinerators, the lead levels in soil have been found to exceed 100,000 ppm (Roels *et al.*, 1980). Each 100 ppm increase in soil lead levels >500 ppm results in mean increases in childhood blood lead levels of 2 μg/dl. Soil exposure rarely causes symptoms of lead toxicity, but subclinical neurotoxicity and intellectual impairment may occur.

Low-Dose Sources

Low-dose sources of lead are the air, food, and water (Landrigan *et al.*, 1987). Two decades ago, these three sources were responsible for an average estimated blood lead concentration of 10 μg/dl. Today, after increasing regulation of environmental lead pollution, these three sources account for about 6 μg/dl.

Air

Lead in air that is inhaled comprises a smaller dose than lead that is ingested, but due to the aerosolized nature of airborne lead, a high percentage of inhaled lead is absorbed into the bloodstream.

Air must contain <1.5 μg lead/m^3 to meet EPA guidelines. Air quality controls have reduced lead content in California air from a mean of 1.2 μg/m^3 in 1975 to a range of 0.1–0.7 μg/m^3 in 1990. Reductions in lead content of gasoline have been largely responsible for the improvement in air lead levels, but in 1 year >1.5 million kg of lead still are dispersed into the atmosphere by gasoline combustion alone.

Lead also is used in many consumer products as part of solder, glass, plastic, and pigment (Silbergeld, 1990). Rarely does lead become bioavailable during consumer use, but upon disposal of these consumer goods, lead may be released into the environment. High-temperature incineration of municipal and hazardous waste is being increasingly utilized by waste disposal facilities. This method produces toxic fly ash particle residues containing lead and other metals (Roels *et al.*, 1980). The particles are more easily transported by wind and water and leach readily into water supplies. The ash is more easily inhaled, ingested, and incorporated into living tissue than lead in its original form. Lead in consumer products can ultimately prove toxic to children exposed to incinerator air and water pollution.

Water

Drinking water usually contains <20 μg lead/dl, but 42 million Americans are exposed to higher concentrations in their tap water (Silbergeld, 1990). Acidic atmospheric pollution problems result in acidic surface waters and water supplies. The low pH of drinking water effectively dissolves lead from plumbing and lead solder into solution. Early-morning first-draw use and intermittent use without adequate flushing can greatly increase lead concentrations in drinking water samples. The scenario of water standing overnight exposed to lead pipe solder before early-morning consumption by children is met by millions of schoolchildren at risk of exposure. The lead levels found in some school water samples are dangerous levels for a child's health and development, although the child may not be acutely symptomatic.

Food

Leafy vegetables absorb lead from the air and soil (Silbergeld, 1990; Landrigan *et al.*, 1987). Lead contamination from pesticide and herbicide residues and by combustion products from leaded gasoline in farm machinery accounts for most of the lead content in food. Children consume foods containing between 20 and 80 μg lead everyday. A small percentage of this dose is absorbed. Lead is no longer permitted in jars and other packaging. In recent decades, baby food was lead-contaminated by leaded lids on jars.

Fetuses and neonates are still exposed to lead circulating in maternal blood and in milk during lactation. The dose is significant because pregnant women mobilize stored bone lead and release it during and after pregnancy (Crocetti and Mushak, 1990). Over 95% of absorbed lead is stored in bone tissue. This maternal bone lead mobilization combined with the mother's ongoing environmental exposure delivers a high cumulative dose of lead to the infant.

Unusual Sources

Uncommon sources of lead exposure in children include metallic objects (e.g., ingested fishing weights and lead shot, injuries due to gunshots), lead-glazed ceramics, old toys and furniture, storage battery casings, leaded paint on farm equipment, poorly soldered and imported canned foods, leaded decorative drinking glasses and food wrappers, folk medicines, leaded stained glass artwork, leaded crystal decanters, cosmetics, antique pewter, parental exposure, and gasoline sniffing and other forms of drug abuse (Landrigan *et al.*, 1987; Trotter, 1990; CDC, 1983; Ali *et al.*, 1978; Baker *et al.*, 1977).

Lead-glazed pottery finds use as cookware among some ethnic groups in the southwestern United States, Mexico, and Central America (Trotter, 1990). Mexican and Central Americans often use earthenware pottery glazed with lead oxide to cook pinto beans, rice, and meat. If these containers are not fired at high enough temperatures, they can later release lead into the food being cooked or stored. Even if properly fired, frequent washing and/or cooking with highly acidic foods can induce the release of lead from the container.

Folk medicines utilize lead-based remedies for the cure of certain conditions (Trotter, 1990). Among Mexican and Central American traditional culture, a lead-based treatment is often employed as a folkloric remedy for *empacho*. Empacho is constipation thought to be induced by eating the wrong food at the wrong time or by forcing children to eat food that they do not enjoy eating, among other reasons. The cure for empacho is believed to be the administration of lead oxide (*greta*) or lead tetroxide (*azarcon*). In one study, between 25 and 96% of Mexican American communities in Texas, New Mexico, and Arizona considered empacho as a true illness. About 20% of these households employed greta or azarcon as treatments. It is estimated that 10% of the children in households treating empacho have been exposed to periodic lead poisoning from this source.

Hmong refugees in Minnesota were found to use a lead-based remedy for common cold symptoms (CDC, 1983). This practice was subsequently traced back to widespread traditional Asian medical practices. In some Arab countries, lead-based substances have been used as astringents applied to the newborn's umbilicus and to aid children with teething.

Cosmetic practices using lead-based compounds are common in Asia, the Middle East, and Nigeria (Ali *et al.*, 1978). Known as *kohl, surma,* and *tiro* in their respective cultures, these substances are used as eye shadow to highlight the beauty of a child's eyes. Children poison themselves when they transfer the eye shadow to their fingers and then subsequently ingest the lead orally.

Some forms of drug abuse serve as sources for exposure to lead. Drug use and abuse in the form of gasoline fume inhalation and cigarette smoking can expose children to lead. Cigarette tobacco, like most agricultural products, contains lead, but the dose delivered by tobacco cigarettes is low compared to the dose delivered by *basuco* cigarettes (Seigel, 1991). The practice of smoking basuco, a cigarette laced with chemical residues from cocaine processing, has been gaining favor among some sectors of Peruvian and Colombian youth. The cocaine-processing wastes in basuco are heavily contaminated with solvents, metals, and other toxic compounds. In addition to the long-recognized problems for youth associated with drug abuse, lead poisoning due to basuco threatens exposed children with irreversible brain damage.

PREDISPOSING FACTORS

Nutritional state, presence of red blood cell disorders, and hand-to-mouth activity (pica behavior) can influence lead toxicity in children (Sachs and Moel, 1989). Deficiencies of iron, calcium, or zinc can lead to increased absorption of a lead dose. Gastrointestinal absorption of lead increases several-fold in children who are not anemic yet are suffering from iron-poor diets. Iron deficiency is considered the most important single predisposing factor for the increased absorption of lead. The prevalence in U.S. children of iron deficiency, and thus increased susceptibility to lead poisoning, may exceed 15%.

Children with sickle-cell trait and thalassemia have been shown to be more susceptible to lead poisoning. Red blood cell distribution width affects absorption and deposition of ingested lead. The high prevalence of the sickle-cell trait among African American children coupled with their disproportionate poverty rate (thus, environmental exposure in dilapidated housing) magnifies the deleterious effects of lead poisoning on this group.

Pica behavior is the process by which some individuals satisfy a craving for unnatural foods such as dirt, dust, or ashes. Pica behavior should not be confused with normal child development. Children at certain ages naturally explore their world by mouthing and tasting nonfood objects. Often these objects are also swallowed with varying effects. Pica behavior can be found in both children and adults. In children, pica exceeds the normal explorations of a developing child and can be thought of as compulsive or habitual. If pica behavior is directed toward lead-based paint chips, the child will obviously be at great risk of lead poisoning.

PREVALENCE OF LEAD POISONING

NHANES II (1978) and the most current (1984) large area stratified survey of lead exposure in U.S. children aged 0.5–5 years estimated a total at-risk population of 13.84 million children (Crocetti and Mushak, 1989, 1990). At the currently defined toxicity blood lead level of 10 μg/dl, *6.4 million children, or 46% of the age group, were poisoned by lead in 1984.*

Crude projections estimate a 25% decline in overall blood lead levels over the past 5 years based on results for mean blood lead levels derived from smaller studies. By this adjustment, *an estimated 4.8 million children in the United States are currently lead-poisoned.*

An African American child in the United States is at 4 times the risk of being lead poisoned than a white child. A child living in poverty faces 7 times the risk of lead poisoning than a more affluent child.

Between 1976 and 1980, the mean blood lead level in preschool-aged children was 16 μg/dl. African American children had mean circulating lead levels of 21 μg/d. The mean blood lead level among white children was 15 μg/dl. Prevalence of high lead levels (in excess of 30 μg/dl) among African American children was 12%. Among white children, 2% experienced dangerously elevated blood lead levels.

Prevalence rates for elevated blood lead levels were highest among poor families (earning less than $15,000/year) and those living in high-population density central city areas. Exposure to lead-based paint chips in dilapidated housing and leaded gasoline combustion products in the urban environment probably explains the higher prevalence of lead poisoning in these groups.

At the time of the 1984 study, the positive toxicity level was defined as any level >25 μg lead/dl blood. With that definition, the overall rate of positive toxicity risk cases was 1.5%. The five highest rates of positive cases occurred in St. Louis, Missouri (11%), Augusta and Savannah, Georgia (9%), Harrisburg, Pennsylvania (4.9%), Washington, D.C. (3.5%), and Merrimac Valley, Massachusetts (3.5%).

If the downward trend in revising toxicity thresholds continues, many million more children may be lead-poisoned. At the 5 μg/dl ceiling, 12.7 million (92%) children would have been considered poisoned in 1984 and 9.5 million would be lead toxic today. As the government recognizes the health effects of ever-lower levels of lead contamination, larger populations of children are defined as lead-poisoned. Many children living in affluent suburbs now fall under risk thresholds that were once ignored by the public, government, and media as health concerns only for low-income, urban, minority group children (Fu, 1990).

Estimates of the numbers of U.S. women of childbearing age whose lead exposure levels present intrauterine risk to their fetuses was estimated in 1984 at 4.47 million (Crocetti and Mushak, 1990). This figure represents 10.82% of the 41.3 million women between the ages of 15 and 44 with blood lead levels of 10 μg/dl. Previous studies have documented long-term neuropsychological impairment in children exposed to such lead levels *in utero*.

About 3.4 million white women of childbearing age (9.65%) were at or above the 10 μg/dl lead level out of 35.22 million women in that race and age group. Among African American women, 1.07 million (17.5%) out of 6.08 million in that age category had blood lead levels that would jeopardize their children *in utero*. While 9.2% of white women in the 15–19-year-old age group and 9.7% of white women in the 20–44-year-old age group exhibited dangerous lead levels, 8.2 and 19.7% of African American women in the same age categories, respectively, were at risk. The high relative risk of lead poisoning for African American children begins in the womb.

Perhaps due to lead poisoning's proxy status for poverty, African Americans sustain a disproportionate share of the lead poisoning burden. Although sensitivity to lead poisoning can be exacerbated by predisposing conditions found disproportionately among African Americans, predisposing factors alone cannot explain the heavy weighting of lead poisoning cases in minority group populations. Because lead poisoning is primarily an institutionally preventable environmental insult, the racial distribution of lead poisoning may well be a reflection of institutionalized racism in America.

Of the estimated 3.6 million pregnancies in 1984, 403,200 women (11.2%) were at or above the 10 μg/dl risk level (Crocetti and Mushak, 1990). Over the course of 10 years, an estimated 4 million fetuses are at elevated risk of *in utero* lead poisoning. Many of these children are at high risk of developing childhood lead poisoning because they will presumably be exposed to the same lead-contaminated environment as their mothers.

A 1991 California study found that 3% of 723 umbilical cord blood lead levels tested exceeded 10 μg/dl (Satin *et al.*, 1991). Interestingly, 14% of all premature babies in the study were associated with elevated umbilical blood lead levels. Lead poisoning of the mother yielded a relative risk for premature birth of 2.9 compared to the risk for premature birth faced by gravid women with low lead exposure (<10 μg lead/dl blood). According to this study, perhaps as much as 47% of premature births can be attributed to excessive lead levels in pregnant women.

EFFECTS OF CHILDHOOD LEAD POISONING

Lead-poisoned children may experience neurologic, metabolic, hematologic, and renal damage (Veerula and Noah, 1990). Pregnant women exposed to lead can suffer sterility, miscarriage, and fetal defects. Acute lead toxicity can be fatal, especially in the 1–3-year-old age group. The significant health risk to millions of lead-exposed children lies in the sometimes subtle neuropsychological impairment resulting from chronic low-level lead toxicity.

The impact of lead poisoning is more pronounced in children than in adults due to several factors (Friedman and Weinberger, 1990). Developing soft tissues are more sensitive to the metabolic changes induced by lead toxicity than mature systems. Long-term effects on cognitive function are thought to be more severe and noticeable when disruption occurs during critical developmental stages of infancy and childhood. The most important factor in children's increased susceptibility to lead poisoning involves differences in lead absorption and retention. Adults absorb only 5–10% of ingested lead and retain only a small percentage of the ingested dose, mostly in bone. Children absorb 40–50% of their lead intake and retain 20–25%, much of it in soft tissue.

Neuropsychological Effects

Lead passes easily across the placental barrier and is delivered through lactation. Fetuses exposed to circulating maternal lead levels are found to have poorer neonatal physical status than unexposed neonates (Dietrich *et al.*, 1990; Bellinger, 1989). Effects of lead exposure include decreased gestational age, delayed fetal maturation, low birth weight, and increased risk of physical anomalies. Some defects in later mental development may be due in part to the secondary effects of lead toxicity in lowering birth weight and gestational maturity. Analysis of NHANES II data found that neonates exposed to moderate lead levels *in utero* exhibited shorter stature, decreased weight, and diminished chest circumference through age 7 years compared to minimally exposed neonates.

Newborns exposed to maternal blood lead levels exhibit several measurable impairments at birth and early infancy (Bellinger *et al.*, 1990, 1991; Lilienthal *et al.*, 1990). Studies of such infants have disclosed abnormal reflex clusters as measured by the Brazelton Neonatal Behavioral Assessment Scale. Soft signs and muscle tonus scores on the Graham/Rosenblith Behavioral Examination of the Neonate are significantly out of normal ranges in lead-exposed infants. Significant negative mental and psychomoter effects of lead exposure have been measured at delivery and at 6-month intervals to 2 years age on the Bayley Scales of Infant Development in lead-exposed neonates. Lead–exposed neonates exhibit poorer perceptual performance, information processing, and linguistic skills as children than do unexposed neonates (Dietrich *et al.*, 1991; Needleman and Bellinger, 1991).

The exact mechanism by which lead disrupts brain cell function and causes neurobehavioral and neuropsychologic changes in exposed children is complex and not fully understood (Wang *et al.*, 1989). Some of lead's neurotoxic effects are secondary to metabolic disturbances, such as disruption of heme synthesis, but lead clearly has direct effects on the nervous system as well. There are, however, no apparent pathologic changes in brain anatomy associated with low-level lead exposure. Several hypotheses exist as to the actual neurophysiological basis for changes caused by chronic low-level lead exposure (Goldstein, 1990).

Lead's direct neurotoxic effects may occur through damage to the blood–brain barrier and subsequent alteration of the homeostatic control processes of the brain. Lead may directly interfere with neuronal activity and/or synaptogenesis. Neurocellular messenger systems are sensitive to lead. The neurologic effects of lead may involve the metal's interference with the binding of neurotransmitters to cell-surface receptors, the transduction processes producing secondary intracellular messengers, or the activation of specific protein kinases. Neurocellular function and gene expression may also be disturbed by lead's phosphorylation of important regulatory proteins.

Learning and cognition depend on the synaptic networks laid down in childhood and on normal neurotransmitter function. Protein kinases are central to both the development of synaptic organization in the developing human brain and the control of neural transmission. Lead disrupts the regulation of protein kinase activity by replacing calcium, an important intracellular messenger. When the synaptic organization and regulation of a developing child's brain is disturbed, both short-term and long-term cognitive and behavioral function will likewise be disturbed.

As a neurotransmitter reaches a cell surface, it binds to a receptor site. A signal that the receptor site is occupied passes through the plasma membrane in the form of a transduction molecule (G-protein). G-protein stimulates an enzyme to produce a soluble molecule (the intracellular second messenger) specific for a type of protein kinase.

Intracellular messengers include cyclic adenosine monophosphate, cyclic guanosine monophosphate, calmodulin, diacylglycerol, inositol triphosphate, and calcium. Protein kinase C, normally complexed with calcium, is especially sensitive to the presence of lead.

In the normal brain, diacylglycerol, in the presence of calcium, activates protein kinase C. Lead is capable of replacing calcium in this reaction sequence (Goldstein, 1990). Such disruption of the normal regulation of protein kinase C severely limits the efficiency of synaptic transmission and modulation.

Another neurotransmitter pathway disrupted by lead involves the activation of calmodulin in the absence of calcium (Goldstein, 1990). Normally, calcium is needed to activate calmodulin and its protein kinase to phosphorylate synapsin, a protein important to enhance appropriate neurotransmitter release. In the presence of lead, the calmodulin–protein kinase complex will activate synapsin even without calcium, thereby disrupting normal neurotransmission.

In the infant's brain, efficient neurotransmission is critical to the accurate formation of complex networks comprising billions of synaptic connections. Neural networks disrupted during the formative process may have no gross pathologic feature to distinguish them from normally formed synaptic connections, but they may result in the type of neuropsychologic impairment exhibited by lead-poisoned children.

Lead can disrupt the blood–brain barrier by accumulating in the brain's endothelial cells (Goldstein, 1990). High-level exposure to lead results in the loss of normal barrier controls, the access of plasma into the brain's interstitial spaces, edema, increased intracranial pressure, loss of cranial perfusion with blood, and irreversible brain damage. Low-level exposure to lead does not result in such encephalopathy but is suspected of altering the blood–brain barrier in less severe ways.

Endothelial cells and astrocytes form the blood–brain barrier. The action of protein kinase C is important to the establishment of endothelial cell differentiation and control of cell growth. Protein kinase C is normally activated at specific developmental stages relevant to the maturation of the blood–brain barrier's endothelial cells. Lead's action in stimulating protein kinase C is suspected of disrupting the normal development of endothelial cells and the selective permeability of the barrier (Goldstein, 1990). Again, no gross pathologic changes are detectable, but normal neuropsychologic development is impaired.

Both the peripheral and central nervous system are damaged by lead (Veerula and Noah, 1990). In peripheral nerves, lead causes segmental demyelination and axonal degeneration. This type of damage results in the classic acute lead-poisoning symptom of extensor muscle palsy with wrist or ankle drop. Motor nerve conduction may be slowed even in asymptomatic cases of lead toxicity.

Clinical manifestations of acute childhood lead poisoning begin with hyperirritability, anorexia, and decreased play activity (Winneke *et al.*, 1990). Lead colic causes sporadic vomiting, intermittent abdominal pain, and constipation. These symptoms precede acute encephalopathy by about 2–4 weeks. Lead encephalopathy is marked by the sudden onset of persistent vomiting, ataxia, impairment of consciousness, coma, seizures, and usually death. Children who survive lead encephalopathy generally suffer recurrent seizures, cerebral palsy, severe learning handicaps, and often blindness due to optic nerve destruction.

Other Health Effects

Chronic nephropathy often resulting in kidney failure is a long-term result of lead poisoning (Winneke *et al.*, 1990). Lead acts on the cells lining the proximal tubules. These cells are similar to the blood–brain barrier's endothelial cells. The proximal tubular cells are responsible for the activation of vitamin D from its precursors. Lead damages these cells by inducing the formation of dense intranuclear lead–protein inclusion bodies. Even very low levels of blood lead severely depress circulating levels of 1,25-dihydroxyvitamin D (vitamin D's bioactive form) by this mechanism (Rosen, 1989). Lead also causes tubular cells to increase reabsorption of uric acid resulting in hyperuremic gout. Hypertension and cerebrovascular accident are secondary effects of lead's action on the kidneys acting in conjunction with lead's direct effect on vascular smooth muscle. (Siegel, *et al.*, 1989)

Other disturbances in biochemical metabolism can be detected in lead-exposed children (Bhattacharya *et al.*, 1990; Landrigan, 1990). Hemoglobin production is especially susceptible to interference by lead. Even very low blood lead levels (<10 μg/dl blood) inhibit δ-aminolevulinic acid dehydratase, an important heme synthesis enzyme (Piomelli *et al.*, 1982; Berlin *et al.*, 1977). The effect of lead on inhibition of this enzyme is dose-related, discernible at 10–20 μg/dl, and nearly complete at 70–90 μg/dl.

Another heme synthesis enzyme inhibited by lead is ferrochelatase. Ferrochelatase, which catalyzes protoporphyrin to produce heme, is inhibited at low levels of lead toxicity. Obstruction of heme synthesis at this juncture causes excretion of coproporphyrin in urine and accumulation of protoporphyrin in erythrocytes. For this reason, erythrocyte protoporphyrin measurements are commonly used in screening programs to identify lead-toxic children.

PREVENTION AND TREATMENT OF CHILDHOOD LEAD POISONING

Treatment

Recommended treatment of childhood lead toxicity depends on four action levels established by the CDC (Daniel *et al.*, 1990; Needleman, 1990). For all lead toxicity cases the first and most important step is to isolate the child from the source of the poisoning. Either the child must be removed from the lead-contaminated house or the house must be thoroughly deleaded, cleaned, and inspected before the child returns.

At the threshold of 10–14 μg lead/dl blood, children should be tested frequently, and secondary preventative measures should be taken at home (i.e., removing paint or other lead sources). (Baker and Lewis, 1990) At the 15–19-μg/dl level, secondary biologic measures should be taken (i.e., dietary modification to limit the damage from lead). At the 20–44-μg/dl level, medical intervention is recommended. Levels >45 μg/dl constitute serious conditions or medical emergencies.

Medical treatment consists of 3–5 days of chelation therapy with 500 mg calcium disodium ethylenediaminetetraacetic acid (CaEDTA) administered twice daily by intramuscular injection (Fu, 1990). Long-term follow-up is always indicated in cases of lead toxicity. Neuropsychologic testing of children should be conducted to evaluate any learning disabilities incurred by exposure to lead. Parents and school authorities should be informed of any special needs for the lead-exposed child.

Prevention and Screening

Prevention of lead poisoning consists of primary environmental measures, primary biologic measures, secondary environmental/biologic measures, and extra-environmental action (Fritz, 1991; Mushak and Crocetti, 1990; Farfel and Chisolm, 1991). Primary environmental measures are the most important and effective solutions to the childhood lead poisoning problem. These preventative steps include the federal governmental actions designed to reduce the amount of lead dispersed in the environment though paints, gasoline, incinerator emissions, soil, dust, water, and food. Commercial dispersion of lead into the environment should be completely eliminated. Residual soil and air contamination will persist indefinitely, entering the food chain and exposing future generations to the lead threat. The safe abatement of lead paint in dilapidated housing already ranks alongside the Superfund cleanup as one of the most challenging and massive-scale public health needs in U.S. history.

Primary biologic prevention consists of nutritional supplementation in the context of community nutrition interventions. Interventions are needed on the scale of the Women, Infants, and Children nutrition program targeting high-risk populations such as those with low incomes, living in urban areas, and with members of minority groups. Dietary calcium and iron are especially important because levels of these nutrients are inversely related to the rate of lead absorption (Roberts, 1987). Nutritional care of at-risk populations to optimum levels would shift higher the level of lead required for toxicity. The risk of exposure would not decrease unless primary environmental prevention measures were concurrently instituted. Nevertheless, community nutrition interventions are important to control the effects of lead poisoning in children. Nutrition supplementation would have multiple benefits in countering problems of anemia and malnutrition in high-risk groups.

Secondary environmental prevention measures consist of lead toxicity screening and case-finding programs (Fritz 1991; Mushak and Crocetti, 1990). The screening instrument is the erythrocyte protoporphyrin (EP) level, a measure of heme synthesis. Positive EP tests require direct blood lead level determination for confirmation because the EP test also detects iron deficiency. Lead screening programs that are funded to conduct comprehensive screening of large populations of children and provide for follow-up are the most effective for early detection and treatment.

The direct cost-effectiveness of screening can be verified by comparing costs in two matched communities, one that conducts lead toxicity screening and the other that hospitalizes acute cases for treatment (Mushak and Crocetti, 1990). The direct benefit : cost ratio of screening has been calculated in this way at 53:1. the indirect cost savings of screening cannot easily be measured. Special education costs, law enforcement and corrections costs, crime victim losses, reduced tax payments, reduced productivity, and, most importantly, the diminution in the quality of life attributable to undetected childhood lead toxicity must be considered in a realistic accounting of the losses incurred by an unscreened lead-poisoned society.

Case-finding by the CDC ended in 1982. In that year, 30% of high-risk children (4.4 million) were screened and 250,000 met that year's toxicity criteria. Federal funding was eliminated and case-finding on a national level was terminated. In 1987, the American Academy of Pediatrics recommended that all children at risk of exposure be tested at 12 months of age and followed up as indicated (Landrigan *et al.*, 1987). Federal funding to meet these needs is unavailable (Zylke, 1991).

Secondary environmental/biologic measures seek to eliminate specific lead threats and institute dietary therapy after individual toxicity cases are identified (Mushak and Crocetti, 1990). After recognition via screening or self-identification, children who are found to be lead-contaminated must be assured a clean and nutritious home environment as part of treatment. Primary measures seek to prevent cases whereas secondary measures follow up on known cases.

Extra-environmental measures are court actions designed to force the removal of known lead hazards. Landlords who do not clean substandard housing in which children have been lead-poisoned are subject to civil action. Incinerators that dump lead into the environment are targeted for court action by environmental and other groups.

The success rate for judicial extra-environmental prevention measures is inconsistent (Mushak and Crocetti, 1990). In St. Louis, 1086 landlords were summoned to court for lead paint ordinance violations in 1985. Only 154 landlords were fined a total of $2447, an average of $16 per violation that reached the court system. The effect of miniscule sanctions on the abatement of the lead hazard is questionable. Nevertheless, the continuing threat of criminal and civil penalties can serve to motivate the appropriate authorities to take corrective action with regard to the lead threat.

CONCLUSION

Social evolution and progress depend on rational leadership and the wise investment of limited resources. The same government that ignored and now underfunds the defense of our nation's children from the domestic lead threat expends trillions of dollars of our wealth on dangerous and unproductive weapons of mass destruction (among many other misuses and corruptions of power). Such unenlightened vision leads to an uncivilized and ultimately unlivable society.

Lead poisoning poses grave risks to the normal development of children. Nearly 5 million American children are currently classified as lead-poisoned according to the CDC. Lead neurotoxicity, evident even at trace blood levels, leads to long-term neuropsychologic impairment. The social costs of lead poisoning place huge burdens on society, but the government has been slow to prevent and correct environmental lead pollution and unwilling to fund necessary national screening programs. Major resources in excess of $100 billion must be allocated to remediate the 44 million lead-contaminated dwellings, screen the 14 million children at risk, and treat the hundreds of thousands of disproportionately poor and minority group children victimized by this environmental disaster.

References

Ali, A. R., Smalls, O. R. C., *et al.* (1978). Surma and lead poisoning. *Br. Med. J.* **3,** 915–916.

Baker, P. O., and Lewis, D. A. (1990). The management of lead exposure in pediatric populations. *Nurse Practitioner* **15**(12), 8–16.

Bellinger, D. (1989). Pre-natal/early post-natal exposure to lead and risk of developmental impairment. *Birth Defects* **25**(6), 73–97.

Bellinger, D., Leviton, A., *et al.* (1990). Antecedents and correlates of improved cognitive performance in children exposed *in utero* to low levels of lead. *Environ. Health Perspect.* **89,** 5–10.

Bellinger, D., Sloman, J., *et al.* (1991). Low-level lead exposure and children's cognitive function in the pre-school years. *Pediatrics* **87**(2), 219–227.

Berlin, A., Schaller, K. H., *et al.* (1977). Environmental exposure to lead: Analytical and epidemiological investigation using the European standardized method for delta-aminolevulinic acid dehydratase activity determination. *Int. Arch. Occup. Environ. Health* **39,** 135–141.

Bhattacharya, A., Shukla, R., *et al.* (1990). Lead effects on postural balance of children. *Environ. Health Perspect.* **89,** 35–41.

Blackfan, K. D., (1917). Lead poisoning in children with special reference to lead as a cause of convulsions in children. *AM. J. Med. Sci.* **155,** 877–881.

Centers for Disease Control. (1983). Folk remedy-associated lead poisoning in Hmong children—Minnesota. *MMWR* **32,** 555–556.

Cohen, M. M. (1970). Toxic neuropathy, *In* "Handbook of Clinical Neurology," Vol. 7 (P. J. Vinken and G. W. Bruyn, eds.), p. 51. American Elsevier, New York.

Crocetti, A. F., and Mushak, P. (1989). Determination of numbers of lead exposed children as a function of lead source: Integrated summary of a report to the US Congress on childhood lead poisoning. *Environ. Res.* **50**(2), 210–229.

Crocetti, A. F., and Mushak, P. (1990). Determination of numbers of lead exposed women of childbearing age and pregnant women: An integrated summary of a report to the US Congress on childhood lead poisoning. *Environ. Health Perspect.* **89,** 121–124.

Daniel, K., Sedlis M. H., *et al.* (1990). Childhood lead poisoning, New York City, 1988. *MMWR–CDC Surveillence Summary.* **39**(4), 1–7.

Dietrich, K. N., Succop, P. A., *et al.* (1990). Lead exposure and neurobehavioral development in later infancy. *Environ. Health Perspect.* **89,** 13–19.

Dietrich, K. N., Succop, P. A., *et al.* (1991). Lead exposure and the cognitive development of urban pre-school children: Cincinnatti lead study cohort at age four years. *Neurobehav. Toxicol. Teratol.* **13**(2), 203–211.

Farfel, M. R., and Chisolm, J. J., Jr. (1991). An evaluation of experimental practices for abatement of residential lead-based paint: Report on a pilot project. *Environ. Res.* **55**(2), 199–212.

Friedman, J. A., and Weinberger, H. L. (1990). Six children with lead poisoning. *Am. J. Dis. Children* **144**(9), 1039–1044.

Fritz, C. J., (1991). New screening guidelines for lead poisoning. *Nurse Practitioner* **16**(7), 14.

Fu, D. J. (1990). Lead poisoning. Cause for alarm. *Hawaii Med. J.* **49**(12), 467–468.

Gibson, J. L., (1904). A plea for painted railing and painted walls of rooms of lead poisoning among Queensland children. *Aust. Med. Gazette* **23**, 149–153.

Goldstein, J. W. (1990). Lead poisoning and brain cell function. *Environ. Health Perspect* **89**, 91–94.

Hammond, P. B., and Dietrich, K. N. (1990). Lead exposure in early life: Health consequences. *Rev. Environ. Contam. Toxicol.* **115**, 91–124.

Hilts, P. J. (1991a). Lower lead limits are made official. *N.Y. Times* **Oct 7**, A7.

Hilts, P. J. (1991b). California to test children for lead poisoning. *N.Y. Times* **Oct 11**, C3.

Landrigan, P. J., DiLiberti, J., *et al.* (1987). Statement on childhood lead poisoning. *Pediatrics* **79**(3), 457–465.

Landrigan, P. J. (1990). Current issues in the epidemiology and toxicology of occupational exposure to lead. *Environ. Health Perspect.* **89**, 61–64.

Lilienthal, H., Winneke, G., *et al.* (1990). Effects of lead on neurophysiological and performance measures: Animal and human data. *Environ. Health Perspect.* **89**, 21–25.

Mushak, P., and Crocetti, A. F. (1990). Methods for reducing lead exposure in young children and other risk groups: An integrated summary of a report to the US Congress on childhood lead poisoning. *Environ. Health Perspect.* **89**, 125–135.

Nadakavukaren, A. (1986). "Man and Environment: A Health Perspective." Waveland Press, Prospect Heights, Illinois, p. 155.

Needleman, H. L. (1990). The future challenge of lead toxicity. *Environ. Health Perspect.* **89**, 85–89.

Needleman, H. L., and Bellinger, D. (1991). The health effects of low-level exposure to lead. *Annu. Rev. Public Health* **12**, 111–140.

Piomelli, S., Seamen, C., *et al.* (1982). Threshold for lead damage to heme synthesis in urban children. *Proc. Natl. Acad. Sci. USA* **79**, 3335–3339.

Roberts, F. B. (1987). Lead poisoning in children. *J. Tenn. Med. Assoc.* **80**(7), 426.

Roels, H. A., Buchet, J. P., *et al.* (1980). Exposure to lead by the oral and pulmonary routes of children living in the vicinity of a primary lead smelter. *Environ. Res.* **22**, 81,94.

Rosen, J. F. (1989). Metabolic abnormalities in lead toxic children: Public health implications. *Bull. N.Y. Acad. Med.* **65**(10), 1067–1084.

Sachs, H. K., and Moel, D. I. (1989). Height and weight following lead poisoning in children. *Am. J. Dis. Children* **143**(7), 820–822.

Satin, K. P., Neutra, R. R., *et al.* (1991). Umbilical cord blood lead levels in California. *Arch. Environ. Health* **46**(3), 167–173.

Schwartz, J., and Levin, R. (1991). The risk of lead toxicity in homes with lead paint hazard. *Environ. Res.* **54**(1), 1–7.

Seigel, J. (1991). Health of Colombian children threatened by potent *basuco*. *Washington Post* **Jan 9**, 24.

Siegel, M., Forsyth, B., *et al.* (1989). The effect of lead on thyroid function in children. *Environ. Res.* **49**(2), 190–196.

Silbergeld, E. K. (1990). Implications of new data on lead toxicity for managing and preventing exposure. *Environ. Health Perspect.* **89**, 49–54.

Thornton, I., Davies, D. I., *et al.* (1990). Lead exposure in young children from dust and soil in the United Kingdom. *Environ. Health Perspect.* **89** 55–60.

Trotter, R. T. (1990). The cultural parameters of lead poisoning: A medical anthropologist's view of intervention in environmental lead exposure. *Environ. Health Perspect.* **89**, 79–84.

Veerula, G. R., and Noah, P. K. (1990). Clinical manifestations of childhood lead poisoning. *J. Trop. Med. Hygiene* **93**(3), 170–177.

Wang, L., Xu, Se, *et al.* (1989). Study of lead absorption and its effects on children's development. *Biomed. Environ. Sci.* **2**(4), 325–340.

Winneke, J., Brockhaus, A., *et al.* (1990). Results from the European Multi-Center Study on lead neurotoxicity in children: Implications for risk assessment. *Neurobehav. Toxicol. Teratol.* **12**(15), 553–559.

Zylke, J. W. (1991). Increased lead poisoning diagnosis may precede possible eradication of problem. *JAMA* **266**(3), 316–317.

IV

Methodological Considerations in Neuroepidemiology

16

The Utility of Stroke Data Banks in the Epidemiology of Cerebrovascular Disease

John F. Rothrock • *Patrick D. Lyden* •*Mark L. Brody*

Stroke data banks have been described as everything from "an attractive means of studying clinical aspects of stroke" (Mohr, 1986, p. 171) to being of " . . . questionable [value], given the predictably high cost of such endeavors and the predictably low-level, descriptive research that such enterprises can support" (McAllister and Chipman, 1987; p. 273). In attempting to evaluate an epidemiologic method that typically requires a massive expenditure of time and effort and has provoked such a wide range of criticisms, one may first be moved to inquire: Why bother? How can the tedious collection, storage, and analysis of data from large numbers of patients with cerebrovascular disease enhance our understanding of that disease and improve clinical management and outcome? In short, why should a stroke data bank be considered necessary? And, such need established, what specific issues can a stroke data bank hope to address?

These are questions that demand plausible responses if we are to accept stroke data banks as a useful epidemiologic tool, and, in sequence, they form the basis of this chapter.

WHY?

Although stroke data banks were developed and used as early as 1935, (Airing and Merit, 1935), the majority of work in this area has occurred only within the last 15 years. Chief among the many forces initially stimulating this effort was simple frustration. Stroke has been (and remains)

Neuroepidemiology:
Theory and Method

Copyright ©1993 by Academic Press, Inc.
All rights of reproduction in any form reserved.

highly prevalent; it is the most common of the truly serious neurologic disorders, and it is the third leading cause of death in the United States (American Heart Association, 1991). Despite this, our understanding of stroke—its causes and pathophysiologic mechanisms—was alarmingly incomplete 15 years ago; and, despite the widespread use of medical agents and surgical procedures for prevention or acute treatment of stroke, often costly and usually accompanied by potential side effects, there have been, until recently, virtually no therapies of *proven* benefit for those purposes (Table I). Diagnosis and treatment of stroke were most often rendered "by anecdote," governed by one's most recent clinical experience and subjective impressions—a process reinforced by medical literature notably lacking in reports from well-designed and conducted clinical trials. Understandably confused by this haphazard approach to a common disease, clinicians often retreated to positions of either therapeutic nihilism or fanatic dedication to a single therapeutic intervention. Management of the individual stroke patient seemed to reflect the physician's personality or current mood more so than any coherent and accessible body of knowledge.

Table I

Stroke Therapies: 1980 and 1991

1980 Therapies widely utilized	1980 Proven Efficacy	1991 Therapies of proven efficacy
Aspirin		
Dipyrimadole	Warfarin[a]	Aspirin[c]
Heparin	?Aspirin[b]	Warfarin[d]
Warfarin		Ticlopidine
Carotid endarterectomy		Carotid endarterectomy[e]
EC/IC bypass surgery		

[a] From comparison against historical controls, warfarin was judged to be superior to no therapy for stroke prevention in patients with rheumatic mitral valve disease and atrial fibrillation. Warfarin also reduces stroke risk in patients with mechanical prosthetic cardiac valves.

[b] ? indicates conflicting results from several large-scale studies involving patients with transient ischemic attack or minor stroke.

[c] Aspirin reduces stroke risk in patients aged 75 or younger with nonrheumatic atrial fibrillation. Recent metaanalyses have convincingly demonstrated that aspirin is similarly beneficial in populations with atherothrombotic transient ischemic attack or minor stroke.

[d] Warfarin also reduces stroke risk in patients of all ages with nonrheumatic atrial fibrillation.

[e] Carotid endarterectomy significantly reduces stroke risk in patients with symptomatic (transient ischemic attack or minor stroke) carotid stenoses of ≥70%.

Abbreviation: EC/IC, extracranial/intracranial.

In response to this chaos, and fueled by impressive technological advancements that improved diagnostic accuracy [in particular, computed brain tomography (CT)], the modern stroke data banks emerged.

WHAT IS SOUGHT AND HOW TO SEEK IT

What

A stroke data bank is simply a registry of stroke patients that contains epidemiologic and clinical data derived from those patients, the complexity of which varies according to the investigator's energy and interests. The information obtained is typically entered into a computer to facilitate data retrieval and analysis. The major requirements for an "ideal" stroke data bank are outlined in Table II, and potential applications of a stroke data bank are listed in Table III.

How

For a stroke data bank to have clinical applicability, it must be both accurate and representative. That the data recorded be true, complete, and transcribed without error is a *sine qua non* of all clinical research, but there are additional requirements unique to a stroke data bank that must be met to ensure utility. To give a specific and important example, any sophisticated attempt to establish a useful stroke data bank must include an effort to identify specific factors that are causing stroke to occur in the population under study.

Virtually all stroke results from one of four basic mechanisms: intracerebral hemorrhage, subarachnoid hemorrhage, embolism, or primary occlusion of a vessel supplying the brain due to an intrinsic process (generally involving thrombosis) that arises within the vessel at that site, but many

Table II
Requirements for Reliability in a Stroke Data Bank

1. Prospective establishment of largely objective diagnostic criteria that optimize sensitivity and specificity.
2. A standardized and objective diagnostic evaluation applied uniformly to all patients.
3. Prospective collection of data directly by the investigators themselves.
4. "At-risk" population clearly representative of a more general population (local, regional, national, or international).

Table III

Potential Applications of a Stroke Data Bank

1. Determine the relative incidences of common stroke etiologies in a given population.
2. Improve diagnostic accuracy (by defining clinical and epidemiologic features of the various stroke subtypes and etiologies) and efficiency.
3. Study diseases associated with (and predisposing to) stroke.
4. Facilitate planning and execution of clinical trials.
5. Assist in prognostication.

specific etiologies may generate each of these mechanisms (Fig. 1). With the advent of CT, it became relatively easy to distinguish between hemorrhagic and nonhemorrhagic (i.e., ischemic) stroke, but further characterization of ischemic stroke, not to mention identification of specific etiologies, has proven more difficult. Because approximately 80% of all stroke is ischemic, and assuming that therapy must to some extent be etiology-specific to be effective, one can easily appreciate the need for more precision in diagnosis. Much of a stroke data bank's potential clinical value, then, will be inextricably linked to its success in unraveling the tangled issue of diagnostic classification.

Diagnostic accuracy within a stroke data bank is primarily a function of the criteria utilized and the process by which information related to diagnosis is obtained. The criteria used for diagnosis of each stroke etiology should be determined prospectively, before initiation of patient entry, and should be as objective, specific, and sensitive as possible. Excessive reliance on subjective criteria will result in a tautology that simply reflects investigator bias, encourages interobserver variability, and perpetuates clinical presumptions that may not be wholly valid. For example, embolic stroke indeed may typically be characterized by maximum neurologic deficit at onset, but to accept only this single clinical course as suitable for diagnosis will effectively eliminate the "atypical" embolic stroke from inclusion in that etiologic category; uniformity is preserved at the expense of accuracy. Alternatively, the diagnostic criteria adopted must not be so relentlessly objective as to become insensitive. A stroke data bank that places the highest percentage of patients in the "stroke, cause unknown" category will obviously be of limited clinical usefulness, despite its admirable diagnostic specificity. Although one must be wary of any stroke data bank that lacks an "unknown cause" group in its analysis of etiologies (thus implying poor specificity), such a group should ideally include only patients whose strokes resist diagnosis despite evaluations at least as thorough as those received by patients whose strokes have been attributed to specific etiologies. While it may be impractical to perform objective testing (e.g., brain scans, arterial imaging) on a routine and nonselective

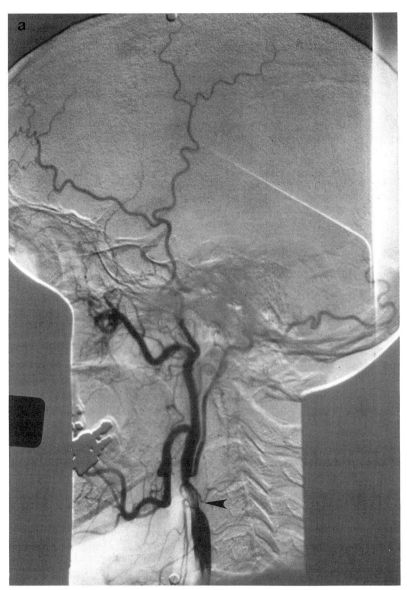

Figure 1 Selective carotid arteriograms performed on five patients with acute stroke and similar neurologic symptoms and signs. All five studies demonstrate complete occlusion of the internal carotid artery (arrows). Responsible etiologies were (a) atherothrombosis, (b) arterial trauma and dissection, (c) migraine-associated vasospasm, (d) methamphetamine inhalation, and (e) cardiogenic embolus. (Figure continues.)

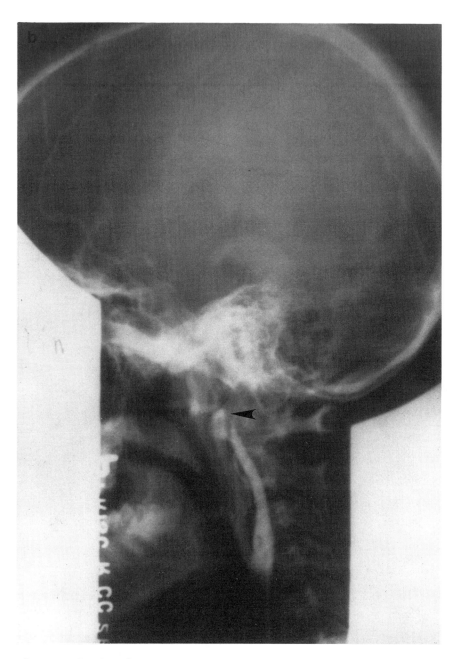

Figure 1 Continued

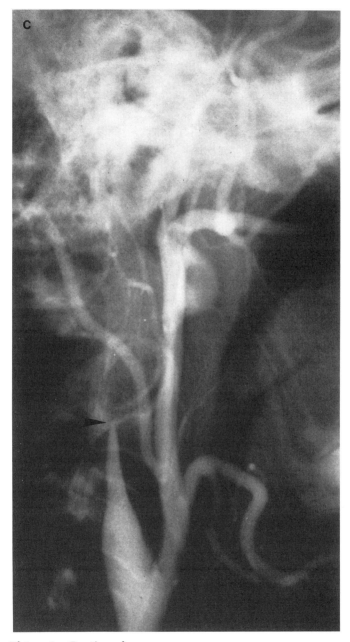

Figure 1 Continued

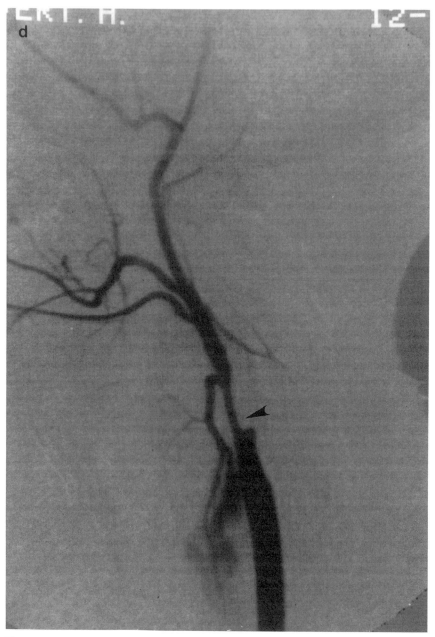

Figure 1 Continued

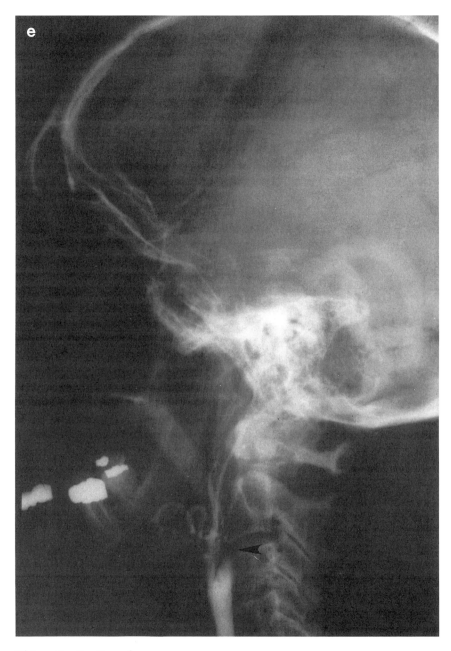

Figure 1 Continued

basis, patients should not be cast into the "unknown cause" category simply because such testing was not performed, especially if an omitted study was likely to have led to a more specific diagnosis. Ideally, a "standardized objective evaluation" may exist that will provide a starting point for diagnostic management of all stroke patients, reduce the number of potentially diagnosable patients in the "stroke, cause unknown" category and identify those patients who require more elaborate diagnostic intervention, without incurring undue financial cost. Until such a standard becomes available, investigators must seek a reasonable balance of subjective and objective criteria that preserves diagnostic sensitivity without sacrificing specificity.

In addition to the establishment of acceptable diagnostic criteria, accuracy demands prospective, "real-time" collection of data by the investigator directly from the patient. As Mohr (1986) has commented, "the farther the source of data gets from the investigator . . . the more limited is the use to which the findings can be put." (p.171). The same may be said for the timing of data collection in relation to the stroke; retrospective accumulation of data will be particularly problematic when subjective diagnostic criteria are heavily utilized, because historical details relating to the acute stroke presentation may be unavailable or distorted by virtue of interval time elapsed.

If its findings are to be generalized to a larger population, a stroke data bank must be, to a high degree, representative of that population; this is particularly critical in a study that purports to calculate relative incidences of stroke etiologies. Selection bias may result from a multitude of factors; racial, economic, and even seasonal variations in study populations and epochs may yield widely divergent results, as may the methods by which stroke patients are recruited for study. A stroke data bank that includes only hospitalized patients potentially introduces a bias in favor of stroke etiologies that tend to cause more severe neurologic deficit. Conversely, a patient accrual process that is largely retrospective and outpatient-based may shift results to favor stroke etiologies that have a more benign prognosis. Any effort to determine the relative incidences of stroke etiologies will optimally involve a patient population that demographically resembles the stroke population at large and a prospective recruitment process that includes *all* patients consecutively evaluated for stroke at the centers involved.

If a stroke data bank is successful in accurately determining stroke etiologies in most of its patients, if that group is representative of the larger stroke population that is under consideration, and, best of all, if the study population at risk (i.e., the population from which the stroke data bank patients accrue) is likewise representative of the general population, then the four remaining potential applications listed in Table III are likely to be realized. The data derived should allow more selective and individualized diagnostic intervention, reducing medical costs by eliminating unnecessary tests and yet improving management by directing the clinician toward procedures more likely to benefit his or her patient. Comparison of stroke data bank patients with a similar but stroke-free group from the same general population should yield information as to what factors, primary (race, sex, ethnicity, age, etc.) or acquired (hypertension, diabetes, smoking, oral contraceptive use, etc.), may influence one's risk of stroke, overall and according to specific etiology. When new potential therapies arise, findings from stroke data banks can assist investigators in formulating experimental protocols, directing their efforts toward those specific patient groups most in need of treatment and most likely to respond; such an approach should help minimize type II error, long the bane of clinical research involving therapies for cerebrovascular disease. Finally, stroke data banks should improve our ability to predict long-term outcome, including recurrent stroke risk, in individual patients, thereby stimulating the implementation of preventative treatment programs tailored to those patients' particular needs.

In the following sections we will describe the University of California, San Diego, Stroke Data Bank, compare and contrast its findings with those from other similar investigations, and offer examples as to how these findings can be applied to clinical practice.

THE UNIVERSITY OF CALIFORNIA, SAN DIEGO, STROKE DATA BANK

Methods

The University of California, San Diego, Stroke Data Bank (UCSD SDB) was established in 1983, and patient accrual began on July 1 of that year. Patients presenting to UCSD Medical Center or the San Diego Veterans Administration Hospital with presumed stroke were acutely, consecutively, and prospectively evaluated; both hospitalized and nonhospitalized patients were entered into the data bank, but patients found by subsequent testing to have subarachnoid hemorrhage from any cause or noncerebrovascular etiologies for their presentations were excluded. A detailed questionnaire recording data on past medical history, acute stroke presentation, physical examination, diagnostic studies, treatment, and clinical course was completed on each patient. When available, follow-up was obtained 1 month, 6 months, and every subsequent 6 months following the initial stroke. All patients were evaluated by a member of the entry team, and all completed questionnaires were reviewed by one of us (J. F. R.) prior to computer entry. Whenever possible, each stroke was assigned a specific etiology according to predetermined diagnostic criteria.

Strengths and Weaknesses

Accuracy (in general and specifically in relation to etiologic classification) was enhanced by our use of diagnostic criteria that were prospectively determined, largely objective, and reasonably well balanced in terms of specificity and sensitivity. A recruitment process that involved all patients (hospitalized and nonhospitalized) consecutively presenting to our facilities and that required acute evaluation of those patients directly by the investigators served to reduce selection bias. On the other hand, our diagnostic evaluations were at times incomplete, failing to supply data that would have fulfilled the criteria needed for specific diagnosis and, thus, resulting in an unfortunate swelling of the ranks of those strokes classified as being of unknown etiology. Furthermore, our study population, while by definition representative of those individuals who seek acute neurologic care at our facilities, cannot be said with any confidence to be representative of the national or regional stroke population. Even the general population served by our facilities may not accurately reflect the demography of the greater San Diego community. Twenty-nine percent of our patients were evaluated within the Veterans Administration system, and those patients tended to be older (mean age 62.4 versus 58.1), more often male (97% versus 54%), and more likely hypertensive (58% versus 50%) or active smokers (47% versus 38%) than patients recruited from the UCSD Medical Center population; and, as UCSD Medical Center serves a higher proportion of indigent and lower-income patients than do most of the other hospitals in the region, further selection bias was inevitable.

Results

Data from the University of California, San Diego, Stroke Data Bank

We have reviewed data from the first 523 patients entered into the UCSD SDB. Of these, 23 (5%) had stroke from intracerebral hemorrhage, and the following analysis will involve only the remaining 500 patients with acute ischemic stroke. Mean age in this group was 60.7 years (range 9–95), and 70 patients (14%) were 45 years of age or younger. Three hundred thirty (66%) were male. There were 324 Whites (65%), 82 Blacks (16%), 64 Hispanics (13%), 20 Asians (4%), and 10 individuals of other racial origins (2%).

Four hundred fifty-eight (92%) were functionally unrestricted by medical disease at the time of stroke. Four hundred thirty-nine (88%) were hospitalized. Brain CT or magnetic resonance imaging (MRI) was performed on 490 (98%), and 122 (24%) underwent cerebral arteriography.

Stroke etiologies for these 500 patients are listed in Table IV. Lacunar stroke was the most common specific etiology identified (133 patients; 27%). Ninety-nine patients (20%) had strokes due to emboli arising in the heart, 57 (58%) had atrial fibrillation, with or without associated valvular lesions, and 19 (20%) had emboli in association with left ventricular thromi. Eighty-one patients (16%) had strokes related to atherosclerotic disease involving the extracranial carotid bifurcation of the intracranial carotid, middle cerebral, vertebral, or basilar artery. Other miscellaneous etiologies for ischemic stroke were identified in 40 patients (8%).

In 117 (23%), no specific etiology for ischemic stroke could be identified. While in some instances this designation resulted from failure to perform a test (most commonly an arterial imaging study) needed to meet the otherwise satisfied criteria for specific diagnosis, in the majority of these cases a diagnosis could not be made despite evaluations typically more extensive than those received by patients in the other etiologic groups.

Data from Other Stroke Data Banks

The relative incidences of ischemic stroke etiologies as reported by a selective sample of other large-scale data banks are outlined in Table V; this sampling does not include studies that categorized stroke only as

Table IV

Ischemic Stroke Etiologies in the University of California, San Diego, Stroke Data Bank

Etiology	No. of patients
Lacunar	133 (27%)
Cardioembolic	110 (22%)
Large vessel	
Atherothrombotic/embolic[a]	88 (18%)
Miscellaneous[b]	52 (10%)
Unknown cause	117 (23%)

[a] Artery of primary involvement: extracranial carotid (81), basilar (3), middle cerebral (2), posterior cerebral (2).

[b] Migraine (19), arterial dissection (8), recreational drug abuse (7), hypercoagulability (5), vasculitis (4), head turning/no obvious dissection (2), tuberculous meningitis (2), eclampsia (2), "paradoxical" emboli (2), mucormycosis (1).

Table V

Relative Incidences of Ischemic Stroke Etiologies Reported from Selected Stroke Data Banks

Study	No. of patients	Large-vessel athero-occlusive	Lacunar	Embolic	Cardioembolic only	Unknown cause
Aring and Merrit, 1935	346	333 (96%)	—	13 (4%)	—	—
Kannel et al., 1965	70	57 (81%)	—	13 (19%)	—	—
Matsumoto et al., 1973	830	701 (84%)	—	76 (9%)	—	53 (6%)
Harvard Registry, 1978[a]	579	233 (40%)	131 (23%)	215 (37%)	112 (19%)	—
National Survey, 1981[b]	1612	592 (37%)	—	93 (6%)	—	927 (57%)
Tilbury (The Netherlands), 1982[c]	443	380 (86%)	—	—	48 (11%)	15 (3%)
Austin (Australia), 1983[d]	580	263 (45%)	140 (24%)	—	51 (9%)	126 (21%)
Kunitz et al., 1984[e]	708	172 (24%)	100 (14%)	200 (28%)	—	236 (33%)
South Alabama, 1984[f]	135	9 (7%)	20 (15%)	42 (31%)	—	64 (47%)
Yatsu et al., 1986[g]	3727	1880 (50%)	—	636 (17%)	—	1240 (33%)
NINDS, 1989[h]	1273	182 (14%)[i]	337 (26%)	—	246 (19%)	508 (40%)
UCSD, 1991	500[j]	88 (18%)[k]	133 (27%)	—	110 (22%)	117 (23%)

[a] See Mohr et al., 1978.

[b] See Walker et al., 1981.

[c] See Herman et al., 1982.

[d] See Chambers et al., 1983.

[e] See Kunitz et al., 1984.

[f] Does not include three unclassified strokes. See Gross et al., 1984.

[g] Specific numbers of patients have been calculated from percentages given in the published report.

[h] Does not include 52 cases classified as "others." NINDS, National Institute of Neurological Disorders and Stroke. See Sacco et al., 1989a.

[i] Number includes 69 cases of "tandem arterial pathology."

[j] Includes 40 cases of stroke from miscellaneous causes.

[k] Includes atherothrombotic and atherothromboembolic cases.

"ischemic" or "hemorrhagic" or surveys that were limited to a specific age group, sex, or race. Even so, as Table V demonstrates, results were widely varied from study to study, and this may in part be due to significant variations in the methods of patient selection, stroke evaluation, and etiologic classification employed by each data bank. Six surveys were either partially or totally retrospective (Airing and Merrit, 1935; Kanuel *et al.*, 1965; Kunitz *et al.*, 1984; Matsumoto *et al.*, 1973; Walker *et al.*, 1981; Yatsu *et al.*, 1986). Six made no attempt to distinguish between large-vessel and small-vessel occlusive stroke (Airing and Merrit, 1935; Herman *et al.*, 1982; Kannel *et al.*, 1965; Matsumoto *et al.*, 1973; Walker *et al.*, 1981; Yatsu *et al.*, 1986); both stroke types were typically grouped together as "cerebral thromboses" or "atherosclerosis" and, so combined, represented the most common cause of stroke in those data banks. In the six studies that attempted to identify small-vessel ("lacunar") occlusive stroke (Chambers *et al.*, 1983; Gross *et al.*, 1984; Kunitz *et al.*, 1984; Mohr *et al.*, 1978; Sacco *et al.*, 1989a; UCSD SDB), the incidence of large-vessel thrombotic stroke ranged from as low as 7% (Gross *et al.*, 1984) to as high as 45% (Chambers *et al.*, 1983).

The degree of diagnostic evaluation undertaken and the criteria used for the determination of stroke etiologies were far from uniform among the data banks. For example, in the data bank constructed by Kunitz *et al.* (1984), cerebral arteriography was performed on 42% of patients whose strokes were attributed to large-vessel atherothrombosis, whereas in the Harvard study this number (at least in the patients with carotid distribution stroke) rises to 74% (Mohr *et al.*, 1978). The survey by Gross *et al.* (1984) employed the strictest criteria of all for diagnosis of atherothrombotic large-vessel stroke, reporting that "the diagnosis of atherothrombosis was based entirely upon a positive angiogram, all nine cases showing occlusion of a major artery"; not surprisingly, then, their reported incidence of this stroke etiology was the lowest among the data banks represented in Table V. Similar variability in the extent of diagnostic intervention and in the sensitivity and specificity of diagnostic criteria employed likely explains the wide range in the reported incidences of embolic stroke as well as cardioembolic stroke. Despite having greater access to brain CT and MRI and noninvasive vascular testing, the more recent stroke data banks tended to record higher incidences of stroke of unknown cause. This may reflect a general trend away from an empirical diagnostic method, which relied more heavily on subjective data and investigator bias, and toward a more rigorous approach employing chiefly objective diagnostic criteria.

The most striking difference between the UCSD SDB results and those from previous studies lies in the higher proportion of lacunar stroke recorded in the former; ours was the only data bank in which lacunar disease was the most common stroke etiology. Although this discrepancy may simply reflect investigator bias and the persisting controversy as to the mechanism(s) of lacunar stroke (Millikan and Futrell, 1990), other factors potentially may have confounded intergroup analysis. For example, lacunar stroke tends to induce less neurologic deficit than most other stroke etiologies, and data banks that recruit exclusively from hospitalized patients will favor those etiologies if the hospitals involved typically choose to evaluate patients with minor stroke on an outpatient basis. Alternatively, a survey that recruits from patients who are initially evaluated in a clinic weeks or months after stroke onset will induce a bias favoring survivors of stroke and, specifically, those survivors who are intact enough to manage a clinic visit. The UCSD SDB attempted to avoid such selection bias by a recruitment process that included consecutively encountered hospitalized and nonhospitalized patients and by restricting entry to only those patients who were acutely evaluated. Finally, brain imaging is generally considered to be integral to the diagnosis of lacunar stroke; stroke data bank studies performed before the advent of CT were thus likely to neglect this etiology and place patients with lacunar stroke in other diagnostic categories (perhaps accounting for the relatively high incidences of large-vessel atherothrombotic stroke recorded in those series), whereas studies that made extensive use of brain MRI, more sensitive than CT in detecting lacunar stroke (Rothrock *et al.*, 1987), would be likely to favor that etiology. Of possible significance in this regard, MRI was performed on 59 (16%) of the 367 UCSD SDB patients with nonlacunar ischemic stroke and on 31 (23%) of the 133 patients with a final diagnosis of lacunar stroke.

APPLICATIONS

Stroke Etiologies

Accurate calculation of the relative incidences of stroke etiologies within a given population may allow identification of subgroups who are at increased risk for particularly virulent forms of stroke, with potential implementation of therapies that may reduce that risk. For example, analysis of findings from the UCSD SDB revealed that nasal inhalation of pulverized methamphetamine is a common cause of stroke in our younger patients (aged 21–35 years) (Rothrock *et al.*, 1988b), and a public information campaign was consequently initiated to desseminate this information to individuals at risk. On the other hand, despite numerous reports demonstrating that racial differences may influence stroke risk (Gross *et al.*, 1984; Hypertension Detection and Follow-up Program Cooperative Group, 1982; Yatsu, 1991), stroke severity (Cooper, 1987), risk of intracerebral hemorrhage (Gross *et al.*, 1986), and even relative incidences of stroke subtypes (Friday *et al.*, 1989), we were unable to find any significant correlation between racial origin and ischemic stroke etiology.

Although the relatively high incidence of lacunar stroke found in our study population may simply reflect an artifact provoked by methodological differences or investigator bias, it's intriguing to speculate that this finding is indeed population-specific. Can it be that stroke etiologies are a heretofore unrecognized degree dependent on the general health of the population under study? Is it possible that our increased awareness of, surveillance for, and treatment of atherosclerotic risk factors has resulted in a disproportionate decline in ischemic stroke directly related to atherosclerotic disease, or at least shifted the clinical expression of that disease from larger to smaller vessels (i.e., from atherothromboembolic large-vessel stroke to classical lacunar stroke)? Even more intriguing, does the reported increase in ischemic stroke of unknown cause over the past decade imply that we may be afflicted by fewer "traditional" atherosclerotic strokes and relatively more strokes of entirely different and, as yet, largely unrecognized origins? While these questions have enormous implications for our understanding and management of cerebrovascular disease, their answers must await results from well-designed surveys that can assess stroke etiologies in different populations simultaneously and over time.

Diagnostic Intervention

Findings from stroke data banks should assist in improving the efficiency of diagnostic management in individual stroke patients. As briefly mentioned earlier, experience with the UCSD SDB has shown that brain MRI is far more sensitive than CT in detecting symptomatic lacunar stroke and should be considered the brain imaging procedure of choice when a lacunar etiology is suspected and confirmation by neuroimaging is desired (Rothrock *et al.*, 1987). UCSD SDB data were indirectly helpful in demonstrating that carotid artery dissection may be diagnosed and followed noninvasively via a combination of MRI and duplex imaging (Rothrock *et al.*, 1989b). Finally, we have found that acute brain CT is of relatively little utility in the management of presumed acute ischemic stroke and, especially, transient ischemic attack (TIA) (Buehning *et al.*, 1989). Routine use of CT in these settings may represent an unwise diversion of health care resources, and given the current crisis in health care cost and delivery, these findings demand confirmation and further elaboration.

Clinical Trials

Data from large-scale stroke surveys can be of invaluable assistance in designing clinical trials intended to evaluate the safety and efficacy of existing and experimental therapies. For example, UCSD SDB findings have indicated that patients with asymptomatic carotid artery stenosis are at low risk for stroke in the distribution of the stenotic vessel, and this holds even for patients who have been symptomatic for stroke or TIA in another vascular distribution in the past (Babcock *et al.*, 1991). Given this relatively benign prognosis, studies investigating the use of prophylactic carotid endarterectomy for asymptomatic carotid artery stenosis will require a large sample size to demonstrate benefit, even if significant benefit exists. Along this same line, we have found a surprisingly high rate of early spontaneous recovery in patients with acute ischemic stroke and especially those with lacunar stroke (Rothrock *et al.*, 1991); studies designed to assess new experimental therapies that may acutely reverse stroke (e.g., tissue plasminogen activator) will need to factor in this confounding variable to avoid potential type II error.

In one recent study, the Stroke Prevention in Atrial Fibrillation Investigators (1990) trial, prospective diagnostic criteria modeled on those from the UCSD SDB were employed in an attempt to determine not just how often ischemic stroke occurred in each treatment arm, but also to characterize what specific types of stroke were and were not being prevented by the therapies under investigation. Interestingly, while both aspirin and warfarin were superior to placebo in preventing stroke in study patients with nonvalvular atrial fibrillation, aspirin's therapeutic effect was seen primarily in the reduction of noncardioembolic stroke, whereas warfarin appeared particularly effective in preventing cardioembolic stroke (Miller *et al.*, 1989). This differential treatment effect provides at least indirect validation of the UCSD SDB diagnostic criteria.

Prognosis

Stroke data banks may yield information that can assist in calculating initial or recurrent stroke risk in patients with conditions predisposing to stroke (e.g., asymptomatic carotid artery stenosis) or acute ischemic stroke itself. Regarding the latter, the National Institute of Neurological Disorders Stroke Data Bank investigators reported an early (first 30 days) recurrent stroke incidence of 3.3% for all ischemic strokes (Sacco *et al.*, 1989b);

among the ischemic stroke etiologies, the highest risk (7.9%) was found in the category of "atherothrombotic" large-vessel stroke, with the lowest risk (2.2%) in the lacunar group and intermediate risks (4.3 and 3%, respectively) in patients with cardioembolic stroke or stroke of unknown cause. These findings are similar to those derived from the UCSD SDB, but two additional points deserve amplification. First, in contrast to previous studies that reported a high rate of early recurrent stroke in patients with acute cardioembolic stroke (Cerebral Embolism Study Group, 1984; Cerebral Task Force, 1986, 1989; Norrving and Nilsson, 1986) and, overtly or by implication, thus called for early therapeutic intervention with anticoagulants, we found a low (2%) incidence of early (first 2 weeks) recurrent stroke in this clinical setting and no clear evidence of benefit from early anticoagulation (Rothrock *et al.*, 1989a). Second, UCSD SDB patients with lacunar stroke suffered a high (15%) incidence of recurrent stroke over the 12 months following initial stroke, but fortunately most of these recurrent strokes were likewise lacunar in origin and rarely inflicted significant, lasting functional impairment (Rothrock *et al.*, 1988a). It thus would appear wise to warn lacunar stroke patients that they are quite likely to experience recurrent symptoms of cerebrovascular disease but to reassure them that their risk of *major* stroke is relatively low.

SUMMARY

As is true in most research, the value of a stroke data bank squarely depends on the quality of the data accumulated. When a stroke data bank is reliable, its findings present a powerful tool for restructuring and developing our knowledge and management of cerebrovascular disease. New technologic advancements will eventually render existing stroke data banks obsolete, but newer and more accurate stroke registries hopefully will arise to enlighten our imperfect understanding of this all too common disorder.

References

Airing, C. D., and Merrit, H. H. (1935). Differential diagnosis is between cerebral hemorrhage and cerebral thrombosis. *Arch. Int. Med.* **56,** 435–456.

American Heart Association. (1991). Stroke facts. American Heart Association, Dallas, Texas.

Babcock, T. V., Rothrock, J. F., Lyden, P. D., Madden, K. P., and Clark, W. M. (1991). Previously symptomatic patients with asymptomatic carotid stenosis: Prognostic implications. *Neurology* **41,**(suppl. 1)126 (abst.).

Buehning, L., Rothrock, J., Ganiats, T., Lyden, P., and Taft-Alvarez, B. (1989). The utility of brain CT scanning in the management of acute stroke. *Stroke* 20, 150 (abstr.)

Cerebral Embolism Study Group (1984). Immediate anticoagulation of embolic stroke: Brain hemorrhage and management options. *Stroke* **15**, 779–789.

Cerebral Embolism Task Force. (1986). Cardiogenic brain embolism. *Arch. Neurol.* **43**, 71–84.

Cerebral Embolism Task Force. (1989). Cardiogenic brain embolism: The second report of the Cerebral Embolism Task Force. *Arch. Neurol.* **46**, 727–743.

Chambers, B. R., Donnan, G. A., and Baldin, P. F. (1983). Patterns of stroke: An analysis of the first 700 consecutive admissions to the Austin Hospital stroke unit. *Aust. N. Z. J. Med.* **13**, 57–64.

Cooper, E. S. (1987). Clinical cerebrovascular disease in hypertensive Blacks. *J. Clin. Hypertension* **3**, 795–845.

Friday, G., Lai, S. M., Alter, M., *et al.* (1989). Stroke in the Lehigh Valley: Racial/ethnic differences. *Neurology* **39**, 1165–1168.

Gross, C. R., Kase, C. S., Mohr, J. P., *et al.* (1984). Stroke in South Alabama: Incidence and diagnostic features—A population based study. *Stroke* **15**, 249–255.

Gross, C. R., Shinar, D., Mohr, J. P., *et al.* (1986). Interobserver agreement in the diagnosis of stroke type. *Arch. Neurol.* **43**, 893–898.

Herman, B., Leyten, A. C. M., van Zuyk, J. H., *et al.* (1982). Epidemiology of stroke in Tilbury, The Netherlands. *Stroke* **13**, 629–634.

Hypertension Detection and Follow-up Program Cooperative Group. (1982). Five-year findings of the Hypertension Detection and Follow-up Program: III. Reduction in stroke incidence among persons with high blood pressure. *JAMA* **247**, 633–638.

Kannel, W. B., Dawber, T. R., Cohen, M. E., *et al.* (1965). Vascular disease of the brain—Epidemiology aspects: The Framingham study. *Am. J. Public Health* **55**, 1355–1366.

Kunitz, S. C., Gross, C. R., Heyman, A., *et al.* (1984). The pilot stroke data bank. Definition, design and data. *Stroke* **15**, 740–746.

Matsumoto, N., Whisnant, J. P., Kurland, L. T., *et al.* 1973). Natural history of stroke in Rochester, Minnesota, 1955 through 1969: An extension of a previous study, 1945 through 1954. *Stroke* **4**, 20–29.

McAlister, N. H., and Chipman, M. (1987). Stroke data banks. *Stroke* **18**, 273 (letter to the editor).

Miller, V. T., Cohen, B. A., Feinberg, W. H., and Rothrock, J. F. (1989). Strokes in patients with nonvalvular atrial fibrillation. *Circulation* **80**,(suppl. 2), 404 (abstr.).

Millikan, C., and Futrell, N. (1990). The fallacy of the lacune hypothesis. *Stroke* **21**, 1251–1257.

Mohr, J. P. (1986). Stroke data banks. *Stroke* **17**, 171–172.

Mohr, J. P., Caplan, L. R., Melski, J. W., *et al.* (1978). The Harvard Cooperative Stroke registry: A prospective registry. *Neurology* **28**, 754–762.

Norrving, B., and Nilsson, B. (1986). Cerebral embolism of cardiac origin; the limited possibilities of secondary prevention. *Acta Neurol. Scand.* **73**, 520 (abstr.).

Rothrock, J. F., Lyden, P. D., Hesselink, J. R., Brown, J. J., and Healy, M. E. (1987). Brain magnetic resonance imaging in the evaluation of lacunar stroke and TIA. *Stroke* **18**, 781–786.

Rothrock, J. F., Chang, C., Lyden, P. D., Taft, B. J., Flores, J., and Wiederholt, W. C. (1988a). Prognosis following lacunar stroke. *Circulation* **78**,(suppl. 2), 602 (abstr.).

Rothrock, J. F., Rubenstein, R., and Lyden, P. D. (1986b). Stroke associated with methamphetamine inhalation. *Neurology* **38**, 589–592.

Rothrock, J., Dittrich, H., McAllen, S., Taft, B., and Lyden, P. (1989a). Acute anticoagulation after cardioembolic stroke: Risk vs benefit. *Stroke* **20**, 730–734.

Rothrock, J. F., Lim, V., Press, G., and Gosnik, B. (1989b). Serial magnetic resonance and carotid duplex studies in the management of carotid dissection. *Neurology* **39**, 686–692.

Rothrock, J. F., Kelly, N. M., Clark, W. M., and Lyden, P. D. (1991). Relative incidences of spontaneous early recovery amongst ischemic stroke sub-types. *Neurology* **41**(suppl. 1), 329 (abstr.).

Sacco, R. L., Ellenberg, J. H., Mohr, J. P., *et al.* (1989a). Infarcts of undetermined cause: The NINCDS Stroke Data Bank. *Ann. Neurol.* **25,** 382–390.

Sacco, R. L., Foulkes, M. A., Mohr, J. P., *et al.* (1989b). Determinants of early recurrence of cerebral infarction. The stroke data bank. *Stroke* **20,** 983–989.

Stroke Prevention in Atrial Fibrillation Investigators. (1990). Preliminary report of the Stroke Prevention in Atrial Fibrillation Study. *N. Engl. J. Med.* **322,** 863–868.

Walker, A. E., Robins, M., and Weinfeld, F. D. (1981). "Clinical findings" in National Survey of Stroke. *Stroke* **12**(suppl. 1), I13–I31.

Yatsu, F. (1991). Strokes in Asians and Pacific-Islanders, Hispanics, and Native Americans. *Stroke* **4,** 560–561.

Yatsu, F. M., Becker, C., McLeroy, K. R., *et al.* (1986). Community hospital-based stroke programs: North Carolina, Oregon and New York. *Stroke* **17,** 276–284.

17

Biostatistics and Neuroepidemiology

Amanda L. Golbeck • Patricia Silva

Some of the contributions that biostatisticians have made to the field of neuroepidemiology will be described in this chapter. Biostatistics involves the "development and application of statistical theory and methods for the study of phenomena arising in the life sciences"; the biostatistician develops stochastic or mathematical models, describing phenomena according to the biological interpretation of the underlying mechanism, defining appropriate random variables, deriving the corresponding probability density functions, and developing mathematics for estimation and other related problems where the required statistical theory does not exist (Chiang, 1985: 771).

Research that has a publication date of 1985 or later will be considered in this review. The first section describes five exemplary studies that involve development and application of stochastic models to illuminate aspects of various neurological disease processes. The second section is a description of research involving development of innovative sampling methods for the study of dementia. Next, stochastic models for medical technology assessment are discussed. The chapter concludes with a brief discussion.

Studies reviewed in this chapter have in common the fact that the model and methods that were developed were motivated by actual neurological disease questions. Omitted from this review are studies that provide an example using data from a neurological disease but otherwise fall under the umbrella of mathematical statistics. Specifically omitted are reviews of articles such as those of Jones and Crowley (1989), who present a general class of nonparametric tests for survival analysis and include a short example using data on low-grade gliomas (brain tumors), and Zeger (1988), who presents a regression model for time series of counts and includes an example using data on polio. Also omitted from this chapter are studies such as that of Kay *et al.* (1987), which involves stochastic

Neuroepidemiology:
Theory and Method

models and neurological diseases but focuses on their behavior in nonhuman populations.

NEUROLOGICAL DISEASES AND STOCHASTIC PROCESSES

Biostatisticians have made significant contributions to the field of neuro-epidemiology in the area of stochastic processes, that is, model building to describe phenomena that are dynamic and time-dependent. This is not surprising, given the view that the future of biostatistics lies in stochastic processes (Chiang, 1985). Different types of stochastic process models—Poisson, queueing, and general Markov process models—have been used to increase understanding of the behavior of neurological diseases such as multiple sclerosis (MS) and epilepsy. Research in this category has resulted from collaborations among researchers at McGill University, the Montreal Neurological Institute, and the Hôpital Neurologique de Lyon.

Natural History of Multiple Sclerosis: Simple Markov Model

A Markov process is a type of probability model that describes movement of individuals among a well-defined set of states over a period of time. Interest centers around the state that an individual is in at time t. Given knowledge about the present state that the individual is in, the conditional probability of movement to the next state is independent of the previous states that the individual has been in. This is called the Markov assumption.

Wolfson and Confavreux (1985) set up a simple Markov model to describe the natural history of MS. The model has three disease states (relapse without sequelae, relapse with sequelae, and progression) and two terminal states (death and censored). The possible movements of patients among these five states are summarized in the form of a transition probability matrix without reference to time, as illustrated in the following matrix. The entries in the matrix show, for example, that a patient in the relapse with sequelae state can move from that state to either the progression, death, or censored states but cannot return to the relapse without sequelae state (transition probability equal to 0), and, for example, that once a patient enters the death state he or she will remain there forever (transition probability equal to 1).

	Destination				
	Relapse without sequelae	Relapse with sequelae	Progression	Death	Censored
Source					
Relapse without sequelae	p_{00}	p_{01}	p_{02}	p_{03}	p_{04}
Relapse with sequelae	0	p_{11}	p_{12}	p_{13}	p_{14}
Progression	0	0	p_{22}	p_{23}	p_{24}
Death	0	0	0	1	0
Censored	0	0	0	0	1

Estimates of the probabilities in a Markov transition matrix may be obtained via the method of maximum likelihood, where the disease course of each patient is assumed to constitute an independent realization of a common Markov process. The authors obtain estimates using patient record data from 278 "definite" and "probable" cases with MS over a 20-year period from the neurology clinic in Lyon. First, the authors estimate the transition probabilities for the entire set of data. Then, they estimate for potential prognostic subgroups of the patient population; they also study separately the distributions of transition times between pairs of states for the various population subgroups.

The authors define five dichotomous variables for study that are potentially prognostic: age at onset (before or after age 35), sex (male or female), initial symptomatology (optic neuritis versus other), mode of onset (mono-versus polysymptomatic), and interval between the first two attacks (less than versus greater than or equal to the observed median). For each of these variables, a χ^2 test is used to compare the two estimated transition matrices, and a log-rank test is used to compare the two distributions of transition times between pairs of states. A prognostic factor is defined to be one that produces a significant result on either statistical test. The authors find that age at onset and sex have a significant effect on the estimated transition matrices, and that number of symptoms and age at onset have a significant effect on the distribution of transition times.

A significance test is applied to check the Markov assumption for the Lyon MS data set. The results provide support for use of the Markov model to describe the global dynamics of the disease of MS in individuals.

There are several limitations to the simple Markov model approach, and the authors delineate these in their article and in subsequent articles (see the following subsection). First, prognostic variables must be considered separately. Second, continuous variables must be grouped into binary categories. Third, interactions between variables can only be investigated using stratification, possibly resulting in small sample sizes for strata and a reduction in power. Fourth, the transition probabilities and the distributions of transition times between pairs of states must be studied separately. Fifth, personalized outcome estimates are unavailable.

Prognosis for Patients with Multiple Sclerosis: Elaborated Markov Model

The elaborated Markov model that is considered in this section falls under the category of stochastic survival models with competing risks and covariates. Wolfson and Confavreux (1987) utilize such a model as they continue their study of the natural history of MS. Their elaborated Markov model has the same states and possible movements among these states as their simple Markov model (cf. the preceding transition probability matrix), except that $p_{03} = p_{13} = 0$; that is, a patient in the relapse states cannot now move directly from those states to the death state.

In stochastic survival models with competing risks and covariates, movements from one state to another are determined by intensity functions. By definition, the intensity function for movement from state j to state k is the probability of making a transition from state j to state k in a very small interval of time $(t, t + \Delta t)$, conditional upon being in state j at time t.

In models such as that used by these authors, there are so-called illness intensity functions and so-called death intensity functions. Let $\nu_{jki}(t)$ denote the *illness* intensity function, for the transition from illness state j to *illness* state k at time t for the ith individual. Similarly, let $\mu_{jki}(t)$ denote the *death* intensity function, for the transition from illness state j to *death* state k at time t for the ith individual. Under the assumption that the intensity functions are independent of time, $\nu_{jki}(t) = \nu_{jki}$ and $\mu_{jki}(t) = \mu_{jki}$.

Let $\mathbf{x}_i$ be a vector of covariates for the ith individual; α', β', δ', ϕ', χ', ε', and γ' are vectors of unknown covariate coefficients to be estimated; and ν_{jk} and μ_{jk} are the underlying illness and death intensity functions, respectively, to be estimated for the transition from state j to state k when covariates have no effect upon this transition. With this notation, the authors' illness intensity function matrix for the ith individual is as follows:

	Destination		
	Relapse without sequelae	Relapse with sequelae	Progression
Source			
Relapse without sequelae	$-(\nu_{01}e^{\alpha'x_i} + \nu_{02}e^{\beta'x_i} + \mu_{01}e^{\chi'x_i})$	$\nu_{01}e^{\alpha'x_i}$	$\nu_{02}e^{\beta'x_i}$
Relapse with sequelae	0	$-(\nu_{12}e^{\delta'x_i} + \mu_{11}e^{\epsilon'x_i})$	$\nu_{12}e^{\delta'x_i}$
Progression	0	0	$-(\mu_{20}e^{\phi'x_i} + \mu_{21}e^{\gamma'x_i})$

The death intensity function matrix for the ith individual is as follows:

	Destination	
	Death	Censored
Source		
Relapse without sequelae	0	$\mu_{01}e^{\chi'x_i}$
Relapse with sequelae	0	$\mu_{11}e^{\epsilon'x_i}$
Progression	$\mu_{20}e^{\phi'x_i}$	$\mu_{21}e^{\gamma'x_i}$

For example, ν_{12i} is the intensity function for the ith individual for the transition from the state of relapse with sequelae to the state of progression, and it has the following form: $\nu_{12i} = \nu_{12e}{}^{\delta'x_i}$.

The important feature of this model is that the intensity functions have an exponential form that depends on any number of discrete or continuous covariates. Notice also that the underlying intensities are constant and the same for each individual. The log-linear form for the covariate adjustment is used for mathematical convenience and to avoid negative intensity functions.

The authors estimate parameters using the method of maximum likelihood for the same set of data as in the previous subsection, although this time the maximum likelihood equations require a computer-intensive solution. The risk of transition between states is written as a function of the five covariates (potential prognostic factors), now treating age at onset and interval between the first two attacks as continuous rather than binary variables. Wald's test is used to evaluate the effect of the covariates on the intensity functions. The authors find that interval between the first two attacks, sex, and mode of onset are significant prognostic indicators.

The preceding formulation allows for an integrated study of transition probabilities and times for transition. The authors stress the advantages of the elaborated Markov model, which were limitations to the simple Markov model approach: the allowing of simultaneous consideration of various prognostic variables, use of continuous variables, and evaluation of possible interactions between variables. Most important, transition probabilities can be estimated for subjects with particular sets of prognostic values: The authors stress that the elaborated model allows one to view MS globally for a set of patients, at the same time allowing a personalized description of MS for each patient; they point out that personalized prognoses for patients can help in selecting appropriate therapies for the patient and can help in appropriate selection of patients for clinical trials.

The authors present less technical descriptions of their research in two additional articles (Confavreux and Wolfson, 1988, 1989). The suggestion is made that an informative way of presenting results from the elaborated Markov model is to plot the changes in probabilities of movement from one state to another over a range of disease duration. Such curves can be drawn for the total set of patients starting from a specified state, for the subset of patients corresponding to any covariate value, or for a set of covariate values specific to any individual patient. The ability to draw this last type of curve corresponds to one of the major advantages of the elaborated Markov model: Estimated transition probabilities are adjustable for an individual patient (i.e., with specific covariates) as he or she passes through the various stages of disease.

The simple Markov model and the elaborated Markov model do not yield identical results. For example, in the simple Markov model, age at onset appears as a significant prognostic variable, whereas in the elaborated Markov model it does not. This demonstrates the importance that the choice of methodology has on prognosis analysis.

The authors discuss two future directions for their research. The first is in the area of refinement: explorations of alternative definitions of disease states, methods to reduce and better handle censoring, definitions and testing of new potential prognostic variables for inclusion in models, etc. The second is in the area of validation: new data sets to be used for estimation and comparisons of estimated prognoses with actual outcomes for the Lyon populations.

Epileptic Seizure Trends: Poisson Process Model

The Poisson process is a simple stochastic model of population growth that has wide applicability. The basic assumption of a simple Poisson process is that the occurrence of a random event at a given moment is independent of both time and the number of events that have previously taken place. In this case, the intensity function can be denoted by the constant λ.

Milton *et al.* (1987) detail how a time series of events, or point process, can be used to examine the timing of seizure occurrence in the general population of patients with epilepsy. The authors studied 24 adults with the disease. Each patient was asked to keep a seizure diary for a minimum of 61 days, indicating when each seizure occurred. The average patient recorded 18 seizures over 237 days. The authors examined five parameters: seizure frequency (number of seizures per day), interseizure interval (number of days between successive seizures), seizure clustering (an increase in the number of days with two or more seizures), differences between successive interseizure intervals, and number of days from the beginning of the seizure diary to the occurrence of a seizure.

The appropriateness of the Poisson process model to the study of epileptic seizure occurrence may be readily examined. For examples using the first three study parameters, the number of seizures per day should be constant, the time between successive seizures should follow an exponential distribution, and the observed number of days with n seizures ($n = 0, 1, 2, 3, \ldots$) should compare to the following equation:

$$ E_n = D \frac{e^{-\lambda}\lambda^n}{n!}, $$

where E_n is the expected number of days with n seizures, D is the number of days of observation recorded in the seizure diary, and λ in disease terms is the mean seizure frequency and is estimated by dividing the total number of recorded seizures by the total number of days observed.

To determine whether or not seizure frequency conformed to a Poisson process, the authors determined if a linear relationship existed between the cumulated number of seizures and the amount of time elapsed since day 1 of the diary. To determine whether or not the interseizure interval conformed to a Poisson process, the authors determined if a linear relationship existed between the natural logarithm of the proportion of interseizure intervals longer than a certain interval length versus that interval length. In both situations, they calculated the slopes using a least-squares linear regression analysis, and the fits were tested by using analysis of variance with F statistics. To determine whether or not the observed number of days with 0, 1, 2, or 3 seizures compared to the number expected by a Poisson process, the authors used a log maximum likelihood ratio test. Statistical tests were performed as well using the remaining two study parameters—differences between successive interseizure intervals and number of days from the beginning of the seizure diary to the occurrence of a seizure—to check how closely seizure occurrence followed a Poisson process.

The authors determined that seizure occurrence followed a Poisson process for one-half of the patients; for the other half, seizure intervals followed an exponential distribution, but other Poisson process assumptions did not hold. The authors point out that there are other processes besides the Poisson that are random, the Poisson being the simplest; showing departure of seizure occurrence from a Poisson process does not mean that the seizures are occurring nonrandomly. On the other hand, failure to show departure does not mean that seizure occurrence is truly Poisson. There may be underlying physiological or psychological parameters strongly correlated with the randomness.

The authors discuss several problems in studies of seizure occurrence. These are phrased here as questions. Should multiple seizures occurring on the first day be counted separately or as a single event? What time unit should be used to express seizure frequency—hour, day, week, etc.? Have enough seizures been observed for each patient in order to make reliable conclusions from statistical tests? The authors counted multiple seizures on day 1 separately, they used the day as the appropriate time unit, and the group of patients that showed departures from the Poisson process had more seizures and higher seizure frequencies. Whether or not, or how, factors such as these may have affected the conclusion reached by the authors—that seizures are occurring randomly in their patients—is unclear.

Distribution of Latent Period of Multiple Sclerosis: Queueing Model

In a queueing system, individuals arrive at certain times (random or patterned) to a location where they receive some kind of service and then depart. A queueing system is characterized by three entities: (1) the input process, which specifies the probability distribution of the pattern of arrivals of individuals in time to the service location; (2) the service process, which specifies the probability distribution of the time to serve an individual; and (3) the queue process, which specifies the number of servers and the order in which individuals are served.

Wolfson *et al.* (1989) use a queueing model to estimate the distribution of the latent period of MS. In their model, the input process is a nonhomogeneous (or time-dependent) Poisson process, in comparison to the homogeneous Poisson process described in the previous subsection; the service process is unspecified; and the number of servers is infinite. This is known in the literature as a $M/G/\infty$ queue.

In disease terms, the arrival of individuals in time to the service location corresponds to the initiation of MS in individuals in time, the time to serve an individual corresponds to the latent period distribution of MS, and the exit of individuals in time from the service location corresponds to the ages at onset of symptoms of MS in individuals. The authors point out that it is appropriate to assume an infinite number of servers because each individual's disease enters its latent period immediately after its initiation.

Previous MS studies have attempted to estimate specific parameters of the latent period distribution, including the mean, median, and support of the distribution. The methods of previous studies have been ad hoc, and hence the range of reported estimates is large. The present paper is the first to try to describe the entire distribution of the latent period in addition to providing estimates of specific parameters of the distribution. Rather than use ad hoc methods, the authors use a more sophisticated approach that involves use of a queueing process stochastic model. They show how the latent period distribution function $F(t)$ can be estimated when only the ages at onset of symptoms of MS are known. Note in this problem that the times of initiation of disease are specifically unknown.

In queueing models such as the one used by these authors, there are so-called input intensity functions and so-called output intensity functions. Let $\lambda(t)$ denote the *input* intensity function, which in this case is one that is associated with a nonhomogeneous Poisson process and which represents the rate of initiation of disease. Let $\gamma(t)$ denote the *output* intensity function, which represents the rate of clinical onset of disease.

The authors assume the following specific form for $\lambda(t)$:

$$\lambda(t) = \begin{cases} 0 & \text{for } t \le \tau_0 \\ \lambda & \text{for } \tau_0 < t \le \tau_1, \\ 0 & \text{for } \tau_1 < t \end{cases}$$

where $\tau_0 \ge 0$ and $\tau_1 > 0$ are fixed constants. In words, the assumption is made that there is a constant rate of disease acquisition in the period of susceptibility.

Start with an empty queue at time $t = 0$: In disease terms, the assumption is made that no one has the disease at time 0. Let $N(t)$ denote the number of customers who have exited the queue by time t: In disease terms, $N(t)$ is the number of individuals who have experienced clinical onset of disease by time t. $N(t)$ has a Poisson distribution with parameter $\Gamma(t)$. $\Gamma(t)$ is known as the mean value function of the Poisson output process. It is related to the input intensity, output intensity, and service time distribution as follows:

$$\frac{d}{dt}\Gamma(t) = \gamma(t) = \int_0^t \lambda(t - u)\, dF(u).$$

Using the specific form of $\lambda(t)$ given earlier for the MS problem, $\gamma(t)$ may be written as follows:

$$\gamma(t) = \begin{cases} 0 & \text{for } t \leq \tau_0 \\ \lambda F(t - \tau_0) & \text{for } \tau_0 < t \leq \tau_1 \\ \lambda[F(t - \tau_0) - F(t - \tau_1)] & \text{for } \tau_1 < t \end{cases}$$

Both nonparametric and parametric estimators are developed for the latent period distribution. Methods involve iterative calculations. A nonparametric estimator of the latent period distribution is derived using the preceding form for $\gamma(t)$. An analogous parametric estimator is derived under the supposition that the incubation distribution depends on a vector of parameters Θ, in which case we have $\gamma(t, \Theta)$ instead of $\gamma(t)$. To be specific, $\gamma(t, \Theta)$ may be written as follows:

$$\gamma(t, \Theta) = \begin{cases} 0 & \text{for } t \leq \tau_0 \\ \lambda F(t - \tau_0, \Theta) & \text{for } \tau_0 < t \leq \tau_1 \\ \lambda[F(t - \tau_0, \Theta) - F(t - \tau_1, \Theta)] & \text{for } \tau_1 < t \end{cases}$$

For the parametric approach both the χ^2 and log-normal distributions were tried.

In applications involving the nonparametric approach, the authors assume that the output intensity function has a mode at 30 years. In applications involving the parametric approach, they maximize the likelihood with respect to the parameter vector, and this procedure does not force the mode to be 30 years.

Methods are applied to patient record data from 528 patients who were seen at the MS clinic at the Montreal Neurological Institute over the most recent 2-year period and who had an approximate date of onset of MS recorded in their patient record. Several susceptibility periods were tried. Nonparametric, χ^2, and log-normal approaches yielded similar results for the 10- to 15-year susceptibility period, leading the authors to conclude that this is the most suitable one. For this susceptibility period, the nonparametric estimates of the average and median latent periods are 18.08 and 16 years, respectively.

Future directions for this research are suggested by the authors. First, a onset intensity that is nonconstant within the susceptibility period would be reasonable to try, if computational problems could be worked out. Second, the data set used in this study is from a mostly nonmigrant population from a country with high prevalence, and it would be useful to try the model on a mostly migrant population and/or a population from a country with low prevalence. Third, it would be useful to estimate the latent period distribution in groups of patients defined by HLA type. The authors conclude by pointing out the inherent limitations of the data.

Rate of Infection of Multiple Sclerosis: Elaborated Queueing Model

Joseph *et al.* (1990) study a queueing process similar to the one discussed in the previous subsection. Assumptions, in review, are that only the output processes are observed, there is a nonhomogeneous Poisson input process, the number of servers are infinite, the observation of output starts at time 0, and no customers are in the system at time 0. Notation will be the same as that used in the previous subsection. Translation of the queueing process model to the MS problem is also the same as in the previous subsection.

The objective of the Joseph *et al.* (1990) study is, however, different from the Wolfson *et al.* (1989) study discussed in the previous subsection. Recall that in the earlier paper, the objective was to estimate the service time distribution after making some assumptions about the shape of the input intensity in the queue over the inferred susceptibility period. In the more recent paper, the situation is reversed: The objective is to develop methods for testing hypotheses about the input intensity after making some assumptions about the shape of the service time distribution. Specifically, the objective is to test hypotheses about the infection rate of MS based on the observed onset rate and knowledge of the latent period distribution.

The χ^2 and Weibull distributions were considered for the service time (or latent period) distribution because they take on contrasting shapes; however, the authors note that the χ^2 distribution is probably the more reasonable choice for the MS problem.

The authors discuss two tests of hypotheses under the one sample case. These are as follows:

1. H_0: $\lambda(t) \equiv \lambda$, a possibly unknown constant
   versus
   H_a: $\lambda(t)$ is increasing

and

2. H_0: $\lambda(t) = \lambda_\alpha(t)$
   versus
   H_a: $\lambda(t) = \lambda_\beta(t)$ for some $\beta > 0$ and all $t \geq 0$,

where $\lambda_\alpha(0) = \lambda_\beta(0)$, $\lambda_\alpha(t)/\lambda_\beta(t)$ is increasing, and $\lambda_\beta(t) > \lambda_\alpha(t)$ for $t > 0$. The authors note that the most often used monotonic input intensities can fit into this framework.

The authors discuss the following test of hypothesis under the two sample case:

H_0: $\dfrac{\lambda_1(t)}{\lambda_2(t)} = c$ for all $t \ \varepsilon \ [0, \infty)$

versus

H_a: $\dfrac{\lambda_1(t)}{\lambda_2(t)}$ is increasing in t.

In this case, two independent displaced Poisson processes are assumed with input intensities $\lambda_1(t)$ and $\lambda_2(t)$; both have service time distribution F, which is unknown.

Let $\{T_i\}$ denote the observed times of departure from the queue. Consider a Poisson input process having $\lambda(t) \equiv 1$, a constant. Let $\Gamma_c(t)$ be the mean value function of the associated Poisson output process. Compute a sequence of transformed times $\{S_i\}$, where $S_i = \Gamma_c(T_i)$. The sequence $\{S_i\}$ forms the occurrence times of a Poisson process.

The authors show how inference about the input process involving $\{T_i\}$ can be transferred to inference about an output process involving $\{S_i\}$. Then, standard test statistics for testing for a constant versus increasing intensity for an observed Poisson process may be employed using the tranformed sequence. "In that context, the Poisson process about which inference is to be made, is actually observed" (Joseph *et al.*, 1990: 341).

The following question is studied: Is MS an infectious disease? Methods are applied to data from 32 individuals (or subsets of these individuals) with MS from the Faroe Islands around 1941, when the British troops arrived. It was assumed that no one had MS before these troops arrived.

One conjecture is that the British troops introduced a virus that caused the spread of MS. If the conjecture is correct, then the Poisson input intensity is an increasing function. Another conjecture would be that the British troops introduced an unknown but noninfectious agent that caused MS. If this conjecture is correct, then the Poisson input intensity is constant. In both cases, the onset rate would have increased, so it is of interest to test whether the Poisson input intensity is increasing or constant.

When tests were carried out on the Faroese data, none were statistically significant. This indicates that the observed increase in the rate of onset of MS on the Faroe Islands after the arrival of the British troops in 1941 does not necessarily indicate that MS is infectious.

A limitation of the Joseph *et al.* (1990) study is that it is impossible to assess the true power of these hypothesis tests. However, the authors perform several simulations to get a rough idea about the misspecification of the shape of the service time distribution on power. The results indicate that it is possible to obtain tests with reasonably high power, particularly when the input intensity increases rapidly.

NEUROEPIDEMIOLOGY AND SAMPLING METHODOLOGY

A cluster sample is one in which the sampling unit is a group (i.e., cluster) of individuals. Ordinary simple single-stage cluster sampling involves taking a simple random sample of clusters and then selecting all individuals within each sampled cluster. Simple two-stage cluster sampling involves taking a simple random sample of clusters and then taking a simple random sample of individuals within each sampled cluster. Higher-stage cluster sampling involves sampling clusters within clusters.

Single-stage cluster sampling is less efficient than multistage cluster sampling. Levy *et al.* (1989) point out specifically that single-stage cluster sampling can fail to be cost-effective when one is interested in identifying and following the same number of individuals in several demographic domains. This is because the number of clusters needed to obtain the target number of individuals in low-frequency domains will produce more than the target number in higher-frequency domains.

The seven authors were interested in identifying and following 1400 individuals in each of the following three age domains: 54–64, 65–74, and 75 years and older. They were studying dementia and planned to take a cluster sample from the 1987 Shanghai population, with clusters consisting of neighborhood groups comprised of households. However, they felt that it was not feasible to take a multistage cluster sample from their particular study population: They felt that individuals who might be selected into a simple random sample within a cluster might feel threatened by being "singled out" and therefore give biased responses or fail to respond.

As a result, the authors decided to take a single-stage cluster sample, but they modified the methodology to make the sampling more efficient. They call their modification a telescopic respondent rule. It is based on the concept that the definition of eligible respondents may vary from cluster to cluster. Its advantage is that it allows one to meet target sample sizes in all domains without sampling extra individuals in the higher-frequency domains.

The following notation will be used to describe the authors' telescopic respondent rule:

N = number of clusters in the population

H = number of domains

m^* = number of individuals to be identified in each domain

M_{ih} = number of individuals in cluster i in domain h ($i = 1, \ldots , N$; $h = 1, \ldots , H$)

$$\overline{M}_h = \frac{\sum_{i=1}^{N} M_{ih}}{N} = \text{average number of individuals per cluster in domain}$$

$h(h = 1, \ldots , H)$

$$\sigma_{M_h}^{2} = \frac{\sum_{i=1}^{N} (M_{ih} - \overline{M}_h)^2}{N}$$

Z_α = the 100αth percentile of the standard normal distribution

n_h = number of clusters required in sample to obtain at least m^* subjects in domain $h(h = 1, \ldots , H)$

n = number of clusters required in sample to obtain at least m^* subjects in all domains

The following result is proven by the authors. Suppose that the number of individuals contained in a cluster in domain h distributes normally over clusters and that clusters are selected by simple random sampling. Then, to have $100(1 - \alpha)\%$ certainty that at least m^* subjects are obtained from domain h, the following number n_h of sample clusters is required:

$$n_h = \left(\frac{|Z_\alpha|\sigma_{M_h}}{\overline{M}_h} + \sqrt{\frac{Z^{\alpha 2}\sigma_{M_h}^{2}}{4\overline{M}_h^{2}} + \frac{m^*}{\overline{M}_h}} \right)^2 \quad \text{for } h = 1,2, \ldots , H$$

The telescopic respondent rule can now be described in a series of steps.

1. Calculate n_h for each domain ($h = 1, \ldots , H$).

2. Order the domains according to increasing required numbers of clusters: $n_{(1)} \leq n_{(2)} \leq \ldots \leq n_{(H)}$. Thus, $n_{(1)}$ denotes the number of clusters for the domain requiring the smallest number of clusters, and $n_{(H)}$ denotes the number of clusters for the domain requiring the largest number of clusters.

3. Take $n = n_{(H)}$. Thus, the sample size required to meet the specifications for the domain requiring the largest number of sample clusters will

ensure that the sample size is met in every other domain as well.

4. Take a simple random sample of n clusters.

5. Randomly designate the n sample clusters as type **1**, type **2**, . . . , type **H** according to the following algorithm:

Cluster type	Number designated
1	$n_{(1)}$
2	$n_{(2)} - n_{(1)}$
.	.
.	.
.	.
h	$n_{(h)} - n_{(h-1)}$
.	.
.	.
.	.
H	$n_{(H)} - n_{(H-1)}$

6. For a type **h** cluster, sample elements in domains (h), $(h + 1)$, . . . , (H) [but not in domains less than (h)]. Thus, for each domain (h), the number of clusters in which elements are sampled in that domain is $n_{(h)}$.

The result of applying the preceeding algorithm is that all clusters have the specified likelihood of meeting the sample size requirements. The overall number of elements sampled is lower than for ordinary single-stage cluster sampling. Cost savings can be expected.

MEDICAL TECHNOLOGY ASSESSMENT AND STOCHASTIC MODELS

Markov models can be used to assist in determining clinical usefulness and cost effectiveness of medical diagnostic tests. Mooney *et al.* (1990) present a decision-analytic model to estimate costs and benefits of ordering immediate magnetic resonance imaging (MRI) versus waiting for a hypothetical patient with mild neurological symptoms possibly suggestive of MS. If an immediate MRI is ordered, there are five possible results: (1) the test is positive for MS, (2) the test is positive for a cerebral infarct, (3) the test is positive for a brain tumor, (4) the test is positive for other pathology, or (5) the test is negative for pathology.

The authors present Markov models for results 1, 2, 4, and 5. Transition probabilities estimated from mortality and incidence rates, costs, and quality-adjusted life expectancies are presented for the various possible health states associated with each result. If the decision is made not to order an immediate MRI, there are also five possible results: (1) the patient dies from unrelated causes, (2) a tumor is missed, (3) the patient suffers a fatal infarct, (4) the patient's condition worsens, or (5) the patient's condition remains unchanged.

Fleming *et al.* (1988) present the case of a woman who suffered neurological complications following a cesarean section with spinal anesthesia. The symptoms worsened following an arteriogram. To assist in deciding whether or not another arteriogram was indicated to rule out an aneurysm, a simple decision tree with associated probabilities for short-term outcomes was developed. Because of the immediacy of the problem, there was not sufficient time to develop a more complex model. The patient chose to undergo another arteriogram, which showed no aneurysm or other problem.

However, at a later point, the authors developed a Markov model to represent different long-term outcomes if any aneurysm were to have been present after the initial bleeding. This would then help them determine the potential benefits of surgery to prevent aneursymal rupture. The model features six health states: well, temporarily okay for the period immediately after an aneurysmal rupture, temporarily disabled for the period immediately after an aneurysmal rupture, okay on a long-term basis after a rupture, disabled on a long-term basis after a rupture, or dead. Their Markov model involves both short-term and long-term time frames.

Electroencephalograms (EEGs) are used by neurologists to assess the electrical activity of the brain. Several authors have shown how stochastic analysis can be applied to EEG phenomena. Jansen and Cheng (1988) describe a method called "structural EEG analysis," which uses Markov modeling, to detect changes in an EEG.

Typical quantitative analysis applies pattern recognition techniques to long segments (10 sec to 1 min) of an EEG strip recording. Such methods fail to take into account how different EEG signals vary with time.

EEGs consist of a series of short patterns. Jansen and Cheng (1988) state that different patterns in an EEG can be considered as states in a Markov chain. Transition probabilities can be calculated between the different patterns. Structural analysis of preseizure EEGs in two adults with confirmed temporal lobe epilepsy "detected more subtle differences between EEG intervals" than traditional methods of analysis.

Jensen and Cheng (1988) point out two limitations with their method. First, interval changes detected by structural analysis may not be seizure-related. Further work is needed to elaborate the nature of identified changes. Second, in theory, their model assumes the transition probabilities within an interval are stationary, but in practice, this assumption may not hold.

Penczek and Grochulski (1989) show how EEG recordings can be broken down into short segments, each of which belongs to a finite set of distinct groups. If each group is identified by a separate symbol, strings of symbols can be examined as a discrete-time Markov process. The authors used such a process to describe the time evolution of epileptic seizures in four brain structures. They induced seizures in rabbits in either the motor sensory cortex, the hippocampus, the ventroanterior nuclei thalmai, or the midbrain reticular formation and compared the states in the stimulated brain structure to the states in the other three brain structures.

DISCUSSION

The stochastic process studies discussed in the first section of this chapter have contributed the following results to knowledge of MS. From Wolfson and Confavreux (1985), where prognostic variables were considered separately, individuals appear to be at a higher risk of transition to a worse disease state if they (1) are older at onset of disease, (2) are female, and (3) have a monosymptomatic mode of onset. From Wolfson and Confavreux (1987), where prognostic variables were considered simultaneously, (1) individuals with a shorter time between the first two attacks appear to be more likely to make the transitions from the relapse without sequalae state to the relapse with sequalae state, and from the two relapse states to the progression state; (2) males appear to be at a higher risk of making a transition from the relapse with sequelae state to the progression state; and (3) individuals with monosymptomatic mode of onset appear to be at increased risk of transition from relapse without sequelae to progression, but a decreased risk of transition from relapse with sequale to progression. From Wolfson *et al.* (1989), there appears to be a 10–15-year susceptibility period, the average latent period in nonmigrant populations from countries of high prevalence appears to be around 18 years, and the median latent period in such populations appears to be around 16 years. From Joseph *et al.* (1990), MS does not appear to be an infectious disease.

The stochastic process studies of the first section have also contributed to our knowledge of epilepsy. From Milton *et al.* (1987), seizures in most epileptic individuals appear to occur randomly rather than cyclically or in clusters, possibly being precipitated by some randomly occurring event like sleep deprivation or increased stress.

Markov models allow one to describe a neurological disease globally for a set of patients. Elaborated Markov models also allow a personalized description of the neurological disease for each patient, which may be useful in selecting appropriate therapies for the patient. Poisson process models can be used to assess whether aspects of neurological disease behavior are occurring at random or in a patterned way. When times of clinical onset are known but times of initiation of neurological diseases are unknown, queueing models can be employed: The idea is to estimate the latent period distribution of the disease after making assumptions about the initiation distribution and inferring the length of the susceptibility period, or to test hypotheses about the rate of initiation after making assumptions about the latent period distribution. Information from the first type of queueing study may be useful in a narrowing down the time frame in which to look for etiologic factors associated with neurological diseases. The second type of queueing study may be useful in inferring some aspects of the nature of the agent that precipitates neurological diseases.

The sampling methodology study discussed in the second section has contributed to the quality of data that are obtainable in surveys involving neurological diseases. Levy *et al.* (1989) demonstrated how a variation of a single-stage cluster sampling plan can be developed for use in a population where multistage cluster sampling is not feasable, simultaneously increasing the response rate, decreasing the response bias, and increasing the general efficiency.

The third section contained sketches of some of the uses of stochastic modeling in assessing the clinical usefulness and cost effectiveness of medical diagnostic tests. The following questions motivated this group of studies. Should a MRI be ordered immediately for a patient with mild neurological symptoms possibly suggestive of MS? Should another arteriogram be ordered to rule out an aneurysm in women who have suffered neurological complications following a ceasarean section with spinal anesthesia? And can structural analysis of EEGs detect subtle differences between EEG intervals and describe the time evolution of epileptic seizures?

The studies reviewed in this chapter have made significant contributions to the understanding of neurological disease processes and how to improve the efficiency of data collection involving such diseases. The research clearly suggests potential developments and applications of stochastic process models to other neurological diseases and other types of medical technology assessment and illustrate the value of such research to the field of neuroepidemiology.

References

Chiang, C. L. (1985). Reader reaction: What is biostatistics? *Biometrics* **41**(3), 771–775.
Confavreux, C. and Wolfson, C. (1988). Multiple sclerosis: Stochastic models of prognosis. *In* "Virology and Immunology in Multiple Sclerosis: Rationale for Therapy" C. L. Cazzullo, D. Caputo, A. Ghezzi, and M. Zaffaroni, eds., pp. 115–124. Springer-Verlag, Berlin.

Confavreux, C. and Wolfson, C. (1989). Mathematical models and individualized outcome estimates in multiple sclerosis. *Biomed. Pharmacother.* **43,** 675–680.

Fleming, C., Wong, J. B., Moskowitz, A. J., and Pauker, S. G. (1988). A peripartum neurologic event: Shooting from the hip. *Med. Decision Making* **8**(1), 55–71.

Jansen, B. H., and Cheng, W.-K. (1988). Structural EEG analysis: An explorative study, *Intl. J. Biomed. Comput.* **23,** 221–237.

Jones, M. P., and Crowley, J. (1989). A general class of nonparametric tests for survival analysis. *Biometrics* **45,** 157–170.

Joseph, L., Wolfson, C., and Wolfson, D. B. (1990). Is multiple sclerosis an infectious disease? Inference about an input process based on the output. *Biometrics* **46,** 337–349.

Kay, B. H., Saul, A. J., and McCullagh, A. (1987). A mathematical model for the rural amplification of Murray Valley encephalitis virus in Southern Australia. *Am. J. Epidemiol.* **125**(4), 690–705.

Levy, P. S., Yu, E. S. H., Liu, W. T., Wong, S.-C., Zhang, M.-Y., and Wang, Z.-Y. (1989). Single-stage cluster sampling with a telescopic respondent rule: A variation motivated by a survey of dementia in elderly residents of Shanghai. *Stat. Med.* **8,** 1537–1544.

Milton, J. G., Gotman, J., Remillard, G. M., and Andermann, F. (1987). Timing of seizure recurrence in adult epileptic patients: A statistical analysis. *Epilepsia* **28**(5), 471–478.

Mooney, C., Mushlin, A. I., and Phelps, C. E. (1990). Targeting assessments of magnetic resonance imaging in suspected multiple sclerosis. *Med. Decision Making* **10**(2), 77–94.

Penczek, P., and Grochulski, W. (1989). Analysis of the multi-channel epileptiform EEG using the Markov chain formations. *Meth. Inf. Med.* **28,** 160–167.

Wolfson, C., and Confavreux, C. (1985). A Markov model of the natural history of multiple sclerosis. *Neuroepidemiology* **4,** 227–239.

Wolfson, C. and Confavreux, C. (1987). Improvements to a simple Markov model of the natural history of multiple sclerosis. *Neuroepidemiology* **6,** 101–115.

Wolfson, C., Wolfson, D. B., and Zielinski, J. M. (1989). On the estimation of the distribution of the latent period of multiple sclerosis. *Neuroepidemiology* **8,** 239–248.

Zeger, S. L. (1988). A regression model for time series of counts. *Biometrika* **75**(4), 621–629.

18

A Case-Control Study of Head Injury to Elementary School Children

Monica Brown • Louise K. Hofherr • Craig A. Molgaard

Twenty-two million children are injured in the United States each year (National Safety Council, 1989). Although the majority are considered minor, between 10 and 20% of these injuries are estimated to occur in and around schools (Sibert *et al.*, 1981).

Head trauma is the most common form of injury in children and accounts for 11% of all emergency room visits, despite the fact that most of these injuries are minor (Rivara, 1984). Parents, educators, and the general public are concerned about minor head trauma because it is associated with the potential for loss of intellectual function, for psychomotor dysfunction, or even for sudden death (Kraus *et al.*, 1986; Snoek *et al.*, 1984).

Epidemiologic studies have shown that injuries among children are nonrandom events and have identifiable factors that may increase the risk of injury. Some of these risk factors include a (1) greater exposure to hazardous environments, (2) decreased ability to avoid hazards, and (3) decreased resistance to injury (Horwitz *et al.*, 1988).

Because children spend a considerable part of their time in school, it appears appropriate to determine the risk of head injury in that environment. Improving our understanding of the epidemiology of childhood head injury in the school environment will focus attention more clearly and precisely on appropriate methods for intervention and prevention.

REVIEW OF THE LITERATURE: RISK FACTORS FOR INJURIES TO CHILDREN AT SCHOOL AND MINOR HEAD TRAUMA

No studies have examined the extent of head injury to children in the school environment nor defined the risk factors for such injuries. This chapter, therefore, treats the topics of injuries in the school environment and head injuries to children separately.

Epidemiology of School Injuries

Incidence

The incidence of injuries to children at school varies greatly. Three Canadian school-based studies in different districts reported incidence rates. These rates ranged from 2.85 to 6.20 per 100 students (Hodgson *et al.*, 1984; Feldman *et al.*, 1983; Sheps and Evans, 1987). Only one U.S. study was conducted on a population sufficiently large to allow a comparison to these injury incidence rates. Boyce *et al.* (1984) described an overall injury rate of 4.9 per 100 student-years in the Tucson, Arizona, school district.

Causes of School-Related Injuries

Falls are consistently reported as the major cause of injury to children at school. Estimates of all school-related injuries that are due to falls range between 57.9 and 66.7% (Langley *et al.*, 1981a,b). Two studies examined the details of injury etiology, and both showed similar results; that is, the majority of the falls were on the same level, followed in frequency by falls from aboveground level from playground equipment. Being struck against or by an object or person was second in incidence to falls (Langley *et al.*,1981a; Sheps and Evans, 1987).

Types of Injuries and Body Parts Affected

Most of the studies reviewed indicated that the head/neck region was the site that sustained injury most often. In a school-based study in Hawaii, Taketa (1984) as well as other researchers (Sheps and Evans, 1987; Dale *et al.*,1969; Pagano *et al.*,1987) found that 43% of all injuries were to the head/neck region, followed by arms (32%) and legs (18%). Sixty-five percent of the injuries were lacerations/abrasions and bumps/bruises, whereas only 25% were sprains/fractures.

Injury Severity

Antedotally, we know that the majority of injuries to children at school are minor. Feldman *et al.* (1983), Hodgson *et al.* (1984), and Dale *et al.* (1969) reported similar results when injuries were examined by severity. In all three studies, it was reported that only about 29% of all injuries were serious. Interestingly, serious injury rates between boys and girls were similar. Minor injuries were more common or more commonly reported in elementary school.

Risk Factors for Injuries at School

Nonbehavioral Risk Factors

From study to study, age and gender are consistently considered major risk factors for injuries to children in all environments. Injury morbidity increases with age throughout the teens (Langley *et al.*, 1987; Fife *et al.*, 1984). Boys are reported to have more injuries than girls at all ages beyond 3 years. This diversity in injury rates increases with age, rates being lowest for boys in their earliest years and lowest for girls in their teens (Rivara *et al.*, 1989; Gallagher *et al.*, 1984; Stallones and Corsa, 1961; Fife *et al.*, 1984; Schor, 1987). Without exception in the studies reviewed, incidence of injuries in boys was greater than in girls (Pagano *et al.*, 1987; Hodgson *et al.*, 1984; Langley *et al.*, 1981b; Taketa, 1984; Boyce *et al.*, 1984; Bell, 1986; Sheps and Evans, 1987; McFadyen *et al.*, 1988).

Age-related data on injuries suggest that as children are able (or encouraged) to venture out, the exposure to risk of injury increases. Moreover, it is suggested that the increase in motor ability is not matched by an equivalent increase in the observance and recognition of hazards. Therefore, researchers postulate that children encounter hazards before they have learned to discern what hazards exist and how to cope with them (Marcus *et al.*, 1960).

Psychosocial

Historically, the study of childhood injuries began through the examination of the child's behavior. Consistent themes in this body of literature are that hyperactive, aggressive, and antisocial behaviors are risk factors for injuries in children (Matheny *et al.*, 1971; Langley *et al.*, 1983a; Bijur *et al.*, 1986; Nyman, 1987). In this literature, age-specific injury rates are related not just to the exposure to hazards and to physiological development but also to emotional maturity.

The close, personal, and intellectual interaction of students in the school environment may offer some special situations that lead to an increase in injuries. In an insightful study on schoolmate interactions and injuries, Bremberg and Gerber (1988) found that 66% of all injuries occurred during "breaks" or recess periods. In the injury pre-event phase, 72% of the students were engaged in peer interaction, in which one-half had been chasing each other or brawling. These interactions were characterized as competitive in 78% of these cases. In the event phase, schoolmates were involved in 48% of the injuries. They contended that injured students were "less connected to other students," felt that their schoolmates did not like them, were less likely to meet schoolmates outside of school, and tended to join schoolmates during breaks less often.

In a study of children in the Seattle public schools, Johnson *et al.* (1974) reported that 15% of all elementary school injuries could be attributed to aggressive behavior. Of those labeled as aggressive, pushing (45%), fights (36%), and throwing objects (18%) were the main components of that behavior.

Risk-Taking behavior

Risk-Taking behavior in young children has been insufficiently explored as a cause of injuries. The common belief is that risk-taking is difficult to assess in early years and prominent expressions of risk-taking are not apparent until adolescence (Zuckerman, 1971; Tonkin, 1987).

In a survey of fifth- through eighth-graders, Lewis and Lewis (1984) found that about 50% of "dares" encouraged problem behaviors that placed the children (and others) at risk of personal injury or held potential for the development of habits hazardous to their health. With increasing age, more dares occurred in the school environment and fewer involved risk of personal injury. Fifth- and sixth-graders reported that personal risk dares were the principle type, especially for boys.

In contrast, in a prospective study of adolescent boys, Padilla *et al.* (1976) stated that willingness to take chances (risk-taking behavior) was not predictive of increased injury frequency. Their explanation for this was the possibility that the risk-taking child may be more experienced and better coordinated. They implied that risk-taking is learned and based on confidence from past experience.

Socioeconomic Status

Several studies have examined the relationship between socioeconomic status (SES) and childhood injuries, but not as related to the school environment. In a New Zealand child development study, Langley *et al.* (1983b) detected no significant relationship between SES and number of injuries to children up to the age of 7. They used three measures to assess

SES: (1) occupation of the father at child's birth, (2) highest level of formal education achieved by both parents by the time the child reached 3 years of age, and (3) type of housing of the family at the child's 6th year.

In contrast, Manheimer *et al.* (1966) noted that children of professionals had greater injury rates, followed by children with no fathers living at home, then children of skilled laborers (clerical and sales), and, finally, children of semiskilled and unskilled laborers, who showed the lowest injury rates. They also reported that African American children had lower injury rates than white children. The distribution of severity of injuries was identical in these two ethnic groups. As a result of this distribution, they concluded that access and use of health care was the same. It should be noted that the African American children in this sample were of a higher SES than in many other similar surveys, because their population was based on those utilizing Kaiser Health Plans.

Parental attitudes on child-rearing, injury prevention practices, and parental stress perception and coping have been shown to influence childhood injuries, and these processes are probably related to SES. Therefore, the inconsistency of findings between SES and childhood injuries reported in the preceding studies may be due to methodological problems or variances within the studies. For example, study populations that are too homogeneous, cover too great a variety of injuries, or allow too much variance in the age range of the children under study may lead to inconsistent findings (Matheny and Fisher, 1984).

Macroenvironment as a Risk Factor

Few studies have tried to address the impact of the school environment on injuries. Boyce *et al.* (1984) found the following ecologic variables to be predictive of injury rates in schools: longer school hours; alternative educational programs, particularly Magnet programs;[1] less-experienced nurses; and lower student : staff ratios. Predictive of rates of serious injury were longer school hours and lower percentages of minority students.

McFayden *et al.* (1988) found that elementary school children who attended Magnet schools and extended-hours programs sustained more injuries and had more visits to the nurse's office than children in regular schools. The author offers three explanations for this: (1) behaviors such as aggressiveness, competition, challenge, and risk-taking may be more prevalent in those settings, (2) the quality and quantity of adult supervision may be less intensive and direct, and (3) parents may place a higher premium on school attendance even when the child is ill.

---

[1]Magnets are defined as programs of study centering on voluntary racial desegregation with an emphasis on programmatic excellence.

Head Trauma to Children

Minor head trauma is defined as an injury to the head with no immediate loss of consciousness and no skull fracture (also called closed head trauma). Most of these head injuries are contusions, lacerations, or simple fractures and are generally inconsequential to the child. True brain injury usually does not occur. A small number of minor or trivial head injuries, however, do result in mental impairment, neuromotor impairment, or even death (Cook, 1972; Levin *et al.*, 1987; Plaut and Gifford, 1976; Rutherford *et al.*, 1977).

Most of the literature on head trauma in children concerns hospital admissions data or emergency room surveillance. In reviewing this literature, it should be remembered that presentation to a hospital depends on environmental and societal factors, which may in turn bias our perception of the causes of or individuals at risk of minor head injuries. Also, the perceived level of severity may be greatly increased by examining this type of data. Three studies were found in this review that utilized an alternate method of studying childhood head injury. These studies used telephone surveys to identify cases but noted that bias and inattention to clinical characteristics were problems (Goldstein and Levin, 1987; Klauber *et al.*, 1981; Kraus *et al.*, 1986).

Incidence of Minor Head Injury among Children

Studies on pediatric head injury have indicated a great range of incidence rates. Annegers (1983) found incidence rates of 220 per 100,000 for children under 15 years. This rate approximates the 230 per 100,000 reported by the National Head and Spinal Cord Injury Survey (Kalsbeek *et al.*, 1980).

Kraus *et al.* (1986) reported 185 per 100,000 children in a study of head injury in San Diego County. Klauber *et al.* (1981) found 295 per 100,000 in a second study in San Diego County. The Klauber study used information from a telephone survey and included head injuries that were not medically treated. In 1986, Casey *et al.* (1986) found that 36% of all accident-related visits to a children's hospital were due to head injuries.

Risk Factors for Minor Head Injury among Children

Risk factors for minor head injury in children appears to be similar if not identical to that of all injuries in children. Boys were injured twice as often as girls (Craft *et al.*, 1972; Jamison and Kaye, 1974; Klonoff and Robinson, 1967; Kraus *et al.*, 1986; Partington, 1960; Snow *et al.*, 1988). There seems to be an age-specific difference in the peak incidence of head trauma for male and female children: Males show an increased incidence starting at age 5, whereas females show a decline throughout the first 15 years. Researchers have suggested that this indicates that males and females differ in both the degree of risk and the kinds of risk for head injury (Frankowski *et al.*, 1985). In contrast to patterns reported in overall injuries to children at school, Kraus noted that nearly 70% of all acute brain injury cases were to males (Kraus, 1980).

Klonoff (1971) found that SES indicators were associated with head injury in school-aged children, such as marital instability and lower occupational status of fathers. Other studies, primarily concerned with adults, support the fact that SES indicators were factors in head injury. Such indicators include the proportion of the population with the lowest income and the highest population density had the highest incidence of head injuries (Fife *et al.*, 1986). Contrary to these findings, the study by Klauber *et al.* (1981) found that income and education were unrelated to the incidence of head injury.

Causes of Minor Head Injury among Children

The major causes of all types of head injuries were falls and recreational activities (regardless of environments) when motor vehicle-related injuries are omitted (Annegers, 1983; Jamison and Kaye, 1974; Kraus *et al.*, 1986; Mlay, 1985; Partington, 1960). There also appears to be a relationship between age and etiology of head injuries in children. Falls predominate as a cause up to age 5 (Annegers, 1983; Kraus, 1987; Rivera, 1984). After age 5, recreational, bicycle, and pedestrian–motor vehicle injuries predominate (Klauber *et al.*, 1981).

Methodological Issues in the Study of Injuries to Children at School

Many of the childhood injury studies described here have methodological shortcomings. These shortcomings influence the usefulness of the resultant information in the formulation of interventions and in how future research should be conducted. Typical problems involved inconsistencies with the classification of injuries and reporting of event-related information.

Some school-based injury studies do not give an injury breakdown by grade or school level, nor is severity of the injury described by grade level (Taketa, 1984; Boyce *et al.*, 1984; Feldman *et al.*, 1983). At times, no attempt to describe injury severity is made.

Few studies are school-based. This could be partly due to difficulty in obtaining information, differences in reporting practices, and the validity of the reported injuries. Researchers have estimated that school injury reporting systems, using a standardized form, underreport injuries by as much as a factor of 4 (Bremberg, 1989; Hodgson *et al.*, 1984). Woodward *et al.* (1984) found that, overall, schools reported 25% less injuries to children than were actually observed. Serious injuries were more likely to be reported; that is, one out of two serious injuries were reported compared to one out of five minor injuries.

   Reasons for differences in reporting practices have been explored by a few studies. Nader *et al.* (1980) found that use of school health facilities could be predicted by ethnicity and family status; African American and Hispanic students used the facilities less than whites or Anglo Americans. Students from single-parent families used the facilities at school less, and these families also used community facilities less than two-parent families. They found the use of health care facilities in the community dependent on SES, family status, and sex. If this is true, then we could hypothesize that underreporting of injuries by non-Anglo ethnicities, single-parent families, and males could present a problem.

Conclusion

This review of the literature suggests several possible risk factors for head injury to young children at school. It provides a basis for exploring the association of many personal and environmental factors with head injury among elementary school children using a case-control methodology.

   The purpose of the present study was to describe personal as well as school-related risk factors for head injury in elementary school children during the 1989–1990 academic year at a large urban school district, and to differentiate the risk factors for these children from those of children who received other types of injuries or no injuries. A case-control analysis, utilizing logistic regression techniques, was carried out utilizing the school district's required injury reporting records, the computerized student information database, and information on individual schools.

METHODS

The Setting

The study was carried out within a large, mostly urban school district with students from a variety of ethnic and socioeconomic backgrounds. In this population, there was a 1989–1990 year-end enrollment of 68,052 kindergarten through sixth-graders in 106 elementary schools, with a student age range of 5–13 years (San Diego City Schools, 1990a).

Study Subjects

The study population consisted of 68,052 elementary school-attending children, in grades prekindergarten to fifth, who possessed a student identification number and were enrolled in school during the 1989–1990 academic year. Cases were defined as children who had sustained a reportable injury to the head region (including facial and dental) while at school.

Controls were comprised of two groups. Control group #1 comprised students who had sustained an injury other than that to the head. Control group #2 comprised those who had sustained no injuries. Students in both control groups were otherwise from the same population as cases. Controls were randomly selected to achieve a power of 95% and detect a relative risk of 3 (Schlesselman, 1982).

Data Sources and Variables of Interest

Data for this study came primarily from four sources: the school district's required standardized Injury Report Form (IRF), the district's Information Services Bureau's computerized student database, the School Accountability Report Card (San Diego City Schools, 1990b) and the School Profiles (San Diego City Schools, 1990c). The school district uses a standardized form for the reporting of school-related injuries for all students, staff, and faculty. The IRF is completed by the adult supervisor (teacher, principal, coach, nurse, or support staff) of the activity area where the injury took place or the first adult supervisor to reach the student, regardless if that adult witnessed the event.

The school district's computerized student database provided information such as the gender, race/ethnicity, and grade of the student. Ethnicity was grouped into four categories: White, Hispanic, African American, and Other.[2] Additional information from this source was whether or not the student was deemed gifted by the school district, whether or not the student participated in the school district's free or reduced-price lunch program, and the number of disciplinary suspensions during the 1989–1990 academic year; the latter two information categories were used as surrogate measures of SES and risk-taking behavior, respectively.

The School Accountability Report Card provided information on student enrollment, average daily attendance, ethnic composition of the school, whether or not the school had Magnet programs,[3] and the degree of student body participation in those programs. The School Profiles was used as a secondary source of information on the 1988–1989 California Assessment Program (CAP) academic achievement measures: reading, writing, and mathematics scores. Students at each school in the school

---

[2]The Other category comprised Indochinese (43%), Filipino (32%), Asian (14%), Alaskan/American Indian (4%), Pacific Islander (4%), and Portuguese (3%).

[3]Magnet schools/programs are defined, specifically in this school district, as specialized academic programs to increase the racial balance of a particular school through voluntary student enrollment. Students elect to attend these schools/programs and are not selected based on intellectual (IQ scoring) or academic ability in the specified subject matter.

district and in the State of California are tested in the third, sixth, eighth, and twelfth grades to determine whether or not learning levels are consistent. These three scores are combined to form a single variable to denote the academic level of the school. Also provided by the CAP was a socioeconomic index[4] and the percentage of limited English-proficient pupils for each school.

Variables from other sources were the staff : student ratio, average number of hours a nurse was on duty per school per week, and the subregional location of the schools within the city.

Analysis

All analyses in this study were carried out using the BMDP (Biomedical Data Processing) statistical programs package (BMDP Statistical Software Inc., 1989). Univariate analysis was carried out using the 1D and the 4F programs, and multivariate analysis utilized stepwise logistic regression.

Independent variables were divided into two categories for model-building analysis: personal and school-related. Models were fit to assess these variable categories' individual ability to predict the risk of head injury.

RESULTS

Population Descriptive Characteristics

There were 2180 injuries among 68,052 elementary students in this school district during the 1989–1990 academic year. The incidence rate of injuries to all district students was 3.6 per 100 students, whereas for elementary children it was 3.2 per 100 students. There were 1220 head injuries to our study population, for an incidence of 1.8 per 100 elementary students. The 1220 head injuries represented 56% of all injuries to this group.

Table I shows the demographic characteristics of the cases and controls. Our sample totaled 1162 students: 837 were cases, 123 were in control group #1, and 202 were in control group #2. The 837 cases represented a census of head-injured elementary students in the school district for the 1989–1990 academic year that met the case criteria.

For all ethnicities, except African Americans, the proportion of those with a head injury was lower than their population proportion in the school district. African American children were head-injured dispropor-

---

[4]The socioeconomic index used by the CAP indicates parental occupations from a sample of third-grade children. The score is as follows: 1 = unknown,, unemployed, and unskilled; 2 = skilled and semiskilled; 3 = semiprofessional and professional.

Table I

Demographic Characteristics of Children Who Sustained Head
Injuries, Injuries Other than to the Head, and No Injuries at School

	Cases	Controls	
		#1	#2
	N (%)	n (%)	n (%)
Ethnicity	837	123	202
White	398 (47.6)	56 (45.5)	82 (40.6)
Hispanic	165 (19.7)	26 (21.1)	48 (23.8)
African American	165 (19.7)	26 (21.1)	36 (17.8)
Other	109 (13.0)	15 (12.2)	36 (17.8)
Gender	835	123	202
Male	536 (64.2)	67 (54.5)	103 (51.0)
Female	299 (35.8)	56 (45.5)	99 (49.0)
Grade	836	123	201
Prekindergarten	12 (15.2)	1 (8.1)	13 (6.5)
Kindergarten	127 (1.4)	10 (0.8)	26 (12.9)
First	164 (19.6)	14 (11.4)	25 (12.4)
Second	134 (16.0)	15 (12.2)	22 (10.9)
Third	131 (15.7)	23 (18.7)	37 (18.4)
Fourth	126 (15.1)	32 (26.0)	38 (18.9)
Fifth	119 (14.2)	26 (21.1)	35 (17.4)
No grade	23 (2.8)	1 (0.8)	5 (2.5
Gifted	836	123	202
No	777 (92.9)	106 (86.2)	193 (95.5)
Yes	59 (7.1)	17 (13.8)	9 (4.5)
SLP	837	123	202
No	406 (48.5)	62 (50.4)	129 (63.9)
Yes	431 (51.5)	61 (49.6)	73 (36.1)
SUSP	837	123	202
0	800 (95.6)	117 (95.1)	199 (98.5)
1–2	34 (4.1)	6 (4.9)	3 (1.5)
>3	3 (0.4)	0 (0.0)	0 (0.0)

[a] Students who sustained injuries other than to the head.

[b] Students who were free of injuries.

Abbreviations: SLP, school's free or reduced-price lunch program participation; SUSP, number of disciplinary suspension for the student.

tionately to their population density in the elementary school population (19.7% of total injured compared to 16.7% of the total population).

About twice the number of males had a head injury compared to females. The greatest number of head-injured children were first-graders; the fewest were in the prekindergarten and special education groups. The greatest number of otherwise-injured students (control group #1) were fourth-graders; the fewest were in the kindergarten and prekinder-garten grades. It appears that there is an inverse distribution by grade to head injuries compared to injuries other than to the head.

The majority of children in all three study categories were not gifted and had no disciplinary suspensions. There was a disproportionate number of children deemed gifted and those who participated in the school's free or reduced-price lunch program who were injured (cases and control group #1) compared to those not injured. In addition, a disproportionate number had received one to two disciplinary suspensions during the study period.

Examination of the descriptive statistics for selected school-related characteristics for the study groups revealed that the school's student enrollment at all grades of the elementary schools, averaged 735 students with a mean staff:student ratio of 1:18. The average daily attendance was 99.2%, this was the percentage of student body that could be officially accounted for. Of the students who were officially not in attendance, only an average of 2.5% were out due to disciplinary suspension.

The ethnic distribution averaged 40% white, 30% Hispanic, 16% African American, and 14% other students. The average number of hours per week that a nurse was on duty at each school was 24, or 3 of 5 full working days.

Using the school background factors at the third-grade level from the CAP, we determined that the average socioeconomic index for our sample was 1.98; this compared to 1.95 for the entire school district (the higher the score, the greater number of children with parents whose occupations can be classified as professional). For percentage of limited English-proficient students, our sample was the same as that of the school district at 17.7%. The mean combined academic achievement scores for the school district was 879; in our sample it was 873.5.

Multivariate Analysis

The Student's Personal Characteristics Variables

The odds ratios and 95% confidence intervals comparing the student's personal characteristics variables potentially associated with head injury are shown in Table II. There was a significant association among gender, ethnicity, grade, and free or reduced-price lunch program participation in those with head injury compared to those with no injury. Though the variable for gifted remained in the model, this measure did not reach statistical significance.

Males were found to have a 1.6 times greater risk for head injury than

Table II

Odds Ratios (95% CI) of Suspected Student Risk Factors for Head
Injury Compared to Those without Injuries and Those with
Injuries Other Than to the Head

		95% CI	
	Ratio	Lower	Upper
No injuries			
Gender, male	1.63	1.18	2.25
Ethnicity (versus White)			
Hispanic	0.43	0.27	0.69
African American	0.73	0.46	1.17
Other	0.52	0.32	0.84
Grade (versus first)			
Second	0.81	0.43	1.52
Third	0.45	0.25	0.81
Fourth	0.48	0.27	0.85
Fifth	0.48	0.27	0.85
Kindergarten	0.77	0.42	1.41
Prekindergarten	0.20	0.07	0.52
Special education	0.70	0.23	2.07
Gifted	2.08	0.98	4.40
SLP	2.39	1.64	3.47
Injuries other than to the head			
Gender, Male	1.53	1.04	2.26
Grade (versus first)			
Second	0.77	0.36	1.66
Third	0.49	0.24	0.99
Fourth	0.34	0.17	0.66
Fifth	0.37	0.19	0.75
Kindergarten	1.07	0.46	2.50
Prekindergarten	1.07	0.13	8.91
Special education	2.02	0.25	16.20

SLP, school's free or reduced-price lunch program participation.

females when compared to children who sustained no injuries. Hispanic
and Other children were at significantly less risk of head injury than white
children. Although white children were also at greater risk than African
American children, this difference was not significant. All other grades
were at significantly less risk of head injury than first-graders, except
second-grade, kindergarten, and special education students.

The relative importance of the variables free or reduced-price lunch,
ethnicity, and gifted when we estimated the risk of a head injury compared to an injury other than to the head was inconsequential. These
variables appear unuseful for discrimination between head injury and

other injuries. Only male gender and grade were found to be statistically significant. Males were at 1.5 times greater risk for head injury than other types of injury. Second- through fifth-graders were at less risk than first graders for head injuries.

School-Related Characteristics Variables

The odds ratios and 95% confidence intervals comparing potential school-related risk factors in those with head injury to those with no injuries and injuries other than to the head is shown in Table III. The following variables were found to be associated with head injury: school's percentage of white, African American, and other students, mean number of nurse duty hours per school per week, percentage of limited English-proficient pupils, degree of magnet program participation, and school's academic achievement as denoted by the CAP.

The risk of head injury was positively associated with the school's staff:student ratio; that is, as the ratio of staff to students decreased, the risk of injury decreased.

Mean number of nurse hours was significantly associated with head injury as every level except the 28–32-hr period. An erratic pattern emerged with the probability of a head injury decreasing with increased number of nurse hours. Mean number of nurse hours were found to be significant at the 12–16-hour level, when head injury was compared to other types of injuries.

Partial school participation in magnet programs was significantly associated with injury to the head. Though the combined CAP scores remained in the model, none were statistically significant. For those with head injuries compared to those with no injuries, the probability of injury was greater for children who attended schools that had scores just above the district's mean than for schools with scores at 1 standard deviation above the mean.

A school's percentage of limited English-proficient students was significantly associated with head injury at every level. A trend was noted that as this percentage increased, so did the risk of injury. Interestingly, white students had a greater risk of head injury than African Americans or other students. School's with 30% of any particular ethnicity were significantly at greater risk of head injuries.

DISCUSSION

An overall injury rate of 3.6 per 100 students was found in this school district for the 1989–1990 academic year. This rate lies between those reported in Canada (Hodgson *et al.*, 1984) and that reported in the Tucson,

Table III

Odds Ratios (95% CI) of Suspected School-Related Risk Factors for Head Injury

	Ratio	95% CI	
		Lower	Upper
No injuries			
MNH (versus 0–8 hr)			
12–16 hr	2.83	1.37	5.84
20–24 hr	2.80	1.38	5.69
28–32 hr	1.94	0.83	4.57
36–40 hr	3.13	1.29	7.61
MS (versus none)			
Most	1.97	1.11	3.49
Some	1.63	0.87	3.04
CCAP (versus 760)			
860	1.79	0.99	3.21
960	1.92	0.96	3.85
>960	1.15	0.51	2.60
LEPP (versus 5%)			
10%	2.85	1.62	5.04
20%	1.80	1.00	3.24
40%	4.01	1.95	8.26
>40%	4.77	1.92	11.90
SRW (versus <10%)			
10–30%	1.12	0.52	2.41
30–60%	4.58	1.70	12.30
>60%	7.89	2.26	27.50
SRAA (versus <10%)			
10–30%	0.83	0.54	1.28
30–60%	2.85	1.15	7.07
SRO (versus <10%)			
10–30%	0.80	0.52	1.23
30–60%	2.49	1.13	5.45
Injuries other Than to the Head			
MNH (versus 0–8 hr)			
12–16 hr	2.99	1.36	6.56
20–24 hr	1.61	0.81	3.21
28–32 hr	1.93	0.83	4.47
36–40 hr	1.80	0.86	3.76

Abbreviations: MNH, mean number of nurse hours per week; CCAP, combined California Assessment Program score; LEPP, percentage of limited English-proficient students; MS, level of magnet program participation; SRAA, school's ratio of African American students; SRO, school's ratio of other students; SRW, school's ratio of white students.

Arizona, school district (Boyce *et al.*, 1984). The percentage of the school district's elementary school children who sustained a head injury compared to all injuries was 56. A similar figure of 43% was reported from the Hawaii Public Schools in 1984 (Taketa, 1984). These discrepancies may be due to many different reasons; geographic differences, differences in child supervision, differing criteria and definitions of what is a reportable injury, or perhaps simply reporting bias.

Risk Factors for Head Injury

Many of the personal and school-related factors hypothesized to characterize the head-injured child were not found on analysis. These results both affirmed prior observations by other researchers and provided some new insights into the epidemiology of childhood head injuries in the school environment.

Student's Personal Characteristics

Gender, grade, participation in the school district's free or reduced-price lunch program, giftedness, and ethnicity were all found to characterize the head injury.

The distributions by gender and grade of head-injured children were consistent with those reported in the literature. The gender-specific head injury ratio was 2:1 (male:female) (Craft *et al.*, 1972; Jamison and Kaye, 1974; Klonoff and Robinson, 1967; Kraus *et al.*, 1986; Partington, 1960; Snow *et al.*, 1988). Being male is predictive of head injuries as well as being of low SES, as denoted by participation in the school's free or reduced-price lunch program. Younger children (prekindergarten through second grade) appeared to have more head injuries than older children (third through fifth grade) in the school district. First-graders were at a significant risk for head injury.

The gender and grade pattern seen in this study are supported by the literature. Younger children are at greater risk for head injury (Frankowski *et al.*, 1985) than for all other childhood injuries. The occurrence of all childhood injuries increased with increasing age (Rivara *et al.*, 1989; Gallagher *et al.*, 1984; Stallones and Corsa, 1961; Fife *et al.*, 1984; Schor, 1987).

Participation in the school district's free or reduced-price lunch program was used as a surrogate measure of SES. The school district gathers information on parental income and number of persons in the household for participants in this lunch program. Participation in this program was, therefore, the best available measure of SES. Few studies have examined the possible relationship between SES and childhood injuries, and support for such a relationship in inconsistent (Langley *et al.*, 1983b; Manheimer *et al.*, 1966; Bourget and McArtor, 1989). Overall, in examining the public's health in this country, SES may be the single most important factor associated with health status (more so than even genetics). Therefore, it is surprising that this factor is not examined more often. In this study, a measure of SES is clearly associated with injury. This association needs further exploration.

The most interesting finding from this study is that being deemed gifted is associated with head injury. The reasons for this association are not clear. It could be conjectured that gifted children are not developmentally equal to children in the same age group or grade regarding motor skills, or perhaps gifted children are participating in activities, either of their own envisage or school-sanctioned, that they are physically not prepared to perform.

Few studies have focused on describing relationships between increased intelligence and motor ability. A report from the National Health Survey on behavior patterns of children in school found that children of above-average intelligence and academic performance were considered "constantly moving" and "more restless" less often than children of average and below-average intelligence by their teachers. Above-average children were ranked between average and below-average children for "quieter than average" behavior (U.S. Public Health Services, 1972).

The paucity of literature on this subject neithers supports nor contradicts an association between advanced or retarded motor development/ability and increased intelligence. Further study is needed to address this subject.

Being of white race/ethnicity is predictive of increased risk of head injury, followed closely by being African American. Many factors are known to contribute to apparent associations between race/ethnicity and health. Perhaps in the school environment, ethnicity is a risk marker for specific kinds of activities or of racially motivated reporting bias.

School-Related Characteristics

Modeling of the school-related factors revealed that staff:student ratio, number of nurse hours per school per week, level of participation of the school in Magnet programs, combined CAP scores or level of academic achievement, percentage of limited English-proficient students, and a school's percentage of white, African American, and other students characterized the head-injured child's environment.

Injuries to children in any environment can be effectively controlled by adult supervision. Thus, it was anticipated that as the number of staff members to students decreases, the risk of injury increases. In contrast, the average number of hours that a nurse is on duty at a school was significantly associated with head injury. This finding supports the suspicion that we may be witnessing reporting bias in the examination of this data, not that supervision is increased. Hypothetically, when a nurse is on duty, the opportunity for more rigorous documentation of injuries (probably minor) is presented.

School's whose level of achievement was above the school district's mean as indicated by the CAP and schools offering a Magnet curriculum not attended by all students were more likely to have injuries. Two studies from the Tucson, Arizona, school district had somewhat contrasting findings. Both found that alternative educational programs, particularly Magnet programs, were predictive of injuries but that lower student:staff ratios were also (McFayden *et al.*, 1988; Boyce *et al.*, 1984). Neither study looked closely at academic achievement level of the school or of the students. In light of other findings from this study (i.e., those associating giftedness with injuries), this would indicate that the possible association between intelligence and injury should be studied further.

A dose–response relationship existed between the percentage of limited English-proficient pupils and head injury; however, the school's ratio of Hispanic students failed to enter the model. The overall effect of the school's percentage of white students and African American students had a greater effect than that of the other students category. Perhaps this is an indication that more attention should be paid to the rising numbers of Indochinese and Filipino students (the majority of the "other" category) in the school system and their rate of injuries.

Limitations of This Study

The primary limitation of this study was that the effect of reporting bias was not assessed. Many of the apparent associations suggested by this study could be in part due to reporting bias. Questions arise concerning possible mechanisms for differential reporting of injuries at school. Are reporting practices influenced by the race/ethnicity, verbal ability, or academic standing of the child? Or are reporting practices a function of the experience level, attitude, or beliefs of school personnel? Although difficult to document, these questions must be answered by future studies of this type.

References

Annegers, J. F. (1983). The epidemiology of head trauma in children. In "Pediatric Head Trauma" (K. Shapiro, ed.), pp. 1–10. Futura, Mount Kisco, New York.

Bell, K. (1986). School accidents. *Health Bull.* **44,** 99–104.

Bijur, P. E., Stewart-Brown, S., and Butler, N. (1986). Child behavior and accidental injury in 11,966 preschool children. *Am. J. Dis. Children* **140,** 487–492.

BMDP Statistical Software, Inc. (1989) Biomedical Data Processing statistical programs package. University of California at Los Angeles, Los Angeles.

Bourget, C. C., and McArtor, R. E. (1989). Unintentional injuries: Risk factors in preschool children. *Am. J. Dis. Children* **143,** 556–559.

Boyce, W. T., and Sobolewski, S. (1989). Recurrent injuries in schoolchildren. *Am. J. Dis. Children* **143,** 338–342.

Boyce, W. T., Sprunger, L. W., Sobolewski, S., and Schafer, C. (1984). Epidemiology of injuries in a large, urban school district. *Pediatrics* **74,** 342–349.

Bremberg, S. (1989). Is school-based reporting of injuries at school reliable?—A literature review and an empirical study. *Accid. Anal. Prev.* **21,** 183–189.

Bremberg, S., and Gerber, C. (1988). Injuries at school: Influence of schoolmate interaction. *Acta Paediatr. Scand.* **77,** 432–438.

Casey, R., Ludwig, S., and McCormick, M. C. (1986). Morbidity following minor head trauma in children. *Pediatrics* **78,** 497–502.

Cook, J. B. (1972). The post-concussional syndrome and factors influencing recovery after minor head injury admitted to hospital. *Scand. J. Rehabil. Med.* **4,** 27–30.

Craft, A. W., Shaw, D. A, and Cartlidge, N. E. (1972). Head injuries in children. *Br. Med. J.* **4,** 200–203.

Dale, M., Smith, M. E., Weil, J. W., and Parrish, H. M. (1969). Are schools safe? Analysis of 409 student accidents in elementary schools. *Clin. Pediatr.* **8,** 294–296.

Feldman, W., Woodward, C. A., Hodgson, C., Harsanyi, Z., Milner, R., and Feldman, E. (1983). Prospective study of school injuries: Incidence, types, related factors and initial management. *Can. Med. Assoc. J.* **129,** 1279–1283.

Fife, D., Barancik, J. I., and Chatterjee, B. F. (1984). Northeastern Ohio trauma study: II. Injury rates by age, sex, and cause. *Am. J. Public Health* **74,** 473–478.

Fife, D., Faich, G., Hollinshead, W., and Boynton, W. (1986). Incidence and outcome of hospital-treated head injury in Rhode Island. *Am. J. Public Health* **76,** 773–778.

Frankowski, R. F., Annegers, J. F., and Whitman, S. (1985). Epidemiological and descriptive studies, Part I: The descriptive epidemiology of head trauma in the United States. *In* D. P. Becker and J. T. Povlishock (eds.) "Central Nervous System Trauma Status Report," pp. 33–43. Triodyne Inc., Niles, Illinois.

Gallagher, S., Finison, K., Guyer, B., and Goodenough, S. (1984). The incidence of injuries among 87,000 Massachusetts children and adolescents: Results of the 1980–81 Statewide Childhood Injury Prevention Program Surveillance System. *Am. J. Public Health* **74,** 1340–1346.

Goldstein, F. C., and Levin, H. S. (1987). Epidemiology of pediatric closed head injury: Incidence, clinical characteristics, and risk factors. *J. Learn. Disabil.* **20,** 518–525.

Hodgson, C., Woodward, C. A., and Feldman, W. (1984). A descriptive study of school injuries in a Canadian region. *Pediatr. Nurs.* **10,** 215–220.

Horwitz, S., Morganstern, H., DiPietro, L., and Morrison, C. L. (1988). Determinants of pediatric injuries. *Am. J. Dis. Children* **142,** 605–611.

Jamison, D. L., and Kaye, H. H. (1974). Accidental head injury in childhood. *Arch. Dis. Childhood* **49,** 376–381.

Johnson, C. J., Carter, A. P., Harlin, V. K., and Zoller, G. (1974). Student injuries due to aggressive behavior in the Seattle Public School during the school year 1969–1970. *Am. J. Public Health* **64,** 904–906.

Kalsbeek, W. D., McLaurin, R. L., Harris, B. S., and Miller, J. D. (1980). The National Head and Spinal Cord Injury Survey: Major findings. *J. Neurosurg.* **53,** S19–S31.

Klauber, M. R., Barrett-Connor, E., Marshall, L. F., and Bowers, S. A. (1981). A prospective study of an entire community—San Diego County, California, 1978. *Am. J. Epidemiol.* **113,** 500–509.

Klonoff, H. (1971). Head injuries in children: Predisposing factors accident conditions, accident proneness and sequelae. *Am. J. Public Health* **61,** 2405–2417.

Klonoff, H., and Robinson, G. C. (1967). Epidemiology of head injuries in children. *Can. Med. Assoc. J.* **96,** 1308–1311.

Kraus, J. F. (1980). Injury to the head and spinal cord: The epidemiological relevance of the medical literature published from 1960 to 1978. *J. Neurosurg.* **53,** S3–S10.

Kraus, J. F. (1987). Epidemiology of head injury. *In* "Head Injury," 2nd ed. (P. R. Cooper, ed.), pp. 1–19. Williams and Wilkins, Baltimore, Maryland.

Kraus, J. F., Fife, D., Cox, P., Ramstein, K., and Conroy, C. (1986). Incidence, severity, and external causes of pediatric brain injury. *Am. J. Dis. Children* **140,** 687–693.

Langley, J., Cecchi, J., and Silva, P. (1987). Injuries in the tenth and eleventh years of life. *Aust. Paediatr. J.* **23,** 35–39.

Langley, J., Silva, P., and Williams, S. (1981a). Primary school accidents. *N. Z. Med. J.* **94,** 336–339.

Langley, J., Silva, P., and Williams, S. (1981b). Accidental injuries in the sixth and seventh years of life: A report from the Dunedin Multidisciplinary Child Development Study. *N. Z. Med. J.* **93,** 344–347.

Langley, J., McGee, R., Silva, P., and Williams, S. (1983a). Child behavior and accidents. *J. Pediatr. Psychol.* **8,** 181–189.

Langley, J., Silva, P., and Williams, S. (1983b). Socio-economic status and childhood injuries. *Aust. Paediatr. J.* **19,** 237–240.

Levin, H. S., Mattis, S., Ruff, R. M., Eisenberg, H. M., Marshall, L. F., Tabaddor, K., High, M., and Frankowski, R. F. (1987). Neurobehavioral outcome following minor head injury: A three-center study. *J. Neurosurg.* **66,** 234–243.

Lewis, C. E., and Lewis, M. A. (1984). Peer pressure and risk-taking behaviors in children. *Am. J. Public Health* **74,** 580–584.

Manheimer, D. I., Dewey, J., Mellinger, G. D., and Corsa, L. (1966). 50,000 Child-years of accidental injuries. *Public Health Rep.* **81,** 519–533.

Marcus, I. M., Wilson, W., Kraft, I., Swander, D., Southerland, F., and Schulhofer, E. (1960). An interdisciplinary approach to accident patterns in children. *In* "Monographs of the Society for Research in Child Development," pp. 1–79. Department of Psychiatry and Neurology, Louisiana State University, New Orleans.

Matheny, A. P., and Fisher, J. E. (1984). Behavioral perspectives on children's accidents. *In* "Advances in Developmental and Behavioral Pediatrics," Vol. 5, pp. 221–264. JAI Press.

Matheny, A. P., Brown, A. M., and Wilson, R. S. (1971). Behavioral antecedents of accidental injuries in early childhood: A study of twins. *J. Pediatr.* **79,** 122–124.

McFadyen, S. C., Boyce, W. T., Sobolewski, S., and Phillips, L. R. (1988). Injuries, absences, and visits to the nurse among children in alternative schools. *J. School Health* **58,** 406–409.

Mlay, S. M. (1985). Head injury in children: A study of 120 cases. *East Afr. Med. J.* **62,** 877–882.

Nader, P. R., Gilman, S., and Bee, D. E. (1980). Factors influencing access to primary health care via school health services. *Pediatrics* **65,** 585–591.

National Safety Council. (1989). "Accident Facts," 1989 ed. National Safety Council, Chicago.

Nyman, G. (1987). Infant temperament, childhood accidents, and hospitalization. *Clin. Pediatr.* **26,** 398–404.

Padilla, E. R., Rohsenow, D. J., and Bergman, A. B. (1976). Predicting accident frequency in children. *Pediatrics* **58,** 223–226.

Pagano, A., Cabrini, E., Anelli, M., Bernuzzi, S., Lopiccoli, S., and Fisher, P. (1987). Accidents in the school environment in Milan, a five year survey. *Eur. J. Epidemiol.* **3,** 196–201.

Partington, M. W. (1960). The importance of accident-proneness in the aetiology of head injuries in childhood. *Arch. Dis. Childhood* **35,** 215–223.

Plaut, M. R., and Gifford, R. R. (1976). Trival head trauma and its consequences in a perspective of regional health care. *Mil. Med.* **141,** 244–247.

Rivara, F. P. (1984). Childhood injuries. III: Epidemiology of nonmotor vehicle head trauma. *Dev. Med. Child Neurol.* **26,** 81–87.

Rivara, F. P., Calonge, N., and Thompson, R. S. (1989). Population-based study of unintentional injury incidence and impact during childhood. *Am. J. Public Health* **79,** 990–994.

Rutherford, W. H., Merrett, J. D., and McDonald, J. R. (1977). Sequelae of concussion caused by minor head injuries. *Lancet* **1,** 1–4.

San Diego City Schools. (1990a). Attendance accounting reports: Pupil accounting, 1989–90 year-end reports. San Diego City Schools, San Diego.

San Diego City Schools. (1990). School accountability report cards. San Diego City Schools, San Diego.

San Diego City Schools. (1990). School profiles for school operations division. San Diego City Schools, San Diego.

Schlesselman, J. J. (1982). "Case-control studies: Design, conduct, analysis. Oxford University Press, Oxford.

Schor, E. L. (1987). Unintentional injuries. *Am. J. Dis. Children* **141,** 1280–1284.

Sheps, S. B., and Evans, G. D. (1987). Epidemiology of school injuries: A 2-year experience in a municipal health department. *Pediatrics* **79,** 69–75.

Sibert, J. R., Maddocks, G. B., and Brown, B. M. (1981). Childhood accidents—an endemic of epidemic proportions. *Arch. Dis. Childhood* **56,** 225–234.

Snoek, J. W., Minderhoud, J. M., and Wilmink, J. T. (1984). Delayed deterioration following mild head injury in children. *Brain* **107,** 15–36.

Snow, W. G., MaCartney, M. S., Schwartz, M. L., Klonoff, P. S., and Ridgley, B. A. (1988). Demographic and medical characteristics of adult head injuries in a Canadian setting. *Can. J. Surg.* **31,** 191–194.

Stallones, R. A., and Corsa, L. (1961). Epidemiology of childhood accidents in two California counties. *Public Health Rep.* **76,** 25–36.

Taketa, S. (1984). Student accidents in Hawaii's public schools. *J. School Health* **54,** 208–209.

Tonkin, R. S. (1987). Adolescent risk-taking behavior. *J. Adolescent Health Care* **8,** 213–220.

U.S. Public Health Service. (1972). Behavior patterns of children in school: United States. U.S. Department of Health, Education and Welfare, Vital & Health Statistics F Series 11-No. 113 HSM 72–1042. Washington, D.C.

Woodward, C. A., Milner, R., Harsanyi, Z., Feldman, W., and Hodgson, C. (1984). Completeness of routine reporting of school-related injuries to children. *Can. J. Public Health* **75,** 454–457.

Zuckerman, M. (1971). Dimensions of sensation seeking. *J. Consult. Clin. Psychol.* **36,** 45–52.

19

The Epidemiology of Alzheimer's Disease and Dementia among Hispanic Americans

Richard L. Hough • *Bohdan Kolody* • *Barbara Du Bois*

Cognitive impairment in the elderly has become a major health problem only in the past few decades as life expectancy has increased. Improved sanitation, public immunization, and antibiotics have decreased the threat of infection while postponing death. Nearly one-half of the people in the United States reach age 75; one-quarter live to age 85. Unfortunately, with longevity comes increased risk of dementia and other degenerative diseases of the elderly, such as stroke and Parkinson's disease. The prevalence and incidence of Alzheimer's disease (AD) and of Parkinson's disease with or without dementia, increase with age; however, the mortality rate for patients with either condition has also declined because of improved medical care, further increasing the number of prevalent cases. Because these factors are not likely to change, the size of the population most at risk for dementia, and the prevalence rates in those populations, will increase. Research findings on the prevalence and incidence rates of dementia therefore has significant implications for the development of appropriate policies and procedures for delivery of health and social services to populations directly or indirectly affected.

Although there has been considerable research on the trends described above for majority populations in the United States, relatively little research has been done on Hispanic populations. Understanding the trends in these ethnic groups is important. The United States has the sixth largest Hispanic population in the world (Perez-Stable, 1987). The official count from the 1990 Census for persons of Hispanic origin was 22,354,000. Of those, some 60% identified themselves as of Mexican origin. Among ethnic minority communities in the United States, the Hispanic population is

Neuroepidemiology:
Theory and Method

not only the most rapidly growing subgroup, but also is projected to become the largest minority group in the country. The number of Hispanics in the country is expected to double, to approximately 46.4 million by the year 2020 (Davis *et al.*, 1983) as a function of higher mean birth rates and migration rates than other minority communities and of improved life expectancy. In the 1980 national population estimates, some 730,000 Hispanics were over the age of 65. California data illustrates the rapidity in growth of this population In 1980, there were an estimated 4.5 million Hispanics California, and by 1990, the number had grown to 7,688,000 (or by 69% from 1980). This is a total population size that was larger than the total population of all but nine states (U.S. Bureau of the Census, 1991).

Not a great deal is scientifically known concerning the epidemiology of neurologic disorders among Hispanic Americans. There is especially little known concerning the prevalence and incidence of differentially diagnosed AD and other dementias. However, several large-scale epidemiologic community surveys provide data on the prevalence of general cognitive impairment, and some treated population data provide some useful information as well. There is also a growing literature on the question of the appropriateness of using standard screening scales and neuropsychological testing procedures to assess the presence of cognitive impairment in Hispanic populations. The first part of this chapter reviews what is known about the prevalence of cognitive impairment from community survey research. The second section considers studies of differentially diagnosed dementias, and the third examines some issues in the cross-cultural assessment of dementia.

COMMUNITY STUDIES OF THE PREVALENCE OF COGNITIVE IMPAIRMENT

Two basic types of community epidemiological studies of cognitive impairment are (1) surveys that use neuropsychological assessment scales with cutpoints to classify the degree of symptomatology and (2) surveys that use clinical diagnosis in addition to neuropsychological tests to establish differential diagnosis of dementia. The former are considered in this section.

Most community studies have relied on the Mini-Mental State Examination (MMSE) (Folstein *et al.*, 1975) to assess cognitive impairment. This brief measure of cognitive functioning was developed to assess cognitive impairment among psychiatric patients. The MMSE was intended primarily to assess the cognitive aspects of mental functioning such as orientation, memory, attention, the ability to name, the ability to follow verbal and written commands, the ability to write a sentence spontaneously, and the ability to copy a figure. It was not intended to be a diagnostic in function nor to measure mood or forms of thinking. The MMSE has been shown to adequately distinguish organic dementia from functional psychiatric disorders and to correlate with verbal and performance scores on the Wechesler Adult Intelligence Scale (Folstein *et al.*, 1975). In addition, test–retest reliability is strong (Folstein *et al.*, 1975; Anthony *et al.*, 1982). The test scores range from 0 to 30 errors, and subjects scoring 13 or more errors are generally regarded as exhibiting severe cognitive impairment.

Two major community surveys have used the MMSE on the Hispanic population. The Los Angeles Epidemiologic Catchment Area (LAECA) research project used the scale on a random sample of just over 1400 Hispanics (Hough *et al.*, 1983; Burnam *et al.*, 1987). The LAECA was one of five sites (New Haven, Connecticut; Baltimore, Maryland; St. Louis, Missouri; the Piedmont area of North Carolina; and Los Angeles, California) in the National Institute of Mental Health (NIMH) sponsored ECA studies. This collaborative research was intended to estimate the prevalence of diagnosable mental disorders and the use of mental health services. Given the difficulty in establishing differential diagnoses of dementias, the MMSE was used to assess levels of cognitive impairment. Second, an ECA-like study of the prevalence of mental disorders was conducted on some 1500 respondents in Puerto Rico (Canino *et al.*, 1987; Bird *et al.*, 1987). The MMSE was similarly employed in this project.

In both studies, a Spanish language version of the MMSE was employed. The LAECA research group developed and tested the reliability of a Spanish language instrument (Karno *et al.*, 1983; Burnam *et al.*, 1983). The translation process was designed to generate an instrument that would represent a fairly literal translation of the English language original to have comparable meaning to Hispanic respondents from a number of Hispanic counties and cultures. The instrument was translated and back-translated with discrepancies resolved in discussion among the translators, backtranslators, and investigators. The instrument was also evaluated by clinicians of Mexican, Cuban, and Puerto Rican background and was then edited to be at least minimally acceptable and usable in each group (Karno *et al.*, 1983).

The reliability of the LAECA Spanish instrument, its equivalence to the English version, and its agreement with clinical diagnoses were then examined in a study of 90 bilingual (English- and Spanish-speaking) and 61 monolingual (Spanish-speaking only) patients from a community mental health center. The study design involved two independent administrations and one independent clinical evaluation of each subject. The standard 13+ cutpoint was used to identify severe cognitive impairment. Severe cognitive impairment did not occur with sufficient frequency in this community mental health center sample for evaluating the MMSE's performance with great confidence, but the findings are suggestive. In terms of test–retest reliabilities, within Spanish language agreement for monolinguals was excellent (96%), but agreement between English and Spanish administration for bilinguals was lower (86%). In terms of agreement with clinician judgement for the entire monolingual and bilingual sample, sensitivity was low (.33) while specificity was acceptable (.88). Sensitivity was even worse for the monolingual subgroup. In general, the MMSE tended to diagnose more subjects as having severe cognitive impairment than did clinicians. This suggests then that, relative to the English version of the MMSE used with English-speaking subjects, the Spanish version of the MMSE may, to some extent, overdiagnose severe cognitive impairment, particularly in respondents whose primary language is Spanish. The issue of the appropriateness of using tests like the MMSE across cultures will be discussed later. The LAECA Spanish translation of the MMSE was slightly modified for the Puerto Rican study.

Several reports from the ECA research program have evaluated factors related to cognitive impairment in designated sites in the United States. The New Haven, Connecticut, ECA program (Yale), reported a 6-month prevalence rate of severe cognitive impairment of 1.3 per 100 individuals (Holzer *et al.*, 1984; Leaf *et al.*, 1984). Among those 65 and older, 3.4% had severe cognitive impairment in the preceding 6-month period (Weissman *et al.*, 1985). Cognitive impairment increased significantly after age 79 and occurred among females more than males. Males had more cognitive impairment up to age 74. The gender differences are suggested to be largely a function of longer survival rates among females.

The LAECA data on prevalence of cognitive impairment among Hispanic respondents is most meaningful when compared to the rates found in Los Angeles and at the other ECA sites for predominantly non-Hispanic populations. Briefly, the prevalence rates and standard errors were as follows (Burnam *et al.*, 1987):

New Haven	1.1 (+0.1)
Baltimore	1.0 (+0.1)
St. Louis	0.9 (+0.1)
Piedmont	3.0 (+0.3)
Los Angeles	
Total	1.2 (+0.2)
Mexican American	1.6 (+0.4)
Non-Hispanic White	0.2 (+0.1)

The LA ECA data showed a prevalence rate of severe cognitive impairment similar to those at the other sites (1.2/100); however, Hispanics were shown to have a higher prevalence rate (1.6) than non-Hispanics (0.2).

In all five ECA sites, a significant relationship was found between cognitive impairment and age (Myers *et al.*, 1984; Burnam *et al.*, 1987; Fillenbaum *et al.*, 1988). Education was also shown to be a significant confounding factor in the MMSE scores. Males also tended to have higher scores than females, and Blacks to have higher scores than Hispanics or non-Hispanic Whites.

Escobar *et al.* (1986) reanalyzed the cognitive impairment data for the LAECA sample. The reanalysis showed that variations in education, ethnicity, and language of the interview appeared to be particularly predictive of errors on the first three orientation items in the MMSE (year, season, and date) and on the serial sevens item (count backward from 100 by 7's). After controlling for these potentially culturally biased items in the MMSE battery, the resulting Mexican American/non-Hispanic white differences were found to be insignificant (Escobar *et al.*, 1986).

In the Puerto Rico study, the prevalence of MMSE scores in the severe cognitive impairment range (13 or more errors) was significantly higher (3% in the 18–64-year-old age group) than in similar U.S.-based studies (Bird *et al.*, 1987; Canino *et al.*, 1987). After controlling for the effects of sex, age, and education; however, the rate decreased to 1.1 (+0.3%), which was not significantly different from the ECA studies. Educational level was the strongest factor associated with errors on total scores of the MMSE.

Although there is some evidence in the Puerto Rican and Los Angeles data reported above that Hispanics may score higher on the MMSE, it should also be noted that the differences tend to disappear when education and other variables are controlled. This would suggest, then, that the differences are more linked to educational status than to culture.

This impression of the relative strength of the relationship between education and ethnic/cultural differences to cognitive impairment is reenforced by a recent analysis of the ECA data (George *et al.*, 1991). This analysis combines the community samples, on which the prevalence estimates reported above were based, with samples of institutionalized respondents who would normally have been resident in each site. "Institutionalized respondents" include individuals resident in board and care homes, nursing homes, mental hospitals, and prisons. The combined community and institutional data were combined across the five sites and standardized to U.S. population characteristics in order to generate national estimates of the prevalence of cognitive impairment (George *et al.*, 1991).

The overall adult population estimates using these methods were similar to those reported above (0.9% with severe and 4.2% with mild cognitive impairment). The comparable prevalence estimates for Hispanic respondents were lower than the total population for severe impairment (0.6%) and higher for mild impairment (7.9%). Non-Hispanic white rates were almost identical for severe impairment (0.5) and significantly lower for mild impairment (3.2). Prevalence estimates for black respondents (2.0 for severe and 9.6 for mild impairment) were significantly higher.

For respondents over 55 years of age, the prevalence of severe impairment was highest for blacks (5.7), lower for Hispanics (2.2), and lowest for non-Hispanic whites (1.4). For mild impairment, the estimated prevalence rates were 27.7 for blacks, 12.9 for Hispanics, and 8.0 for non-Hispanic whites.

In addition to differences by age and ethnicity, the analyses also found significant variations by education. Overall, for respondents over the age of 55, the prevalence of both mild and severe cognitive impairment decreased with higher education at approximately the same rate for Hispanic and non-Hispanic white respondents. For both the groups, 3.6% of subjects with less than 9 years of education were severely impaired. For those with more than 9 years of education, the rates for both groups were consistently far below 1%. Similarly, for mild impairment, the estimates for Hispanics and non-Hispanic whites were similar (20.0 and 19.1, respectively). For respondents with 9–11 years of education, the same estimates were 5.8 and 5.1; for 12 years of education, 0.0 and 3.0; and for more than 12 years of education, 0.0 and 1.0.

Thus, the data tend to support the notion that performance on this screening test is more strongly related to educational factors than to ethnic or cultural variations—at least in reference to Hispanic/non-Hispanic white differences. Hispanics and non-Hispanic whites apparently have very similar rates of severe cognitive impairment, and rates vary significantly by education within both groups. Strong racial differences do appear in that black respondents reflect significantly higher prevalence of severe impairment than both Hispanics and non-Hispanic whites even with education controlled.

Certainly, however, the ECA analyses do not conclusively demonstrate that there are no significant ethnic or cultural differences on cognitive impairment. There is the fact that Hispanics, in the ECA analyses reported earlier (Fillenbaum *et al.*, 1988; Escobar *et al.*, 1986), do report rates of mild cognitive impairment higher than non-Hispanic whites and almost as high as blacks.

At least four other factors limit the importance of the ECA analyses. First, only approximately 300 Hispanics over the age of 55 were in the analyses. The prevalence estimates are therefore unstable compared to those for the more numerous black and non-Hispanic white respondents. Second, the "Hispanic" respondents, while mainly Mexican American, include a number of non-Mexican Hispanics from the Los Angeles and other ECA sites. How any possible variations in the prevalence of cognitive impairment across Hispanic subgroups might have affected the outcomes is not known. Third, there are relatively few severely unacculturated respondents in the 300 Hispanics over the age of 55. The real concern about the appropriateness of using the MMSE across cultural groups is focused on the more severely unacculturated segments of the Hispanic population. Fourth, the major concern with potential interaction of education and cultural affects on cognitive impairment revolves around the issue of how relatively uneducated and even illiterate segments of culturally different populations may perform on the MMSE or similar tests. The ECA studies cannot address these questions.

STUDIES OF DIFFERENTIALLY DIAGNOSED DEMENTIAS

Prevalence estimates for differentially diagnosed dementias, as opposed to general cognitive impairment, have been based on studies of either treated populations or community surveys. Although the strength of clinical data enhances the possibilities for making an accurate differential diagnosis of AD and other forms of cognitive disorder, such data are generally weak in terms of estimating general population prevalence rates due to selection bias. Of course, community-based population surveys can reveal true prevalence rates, but they are subject to problems related to diagnostic reliability.

Studies of Treated Populations

No studies of treated Hispanic populations have provided a base for estimating prevalence of AD or other dementias for this population. Generally, researchers studying the institutionalized elderly have estimated that as many as two-thirds suffer from some degree of cognitive impairment, the majority of those at severe levels. The greatest proportion of those with severe impairment can be classified as having probable AD (e.g., Larson *et al.*, 1986; Bland *et al.*, 1988). Among clinically treated geriatric patients with some cognitive impairment, some 60–70% appear to suffer from AD with much smaller proportions exhibiting dementias more related to Parkinson's disease, depression, head injury, or other conditions (e.g., Larson *et al.*, 1984a,b, 1985). Lacking comparable data, one must assume that rates for Hispanics are similar to those noted earlier for non-Hispanics.

Community Epidemiological Surveys Using Clinical Diagnosis

Epidemiological studies that incorporate second-stage clinical assessments for case identification following initial neuropsychological screening surveys are the second type of means for estimating prevalence of differentially diagnosed dementias. Again, there has been no diagnostic-level epidemiologic data on community samples to allow us to examine possible differences in prevalence rates between Hispanics and others.

Several studies, however, illustrated the method and may suggest the prevalence rates that might be found among Hispanics. For example, data from Shanghai, China, reported a 4.6% prevalence rate for dementia in those over 65 (Zhang *et al.*, 1990). Clinical examinations based on functional assessments, psychiatric interview, medical/neurological examinations, mental status, and psychometric status tests determined that 65% of dementia subjects had AD, or two out of every three persons suffering from dementia. After controlling for the effects of low education, data indicated that gender (being female) was significantly related to AD after the age of 65 (Yu *et al.*, 1989).

The China data contrast sharply to the results of a similar study in Boston, which established a significantly higher prevalence rate of 10.3% in those over age 65 (Evans *et al.*, 1989). The Boston data showed age-specific rates of 3% in those 65–74, 18.7% in those 75–84, and 47.2% in those 85 +, thus indicating a strong age relationship. Rates also occurred more commonly in females than in males.

Incidence rates are an important aspect of the epidemiologic understanding of a disorder. Again, no data are available on incidence rates of differentially diagnosed dementias among Hispanics. The Baltimore Longitudinal Study examined incidence rates of AD using abstracts from medical records of a clinic population of reasonably well-educated white older men (Sayetta, 1986). Records were reviewed by two psychiatrists and algorithmic criteria were applied to identify incident cases and dates of onset. An AD diagnosis was thus presumptive by excluding other conditions showing similar presentations. The age-specific incidence rates were 0.43% for those between ages 60 and 64 and 3.3% for those over age 80. The incidence rate is less than 1 per 1000 for those age 60 in contrast to 54 per 1000 for those age 90, and may exceed 50% of cohort members for those 95 and older (Sayetta, 1986). Although the study was criticized due to small study size of white males ($N = 27$), it remains one of the few incidence studies of AD.

METHODOLOGICAL ISSUES IN THE CROSS-CULTURAL ASSESSMENT OF COGNITIVE IMPAIRMENT AND DEMENTIA

Sociocultural factors of race, ethnic membership, immigration status, social class, and education may all play important roles in predisposing individuals to AD or other dementias, or they may impact the reliability of a diagnosis (Gurland, 1981). When using an instrument such as the MMSE across categories of racial/ethnic background or education, for example, it is often difficult to sort out whether the differences or similarities in rates of severe cognitive impairment may be a function of the true rates within the subgroups or may be an artifact of a measurement procedure that does not adequately reflect the same phenomenon in each setting. Developing culture-fair instrumentation for the assessment of dementia is obviously crucial for cross-cultural research.

An example of the difficulty inherent in developing a culture-fair instrument is an attempt recently made to construct a culture-fair version of the MMSE. The Hispanic Alzheimer's Research Project (HARP) was a collaborative NIMH-funded venture between investigators at San Diego State University (Drs. Ray Valle, Richard Hough, and Bohdan Kolody) and the Alzheimer's Disease Research Center (ADRC) at the University of California, San Diego (UCSD) Medical School (Valle *et al.*, 1991). The project attempted to develop culture-fair versions of several standard neuropsychological measures of cognitive impairment, but only their work on the MMSE will be reported here.

The HARP project attempted to develop a version of the MMSE that would remain equivalent in Spanish and English on four dimensions. First, the items and instruments as a whole would be equivalent in meaning. Obtaining an exact fit in meaning across languages and cultures is not an easy process and sometimes is impossible. Second, the items and instruments as a whole would be equivalent in construct. Sometimes an item can be easily translated from one language or culture to another, but the original intent of the specific item or the measure as a whole can be lost. An example is the "no ifs, ands, or buts" phrase that respondents are asked to repeat in the MMSE. The phrase can be directly translated into Spanish, but it has no real idiomatic meaning in that language as it does in English. Similarly, the phrase, when literally translated into Spanish, is not nearly as difficult to repeat as it is in English.

Third, items and instruments would be equivalent in scale requirements. That is, if meaningful comparisons are to be made across cultures,
the same general scale parameters (e.g., total number of points possible,
scoring procedures) would need to be retained. Fourth, the items and
instruments would be equivalent in technical demands of difficulty.

The first task was to translate the MMSE items into Spanish. This was
accomplished by typical translation, backtranslation, and group resolu-
tion of the discrepancies. For the most part, fairly literal translation of
the original items appeared, on face value, to be culturally appropriate.
However, several items required more careful consideration. The primary
example was the "no ifs, ands, or buts" phrase previously mentioned. A
literal translation is not a meaningful phrase in Spanish and does not
satisfy the intent of having a phrase with (a) labials and syllibants and
(b) conjunctions and prepositions. The phrase used in the HARP study
was *"si no bajo, entonces Usted suba"* (if I do not come down, then you
come up). Similarly, two items in the spatial orientation question of the
MMSE ask the respondent to identify the hospital, clinic, or nursing home
they are in and what floor they are on. In the HARP Spanish language
version, directed at subjects living in the community, the item "where is
it that I am interviewing you" was substituted for the former and "in what
room/living area are we" was substituted for the latter. The rest of the
MMSE items were translated directly into Spanish.

The next step in the HARP research process was to determine which
items might require alternative phrasing or content to be culturally fair.
Alternatives were developed for four items. Asking respondents to identify
the "season of the year" is easily translated into Spanish, but appropriate
answers might vary from those of English. A Mexican American with good
cognitive abilities might well answer in terms of a holiday season (e.g.,
Christmas time), a religious season, or an agricultural season instead of
the expected answer of fall, spring, summer, or winter. Similarly, it was
thought that Mexican Americans may be more likely to identify the city
they live in with the name of a *barrio*, a *colonia*, or some other local
community name than the name of the larger city.

Two other items were felt to be potentially "culturally unfair" because
they rely on reading and writing skills. Among elderly Mexican American
respondents, there may well be less lifetime practice at reading and
writing than among non-Mexican Americans. A significant minority may
even be essentially illiterate. Therefore, an alternative to asking the respondent to write a sentence was to ask them to "say" a sentence. Similarly,
the alternative to asking the respondent to read and follow a command
was to ask them to imitate the action being portrayed in a picture.

A final item that was thought might not be culturally fair is the drawing of a pentagon. Elderly Mexican American respondents may have much less practice, through their lives, in the use of a pencil and in drawing than comparable non-Mexican American respondents. However, no reasonable alternative was devised for this question.

The original and alternative items were then given to 72 community-dwelling Hispanics over the age of 65 in San Diego County. Subjects were recruited by contacting a wide range of service organizations and medical professionals who work with the Mexican American elderly and through solicitation of volunteers through the Spanish language mass media. Subjects were sampled to a matrix of education and Blessed scores to ensure a range for both variables.

A clinical diagnosis of probable or possible AD or other dementia was used as the criterion against which the performance of the items and their alternatives could be judged. The clinical diagnosis was established by neurologists at the UCSD ADRC. The protocol was to use the physical and neurologic examinations typically employed by the ADRC in their research, along with the administration of several of the neuropsychological tests normally employed in the center. In addition, a standardized neuropsychiatric examination was developed for use with Hispanics. All of these instruments were administered in Spanish. As in the ADRC protocol, the information from all sources was summarized and reviewed by neurologists and final diagnoses were generated. Some 42 subjects were diagnosed as normals and 30 as demented, most with AD.

The sensitivity, specificity, percentage of correctly classified, and other characteristics of the individual dichotomous items were examined with the clinical diagnosis as a criterion to determine whether or not the alternative items were more accurate predictors than the originals. Items were examined separately for the demented and nondemented segments of the study population. The polychotomous variables were examined to determine whether or not the alternative items produced fewer numbers of errors than did the originals.

Rather than trying to generate a maximally predictive Spanish language screening scale, the researchers tried to identify items and scoring procedures that would predict dementia at about the same levels as the English version of the same items when used in English-speaking populations. For this purpose, results from a matched sample of 29 HARP and 29 UCSD ADRC subjects were compared. This comparison was not maximally informative because matches in the ADRC data could not be found for many of the lower-education HARP subjects, and few high-education HARP subjects could be found to match the large number of ADRC clients in that category.

By and large, it was found that the alternative items were slightly more likely to be predictive of clinically diagnosed dementia and to produce proportions correctly classified that were more similar to ADRC English-speaking, non-Mexican American clients than the originals (for the detailed analyses, see Valle *et al.*, 1991).

Finally, MMSE scale scores were computed using the Spanish language version of the original items and, alternatively, with the alternatives. In computing the alternative, purportedly more culture fair scores, the algorithm used was to count the item as an error only if the original version was answered incorrectly *and* the alternative version was also answered incorrectly.

Using the original cutpoint of 13 or more errors to represent severe cognitive impairment, the sensitivity of the original scale was .57, the specificity .98, and 81% correctly classified (PCC). The alternative scale fared no better with a sensitivity of .53, and specificity of .98 and a 79 PCC. Both versions produced a 79 PCC when examined in the matched HARP/ADRC subsample as compared to a 69 PCC in the ADRC group. Using the standard cutpoint of 7 or more errors to represent mild and severe cognitive impairment, the original items produced a sensitivity of .83, specificity of .79, and 81 PCC. The alternative version produced .80 sensitivity, .83 sensitivity, and 82 PCC. The PCC for the original scale in the matched subsample was 83 and 79 for the alternate as opposed to a 79 PCC for the English-speaking ADRC group.

Other scoring algorithms are currently being tried to see whether or not the alternative version might produce more dramatic differences, but this initial data suggests that there may be little gain from using the culturally fair alternative items and scales. Certainly, however, the scale construction and testing process illustrates the difficulty in establishing culture-fair instrument for cross-cultural assessment of dementia.

RISK FACTORS

A very important aspect of epidemiologic investigation of any physical or mental disorder is the identification of risk factors. Aside from the data from the ECA and Puerto Rican studies reported on age, sex, racial/ethnic identity, and education, little is known concerning whether or not specific risk factors may differentially exist for Hispanic populations.

According to most previous reviews of risk factors (e.g., Cross and Gurland, 1981; Katzman, 1986), the demographic risk factors most commonly associated with AD are age, sex, education, and sociocultural factors. These factors were explored, on a preliminary basis, in the ECA and Puerto Rican data cited earlier. Gender did not appear to be a significant risk factor for severe cognitive impairment among Hispanics in those studies. However, reviews of the general literature suggest that although males are more likely to get AD up to age 75, most increases in prevalence occur among women after age 75. After age 75, women have nearly a threefold greater chance of acquiring AD than men. This is largely a function of the increase longevity of older women but may also indicate higher levels of susceptibility that may be related to risk factors that have yet to be clearly defined.

A recent supplement to the *International Journal of Epidemiology* (Van Duijn *et al.*, 1991a,b) nicely summarizes much of the literature on risk factors for AD and reports on the EURODEM Risk Factors Research Group collaborative analysis of 11 case-control studies of risk factors. Among the most significant risk factors was the presence of a family history of AD, Down's syndrome, or Parkinson's disease among first-degree relatives. Relative risk was particular high if more than one first-degree relative reported such a history (Van Duijn *et al.*, 1991b).

Maternal age over 40 was a significant risk factor for women but was less important for men (Rocca *et al.*, 1991). On the other hand, head trauma with unconsciousness was significant for men but was less so for women (Mortimer *et al.*, 1991). Generally, none of a wide range of medical problems evaluated were convincingly associated with AD, but it was felt that hypothyroidism, epilepsy, and encephalitis deserved further attention (Breteler *et al.*, 1991). There was no excess estimated risk of AD for alcohol assumption. Smoking appeared to be a "negative risk factor." (Graves *et al.*, 1991a). History of psychiatric disorder did not appear to be important except for depression as a risk factor for late-onset cases. No association was found with environmental factors such as occupational exposures to solvents and lead (Graves *et al.*, 1991b).

There may be some reason to believe that the prevalence of at least some of these risk factors may be higher in Hispanics than in others. No evidence indicates that Hispanics might have exceptionally high rates of a family history of Down's syndrome or Parkinson's disease. However, it might be reasonable to hypothesize that larger proportions of Hispanics than non-Hispanic Whites may have maternal age over 40 or head trauma. Research is needed to clarify the relative risk for Hispanics.

Of these "risk factors," the role of education may be the most difficult to understand. Higher education of the respondents is consistently related to better performance on neurological assessment batteries; hence, the presumed prevalence rates of AD may in fact be artifacts of higher or lower educational effects. However, the increased mental activity associated with higher education and the more intellectually demanding kinds of work that better educated people do may provide some buffering for the individual against the development of dementia.

A risk factor that seems particularly salient for cognitive impairment in the Hispanic elderly and that has not been well studied is pesticide exposure. Mexican American populations in the Southwestern United States may be at high risk for cognitive impairment in later life as a consequence of their disproportionate exposure to pesticides in rural areas. Although the long-term health effects of exposure to insecticides have not been well characterized, it is known that Mexican-origin farmworkers experience a high frequency of acute poisoning.

SUMMARY

The few completed community survey studies of Mexican American and Puerto Rican communities suggest little difference in the prevalence of severe impairment between Hispanic and non-Hispanic populations, although higher levels of mild impairment may be found among Hispanics. These studies are far from conclusive. They have explored only the aspects of dementia covered in the MMSE, and they have not provided data concerning Cuban, Central American, or other Hispanic groups.

Certainly, very little is known about the prevalence of differentially diagnosed AD and other cognitive impairments in Hispanic communities. Some tentative evidence indicates that Hispanics may exhibit higher rates of cognitive impairment than non-Hispanics. For example, Lopez-Aguires *et al.* (1984) indicated that Spanish-speaking elderly over the age of 60 had higher rates of cognitive impairment and depression than non-Latino elderly. Whether these higher rates, if they are confirmed in other studies, are a function of lower educational level, lower socioeconomic status, culturally patterned risk factors present in Latino communities, or genetic predisposition/family aggregation, or indicate actually higher rates of impairment is an area that warrants further scrutiny. There is little reason to assume at this point, however, that rates of cognitive impairment among the Hispanic population exceeds or is lower than that established for the elderly in general.

Estimates of the proportion of elderly populations (age 65 +) with AD range from 5 to 20%, with the prevalence rising to 25–50% in the population over 85 (Larson *et al.*, 1984a; Mortimer *et al.*, 1981). Similar proportions might be expected among Hispanics. However, whatever the current prevalence, the number of Hispanics with AD or other cognitive impairment is projected to increase rapidly and to make increasing demands on a health care system that may not have culturally appropriate diagnostic, treatment, or case-management procedures. There is great need, then, for the development of appropriate assessment tools for screening dementia among Hispanics and for data concerning prevalence, incidence, course of the disease, differential diagnosis, and etiology that would enable health care planners and policymakers to develop appropriate systems of care.

In summary there is need for careful epidemiologic estimates of the prevalence and incidence of AD and other cognitive impairments in the Hispanic elderly, for prospective examination of the characteristics of the disorder in these populations and for development of protocols for differential diagnosis of AD and cognitive impairments and their linkages to putative risk factors.

References

Anthony, J. C., LeResche, L., Nisz, U., *et al.* (1982). Limits of the "Mini-Mental State" as a screening test for dementia and delirium among hospital patients. *Psychol. Med.* **12,** 397–408.

Bird, H. R., Canino, G., Stipec, M. R., *et al.* (1987). Use of the Mini-Mental State Examination in a probability sample of a Hispanic population *J. Nerv. Ment. Dis.* **175,** 731–737.

Bland, R. C., Newman, S. C., and Orn, H. (1988). Prevalence of psychiatric disorders in the elderly in Edmonton. *Acta Psychiatr. Scand.* **77,** 57–63.

Breteler, M. M. B., Van Duijn, C. M., Chandra, V., *et al* (1991). Medical history and the risk of Alzheimer's disease: A collaborative re-analysis of case-control studies. *Int. J. Epidemiol.* **20**(2; suppl. 2), S36–S42.

Burnam, M. A., Karno, M., Hough, R. L., and Escobar, J. I. (1983). The Spanish Diagnostic Interview Schedule: Reliability and comparison with clinical diagnoses. *Arch. Gen. Psychiatry* **40,** 1189–1196.

Burnam, M. A., Hough, R. L., Timbers, D. M., *et al.* (1987). Current psychiatric disorders: Mexican Americans and Nonhispanic Whites in Los Angeles. *Arch. Gen. Psychiatry* **44,** 687–694.

Canino, G. J., Bird, H., Shrout, P., *et al.* (1987). Prevalence of specific psychiatric disorders in Puerto Rico. *Arch. Gen. Psychiatry* **44,** 727–735.

Cross, P., and Gurland, B. J. (1986). The epidemiology of the dementing disorders. *In* "Losing a Million Minds' Confronting the Tragedy of Alzheimer's Disease and Other Dementias," OTA-BA-323. Office of Technology Assessment, Washington, D.C.

Davis, C., Haub, C., and Willett, J. (1983). U.S. Hispanics: Changing the face of America. *Pop. Bull.* **38,** 3–43.

Escobar, J. I., Burnam, M. A., Karno, M., *et al.* (1986). Use of the Mini-Mental State Examination (MMSE) in a community population of mixed ethnicity. *J. Nerv. Ment. Disorder* **174,** 607–614.

Evans, D. A., Fundenstein, H. H., Albert, M. S., *et al.* (1989). Prevalence of Alzheimer's disease in a community population of older persons: Higher than previously reported. *J. Am. Med. Assoc.* **262,** 2551–2556.

Fillenbaum, G. G., Hughes, D. C., Heyman, A., *et al.* (1988). Relationships of health and demographic characteristics to Mini-Mental State Examination scores among community respondents. *J. Am. Med. Assoc.* **236,** 2767–2769.

Folstein, M. F., Folstein, S. E., and McHugh, P. R. (1975). Mini-Mental State: A practical method for grading the cognitive status of patients for the clinician. *J. Psychiatr. Res.* **12,** 189–198.

George L. K., Landerman, R., Blazer, D. G., *et al.* (1991). Cognitive impairment. *In* "Psychiatric Disorders in America: The Epidemiologic Catchment Area Study" (L. N. Robins and D. A. Regier, eds.), pp. 291–327. The Free Press, New York.

Graves, A. B., Van Duijn, C. M., Chandra, V., *et al.* (1991a). Alcohol and tobacco consumption as risk factors for Alzheimer's disease: A collaborative re-analysis of case-control studies. *Int. J. Epidemiol.* **20**(2; suppl. 2), S48–S57.

Graves, A. V, Van Duijn, C. M., Chandra, V., *et al.* (1991b). Occupational exposures to solvents and lead as risk factors for Alzheimer's disease: A collaborative re-analysis of case-control studies. *Int. J. Epidemiol.* **20**(2;suppl. 2), S58–S67.

Gurland, B. (1981). The borderlands of dementia: The influences of socio-cultural characteristics on rates of dementia occuring in the senium. *In* "Clinical Aspects of Alzheimer's Disease" (N. Miller and G. Cohen, eds.). pp. 61–84. Raven Press, New York.

Holzer, C., Tischler, G., Leaf, P., *et al.* (1984). An epidemiologic assessment of cognitive impairment in a community population. *Res. Comm. Ment. Health* **4**, 3–32.

Hough, R. L., Karno, M., Burnam, M. A., *et al.* (1983). The Los Angeles Epidemiologic Catchment Area Research Program and the epidemiology of psychiatric disorders among Mexican Americans. *J. Operation. Psychiatry* **14**, 42–51.

Karno, M., Burnam, A., Escobar, J. I., Hough, R. L., and Eaton, W. W. (1983). Development of the Spanish-language version of the National Institute of Mental Health Diagnostic Interview Schedule. *Arch. Gen. Psychiatry* **401**, 1183–1188.

Katzman, R. (1986). Differential diagnosis of dementing illnesses. *Res. Comm. Ment. Health* **4**, 3–32.

Larson, E. B., Burton, M. P. H., Reifler, B. V., *et al.* (1984a). Dementia in elderly outpatients; A prospective study. *Ann. Intern. Med.* **100**, 417–423.

Larson, E. B., Reifler, B. V., Canfield, C., *et al.* (1984b). Evaluation elderly outpatients with symptoms of dementia. *Hosp. Comm. Psychiatry* **35**, 425–428.

Larson, E. B., Reifler, B. V., Sumi, S. M., *et al.* (1985). Diagnostic evaluation of 200 elderly outpatients with suspected dementia. *J. Gerontol.* **5**, 536–543.

Larson, E. B., Lo, B., and Williams, M. E. (1986). Evaluation and care of elderly patients with dementia. *J. Gen. Intern. Med.* **1**, 116–126.

Leaf, P. J., Weissman, M. M., Myers, J. K., *et al.* (1984). Social factors related to psychiatric disorder. The Yale Epidemiologic Catchment Area Study. *Soc. Psychiatry* **19**, 53–61.

Lopez-Aqueres, L., Kemp, B., Plopper, M., and Stables, F. R. (1984). Health needs of the Hispanic elderly. *J. Am. Geriatr. Soc.* **32**, 191–198.

Mortimer, J. A., Schulman, L. M., and French, L. R. (1981). Epidemiology of dementing illness. *In* "The Epidemiology of Dementia" (J. A. Mortimer and L. M. Schulman, eds.). Oxford University Press, New York.

Mortimer, J. A., Van Duijn, C. M., Chandra, V., *et al.* (1991). Head trauma as a risk factor for Alzheimer's disease: A collaborative re-analysis of case-control studies. *Int. J. Epidemiol.* **20**(2; suppl. 2), S28–S35.

Myers, J. K., Weissman, M. M., Tischler, G. I., *et al.* (1984). Six-month prevalence of psychiatric disorders in three communities. *Arch. Gen. Psychiatry* **41**, 959–967.

Perez-Stable, E. J. (1987). Issues in Latino healthcare-medical staff conference. *Western J. Med.* **146**, 213–218.

Rocca, W. A., Van Duijn, C. M., Clayton, D., *et al.* (1991). Maternal age and Alzheimer's disease: A collaborative re-analysis of case-control studies. *Int. J. Epidemiol.* **20**(2;suppl. 2), S21–S27.

Sayetta, R. B. (1986). Rates of senile dementia–Alzheimer's type in the Baltimore Longitudinal Study. *J. Chem. Disorder* **39**, 271–286.

U.S. Bereau of the Census (1991). Race and Hispanic origins. 1990 Census Profile, Vol. 2, June 1991.

Valle, R., Hough, R., Kolody, B., *et al.* (1991). The validation of the Blessed Mental Status Test and the Mini-Mental Status Examination with an Hispanic population: A final report. Final report on NIMH grant RO1 MH43390. The Hispanic Alzheimer's Research Project, San Diego State University, San Diego.

Van Duijn, C. M., Clayton, D., Chandra, V., *et al.* (1991a). Familial aggregation of Alzheimer's disease and related disorders: A collaborative re-analysis of case-control studies. *Int. J. Epidemiol.* **20**(2; suppl. 2), S13–S20.

Van Duijn, C. M., Stijnen, T., and Hofman, A. (1991b). Risk factors for Alzheimer's disease: Overview of the EURODEM collaborative re-analysis of case-control studies. *Int. J. Epidemiol.* **20**(2; suppl. 2), S4–S12.

Weissman, M. M., Myers, J. K., Tischler, G. I., *et al.* (1985). Psychiatric disorders (DSM-III) and cognitive impairment in the elderly in a U.S. urban community. *Acta Psychiatr. Scand.* **71**, 366–379.

Yu, E. S. H., Liu, W. T., Levy, P. S., *et al.* (1989). Cognitive impairment among the elderly in Shanghai, China. *J. Gerontol. Soc. Sci.* **44**, S97–S106.

Zhang, M., Katzman, R., Jin, H., *et al.* (1990). The prevalence of dementia and Alzheimer's disease (AD) in Shanghai, China: Impact of age, gender and education. *Ann. Neurol.* **27**, 28–37.

Index

Aborigines, and WKS, 155
Acute toxicity in lead poisoning, symptoms, 264
AD. See Alzheimer's disease
ADL scales, limitations, 102
Adult T-cell leukemia-lymphoma (ATLL), 109
Air, as source of low-dose lead poisoning, 269
Alcoholic cerebellar degeneration, 159–160
Alcoholic dementia, 158
Alcoholism, WKS and related disorders due to
    current research topics, 157–158
    continuity hypothesis, 157–158
    relationship of WKS to other alcoholic disorders, 158–159
    descriptive studies, review, 151–157
    public health intervention, 161–162
    research, future, 160–161
    Wernicke's encephalopathy (WE), 149–150
    women, effects of alcohol in, 159–160
Alien hand
    anatomy and etiology, 186–187
    disease models, 181
    phenomenology, 182–186
        apraxia, 183
        ataxia, 183–184
        grasp reflex and motor preservation, 182–183
        movement disorders, 184–185
        psychomotor disturbance, 185–186

questions, unanswered, 191–192
    sociocultural aspects, 187–191
        alien hand as folk illness, 189
        prehistory, 187–189
        signs versus syndromes, 189–190
        social construction, 191
    α-amino-β-methylaminopropionic acid, 82–83
ALS. See Amyotrophic lateral sclerosis
ALS-PDC. See Amyotrophic lateral sclerosis in Western Pacific
Alzheimer's disease (AD), 9–10
    assessing risk factors for, 10
Alzheimer's disease among African Americans
    concerns for conducting dementia research in African American community, 206–208
        caregiving support, 207–208
        problem of misdiagnosis, 206–207
    conclusions, 208
    dementia and culture, 197–198
    dementia in African American population, 198–206
        demographics, 199–200
        prevalence rates of, 200–206
    research interest, 195–196
Alzheimer's disease and demential among Hispanic Americans, epidemiology
    cognitive impairment in elderly, 351–352
    community studies of prevalence of cognitive impairment, 352–357

differently diagnosed dementias,
    studies, 357–359
community epidemiological
    surveys using clinical
    diagnosis, 358–359
treated populations, 357–358
methodological issues in cross-
    cultural assessment of cognitive
    impairment and dementia,
    359–362
risk factors, 362–364
summary, 364–365
Alzheimer's Disease and Related
    Disorders Association (ADRDA),
    9, 58
Alzheimer's Disease (AD) in People's
    Republic of China, epidemiology
AD, 53–54
background, 54–55
discussion, 62–68
methods, 55–59
    data collection, 56–58
        case identification, 57–58
        screening, 56–57
    diagnostic criteria and procedures,
        58–59
    sample, 55–56
results, 59–62
Alzheimer's Disease Research Center
    (ADRC), 9, 53–54
Amyotrophic lateral sclerosis (ALS), 1,
    8–9
Amyotrophic lateral sclerosis (ALS) in
    Western Pacific, update on
    epidemiology
ALS, 73
data from Guam and Mariana
    Islands, 75–80
environmental considerations, 81–84
patterns of distribution and etiologic
    implications, 80–81
Western Pacific ALS, 73–74
Anencephaly
and spina bifida by outcome type in
    San Diego County and
    California, 225, 226

and spina bifida by race in California,
    229
by sex in San Diego County and
    California, 228
Anxiety, forms of following stroke,
    103–104
Apraxia, 183
Ataxia, 183–184
Atomic bomb survivors, neurological
    endpoints studied in, 249–251
Atomic Bomb Casualty Commission
    (ABCC), 241
Atomic bomb survivors
head circumference and mental
    retardation among atomic bomb
    survivors with radiation
    exposure, early studies, 242–244
mental retardation and IQ among
    atomic bomb survivors with
    radiation exposure based on
    DS86 dosimetry, 247–249
T65DR dosimetry, studies of head
    circumference among atomic
    bomb survivors, with radiation
    exposure based on, 245–247
Australia, cerebrovascular disease
    study in, 93–94

•

Barthel Index of self-care ADL, 96
β-N-methylamino-L-alanine (BMAA),
    82–83
Biostatistics and neuroepidemiology
discussion, 325–326
medical technology assessment and
    stochastic models, 323–325
neurological diseases and stochastic
    processes, 310–321
    distribution of latent period of MS,
        queueing model, 316–319
    epileptic seizure trends, Poisson
        process model, 314–316
    natural history of MS, simple
        Markov model, 310–312

prognosis for patients with MS, elaborated Markov model, 312–314

rate of infection of MS, elaborated queueing model, 319–321

research, 309

sampling methodology and neuroepidemiology, 321–323

studies, 309–310

Blacks, AD and related disorders among. *See* Alzheimer's disease among African Americans

Brain tumors, 15–16

British occupation, and transmission of MS in Faroe Island, 40–41

•

California birth cohort perinatal files (CBCPF), 221–222

California Code of Regulations, 233

California Health and Safety Code mandates, and LOC, 234

California, prevalence of NTDs in at birth. *See* Neural tube defects

Central nervous system (CNS), and poliomyelitis, 3–4

Cerebral malaria in Ghana, childhood convulsions associated with

background, 257–258

discussion, 261–262

methods, 259

results, 259–261

Cerebral palsy, 12–13

Cerebrovascular disease (CVO), and smoking

analytical studies, 166

introduction, 166

prospective studies, 170–175

retrospective case-control studies, 168–170

retrospective studies, 166–168

causation, 175–176

conclusion, 177

stroke, as manifestation of CVO, 165–166

Cerebrovascular disease, utility of stroke banks in epidemiology

applications, 303

clinical trials, 304

diagnostic intervention, 303–304

prognosis, 304–305

stroke etiologies, 302–303

description of, 289–297

potential applications of, 290

requirements for reliability in, 289

stroke data banks, 287–289

stroke therapies, 288

summary, 305

University of California, San Diego stroke data bank, 297–302

methods, 297–298

results, 298–302

data from other stoke data banks, 299–302

data from UCSD data bank, 298–299

strengths and weaknesses, 298

Cerebral vascular diseases, 90

Charcot, and MS, 7

Childhood lead poisoning. *See* Lead poisoning, childhood, epidemiology

Children, elementary school, head injury to. *See* Head injury to elementary school children

Children, head trauma to, 334–336

causes of minor head injury, 335

incidence, 334

methodological issues in study of injuries to children at school, 335–336

risk factors for minor head injury, 334–335

China, AD in. *See* Alzheimer's Disease in People's Republic of China, epidemiology

Chinese Mini-Mental State Examination (CMMSE), 56, 57–58

Chronic headache, 139–142

clinic, satisfaction with, 141–142

expectations and concerns, 140–141

introduction to study of patients
consulting, 139–140
CNS development, proposed
mechanism for radiation effects
on, 251–253
Cognitive impairment and dementia,
cross-cultural assessment of,
methodological issues in 359–362
Cognitive impairment, prevalence of by
age, race/ethnicity and education,
202
among those aged 55 and older, 203
Cognitive impairment in Hispanic
elderly, 351–352
community studies of prevalence of,
352–357
Community epidemiological surveys
using clinical diagnosis, 358–359
Confounders and contributors to
differences in mental retardation
between Hiroshima and Nagasaki,
253–254
Congenital malformations in California,
types of, 224
Consciousness, lapse of. *See* Lapse of
consciousness
Continuity hypothesis, 157–158
Coronary heart disease (CHD), 167
Creutzfeldt-Jakob disease (CJD), 1, 4, 14
Cross-cultural assessment of cognitive
impairment and dementia,
methodological issues in 359–362
Cycas circinalis, toxins of and ALS,
81–82
toxicity, 83

•

Dementia and AD
age-specific prevalence by age,
education and gender, 61, 62
prevalence of, 65
prevalence of in percentage by age
groups and gender, 60
Dementia and cognitive impairment,
cross-cultural assessment of,
methodological issues in 359–362

Dementia of Alzheimer's type, 9–10.
See also Alzheimer's disease
Dementia research in African American
community, concerns for
conducting, 206–208
caregiving support, 207–208
problem of misdiagnosis, 206–207
Dementias, studies of differently
diagnosed, 357–359
community epidemiological surveys
using clinical diagnosis, 358–359
studies of treated populations, 357–358
Dementia syndrome
and black culture, 197–198
in African American population,
198–206
demographics, 199–200
prevalence rates of, 200–206
Depression, cumulative incidence of, in
stroke survivors, 89–90
Diagnostic Interview Schedule (DIS),
54, 58
Depression Section, 58
Diagnostic and Statistical Manual, 3rd
Edition (DSM-III), 9
criteria for diagnosing dementia, 9,
58, 59
standard psychiatric classifications
in, 97
Dietary intake studies of factors of NTD
births, 218–219
Digit Span test, 59
Diphtheria, neurological illness
associated with, 12
Disease expression in HTLV-1, 117
DS86 dosimetry, mental retardation
and IQ among atomic bomb
survivors with radiation exposure
based on, 247–249
DSM-III, *see Diagnostic and Statistical
Manual*

•

Education, significance of lack of in
course of developing AD in China,
66–67

Elaborated queueing system, and rate of infection of MS, 319–321
Elaborated Markov model, and prognosis for patients with MS, 312–314
Elementary school children. *See* Head injury to elementary school children
Emotional disorders, and stroke, 98–99
  pathological emotionalism, 103
  problems following stroke, 102
Endrin poisoning, 239
Environmental considerations of ALS in Western Pacific Islands, 81–84
Epidemic of MS in Faroe Islands
  epitome of, 24–26
  fourth, 47–49
  three epidemics, as alternative view, 38–40
Epidemiologic characteristics of NTD births, 214–220
  environmental or nongenetic factors, 214–219
    dietary intake studies, 218–219
    fertility drugs, 219
    geographic variation, 214–218
    maternal age and parity, 217–218
    seasonal variation, 216–217
    socioeconomic status, 218
  genetic or nonenvironmental factors, 219–220
    distribution by sex, 220
    ethnic/racial differences, 219–220
Epidemiological Catchment Area (ECA) studies, 197–198
Epidemiology of MS in Faroe Islands, epitome of, 24–26
  geographic distribution of MS, 24
  migrations studies, 25
Epilepsy, 132–235
  definition of, 15
  quality of life and, 133–134
  label of and experiences of health care, 134–135
  sufferer's perceptions, study of, 132

Epileptic seizure trends, Poisson process model, 314–316
Ethnic/racial differences of NTD births, 219–220
Eurage Group on Aging of the Brain and Senile Dementia, 9

•

Falciparum malaria, 258
Familial aggregation of ALS-PDC on Guam, 80–81
Faroe islands, 26–28
  general features of, 26–27
  medical facilities, 28
  nature of MS in Faroes, 49–50
    from Faroese experience, 50
    summation of MS in Faroes, 49–50
  parishes and populations, 44–45
  primary MS affection (PMSA), 43
  published resident series, 34–40
    incidence rates, 36–38
    three epidemics, as alternative view, 38–40
Faroe Islands, and study of MS, 2
Fertility drug intake, and NTD births, 219
First-pass metabolism of alcohol, 160
Food, as source of low-dose lead poisoning, 169–270
Fuld Object Memory Test, 58

•

Gender, as risk factor for AD, 63–64
Genetic factor, as risk for AD, 67
Genetic or nonenvironmental factors of NTD births, 219–220
  distribution by sex, 220
  ethnic/racial differences, 219–220
Geographic variation of NTD births, 214–218
Grasp reflex and motor preservation of alien hand, 182–183
Guam, data on ALS from, 75–80
Guamanian ALS, 8
Guillaine-Barre syndrome and swine flu vaccine, 13–14

•

*Handbook of Geographical and
Historical Pathology*, 2
Harp project, 359
Head circumference and mental
retardation among atomic bomb
survivors with radiation exposure,
early studies, 242–244
based on T65Dr dosimetry, 245–247
Head injury, 14–15
Head injury to elementary school
children, study
discussion, 342–346
limitations of study, 346
risk factor for head injury, 344–346
school-related characteristics,
345–346
student's personal
characteristics, 344–345
literature, review, 330–336
conclusion, 336
epidemiology of school injuries,
330–331
causes of school-related injuries,
330
incidence, 330
severity, 331
types of injuries and body parts
affected, 330–331
head trauma to children, 334–336
causes of minor head injury, 335
incidence, 334
methodological issues in study
of injuries to children at
school, 335–336
risk factors for minor head
injury, 334–335
risk factors for injuries at school,
331–333
macroenvironment as risk
factor, 333
nonbehavioral risk factors, 331
psychosocial, 331–332
risk-taking behavior, 332
socioeconomic factors, 332–333

methods, 336–338
analysis, 338
data sources and variables of
interest, 337–338
setting, 336
study subjects, 336–337
results, 338–342
multivariate analysis, 340–342
school-related characteristics
variables, 342
student's personal
characteristics variables,
340–342
population descriptive
characteristics, 338–340
studies, 329
Health effects of lead poisoning, other,
277–278
Heart Disease Epidemiology
(Framingham Study), 172
Heterosexual transmission of HTLV-1,
117
Hiroshima and Nagasaki, confounders
and contributors to differences in
mental retardation between,
253–254
Hispanic Americans, Alzheimer's
disease and dementia among,
epidemiology
cognitive impairment in elderly,
351–352
community studies of prevalence of
cognitive impairment, 352–357
differently diagnosed dementias,
studies, 357–359
community epidemiological
surveys using clinical
diagnosis, 358–359
treated populations, 357–358
methodological issues in cross-
cultural assessment of cognitive
impairment and dementia,
359–362
risk factors, 362–364
summary, 364–365

Human immunodeficiency virus (HIV), 109
Human T-cell lymphotrophic virus-1 (HTLV-1), 2, 113–115
Human T-cell lymphotrophic virus-1 (HTLV-1), neuroepidemiology
  clinical features associated with myelopathy-tropical spastic paraparesis, 119–121
  conclusions, 122
  diagnosis, 118
  epidemiology associated with myelopathy-tropical spastic paraparesis, 116–118
  HTLV-1-associated myelopathy, 111–112
  human t-cell lymphotrophic virus-1, 113–114
  infection, epidemiologic pattern of, 114–115
  isolation of, 112–113
  other human T-cell viruses, 121–122
  retroviruses, 109
  transmission of, 115
  tropical neuropathies, 109–111
Huntington's disease, 10

●

In utero effects of radiation exposure, 241–242
Infection, epidemiologic pattern of, 114–115
Injuries to children at school. *See* Head injury to elementary school children
International Journal of Epidemiology, 363
Intrauterine radiation exposure, neuroepidemiology
  conclusions, 254–255
  confounders and contributors to differences in mental retardation between Hiroshima and Nagasaki, 253–254
  effects of *in utero*, 241–242

head circumference and mental retardation among atomic bomb survivors with radition exposure, early studies, 242–244
based on T65Dr dosimetry, 245–247
mental retardation and IQ among atomic bomb survivors with radiation exposure based on DS86 dosimetry, 247–249
neurological endpoints studied in atomic bomb survivors, 249–251
proposed mechanisms for radiation effects on CNS development, 251–253
summary, 254–255
IQ and mental retardation among atomic bomb survivors with radiation exposure based on DS86 dosimetry, 247–249

●

Kuru, 4

●

Lapse of consciousness (LOC), impact of litigation on surveillance in defined population
  conclusions, 238–239
  methods, 234–235
    case definition, 234
    data collection and analysis, 234–235
  results, 235–238
  surveillance systems, 233
Lead poisoning, childhood, epidemiology acute toxicity, symptoms, 264
  background, 263–271
    history, 264–265
    sources of poisoning, 267–271
      low-dose, 268–270
      paint, 267–268
      soil, 268
      unusual sources, 270–271

symptoms of acute toxicity, 264
conclusions, 280–281
effects of, 274–278
  neuropsychological effects,
    274–277
  other health effects, 277–278
predisposing factors, 271–272
prevalance of, 272–274
prevention, 278–280
  and screening, 278–280
treatment, 278
LOC. *See* Lapse of consciousness
Los Angeles Epidemiological
  Catchment Area (LAECA) research
  project, 353
  data on prevalence of cognitive
    impairment among Hispanics,
    354–355
Low-dose lead poisoning, 268–270
  air, 269
  food, 169–270
  water, 269

•

Macroenvironment as risk factor for
  school-related injuries, 333
Malaria, definition of, 258. *See also*
  Cerebral malaria
Mariana Islands, data on ALS from,
  75–89
Markov model
  elaborated, and prognosis for
    patients with MS, 312–314
  simple, and natural history of MS,
    310–312
Maternal age and parity of NTD births,
  217–218
Medical technology assessment and
  stochastic models, 323–325
Mental retardation
  differences in between Hiroshima
    and Nagasaki, 253–254
  and head circumference among
    atomic bomb survivors with
    radiation exposure, based on

distance from epicenter, early
  studies, 242–244
based on T65DR dosimetry,
  245–247
and IQ among atomic bomb survivors
  with radiation exposure based
  on DS86 dosimetry, 247–249
Mercury poisoning and Minimata's
  disease, 4–5
Mexican Americans, data on cognitive
  impairment among, 355, 356,
  360–361, 364
  Spanish instrument, 353–354
Migrant MS, excluded, 32–34
  occurrence of, 23–24
Mini-Mental State Examination
  (MMSE), 352–353, 354, 357, 359
  in Spanish, 360
Minimata's disease, 4–5
Minor head injury
  causes of, 335
  risk factors, 334–335
Movement disorders, 184–185
MS. *See* Multiple sclerosis
MTPT, discovery of, 6
Multiple sclerosis (MS)
  distribution of latent period,
    queueing model, 316–319
  natural history of MS, simple Markov
    model, 310–312
  prognosis for patients with MS,
    elaborated Markov model,
    312–314
  rate of infection of MS, elaborated
    queueing model, 319–321
Multiple sclerosis (MS), 1, 2, 7–8,
  136–139
  as autoimmune malfunction, 8
  coping with problems, 137–139
  experiences leading to diagnosis,
    136–137
Multiple sclerosis (MS), in Faroe Islands
  case ascertainment, 28–30
  case definition, 30–31
  epidemiology, epitome of, 24–26
  geographic distribution of MS, 24

migrations studies, 25
Faroe islands, 26–28
  general features of, 26–27
  medical facilities, 28
  grouping and inclusion criteria,
      31–32
  introduction and transmission,
      40–49
    British occupation, 40–41
    fourth epidemic, 47–49
    transmission of MS and models
        thereof, 41–47
    Faroe Islands parishes and
        populations, 44–45
    primary MS affection (PMSA), 43
  migrant MS, excluded, 32–34
  nature of MS, 49–50
    from Faroese experience, 50
    summation of MS in Faroes, 49–50
  occurrence of, 23–24
  published resident series, 34–40
    incidence rates, 36–38
    three epidemics, as alternative
        view, 38–40
Multivariate analysis of head injury in
    elementary school children,
    340–342
  school-related characteristics
      variables, 342
  student's personal characteristics
      variables, 340–342
Muscle atrophy and weakness and
    degeneration of motor neurons, 82
Myelopathy, HTLV-1-associated,
    111–112
Myelopathy-tropical spastic
    paraparesis, clinical features of
    HLTL-1 associated with, 119–121
  epidemiology of HTLV-1 associated
      with, 116–118

•

Nagasaki and Hiroshima, confounders
    and contributors to differences in
    mental retardation between,
    253–254

National Childhood Encephalopathy
    Study, 12
National Institute of Neurological and
    Communicative Disorders and
    Stroke (NINCDS), 6, 58, 59
National Institute of Neurologic Disease
    and Stroke (NINDS), 77
Neural tube defects (NTDs), 10–11
Neural tube defects (NTDs) in
    California, prevalence at birth
  discussion, 228–231
  epidemiologic characteristics of NTD
      births, 214–220
    environmental or nongenetic
        factors, 214–219
      dietary intake studies, 218–219
      fertility drugs, 219
      geographic variation, 214–218
      maternal age and parity, 217–218
      seasonal variation, 216–217
      socioeconomic status, 218
    genetic or nonenvironmental
        factors, 219–220
      distribution by sex, 220
      ethnic/racial differences,
          219–220
  etiology, 213
  frequency of NTD births in the United
      States, 214
  methods, 221–223
    California birth cohort perinatal
        files, 221–222
    statistical analysis, 223
    study design and case definition,
        222–223
    subjects an setting, 221
  results, 223–228
Neuroepidemiology
  amyotrophic lateral sclerosis, 8–9
  brain tumors, 15–16
  cerebral palsy, 12–13
  conclusions, 16
  Creutszfeldt–Jakob disease, 14
  dementia of Alzheimer's type, 9–10
  epilepsy, 15
  field, 1–2

Guillaine-Barre syndrome and swine
  flu vaccine, 13–14
head injury, 14–15
Huntington's disease, 10
kuru, 4
Minimata's disease, 4–5
multiple sclerosis, 1, 7–8
neural tube defects, 10–11
Parkinson's disease, 5–6
pertussis vaccination, 11–12
poliomyelitis, 3–4
stroke, 6–7
Neurological diseases and stochastic
  processes, 310–321
  distribution of latent period of MS,
    queueing model, 316–319
  epileptic seizure trends, Poisson
    process model, 314–316
  natural history of MS, simple Markov
    model, 310–312
  prognosis for patients with MS,
    elaborated Markov model,
    312–314
  rate of infection of MS, elaborated
    queueing model, 319–321
Neurological endpoints studied in
  atomic bomb survivors, 249–251
Neuropsychological effects of lead
  poisoning, 274–277
Nonbehavioral risk factors for school-
  related injuries, 331
NTDs. *See* Neural tube defects

•

Paint, lead poisoning in, 267–268
Parkinson's disease, 1, 5–6
Parkinsonian-dementia complex (PDC)
  and ALS in Western Pacific, 73,
  78–79
Passive surveillance systems, 239
Pathological emotionalism, 103
Patient-based assessment of health
  status and outcome for
  neurological disorders
  chronic headache, 139–142
    clinic, satisfaction with, 141–142

expectations and concerns,
    140–141
  introduction to study of patients
    consulting, 139–140
  discussion, 143–145
  epilepsy, 132–135
    and quality of life, 133–134
    label of and experiences of health
      care, 134–135
    sufferer's perceptions, study of, 132
  multiple sclerosis, 136–139
    coping with problems, 137–139
    experiences leading to diagnosis,
      136–137
  neurological disorders, 131–132
Pediatric convulsions
  age- and sex-specific frequency, 260
  etiology of, 260
  treatment of patients, outcome, 231
People's Republic of China, AD in. *See*
  Alzheimer's disease in People's
  Republic of China, epidemiology
Perth community stroke study, 94–105
  aims and methods, 94–97
    ascertainment of cases, 95
    assessment instruments, 96–97
    follow-up schedule, 95–96
  discussion, 101–105
  results, 97–101
    emotional disorders, 98–99
    physical disability, 97–99
    residence, 101
    social activities, 99–101
Pertussis vaccination, 11–12
Physical disability, and stroke, 97–98
Poisson process model, and epileptic
  seizure trends, 314–316
Poliomyelitis, 3–4
Post-polio syndrome, 3–4
Predisposing factors of lead poisoning,
  271–272
Present State Examination (PSE), 54
Prevention of lead poisoning, 278–280
  and screening, 278–280
  treatment, 278
Psychiatric Assessment Schedule (PAS), 96

Psychomotor disturbance, 185–186
Psychosocial risk factors for school-related injuries, 331–332
Public health intervention for alcoholism, 161–162

•

Quality of life and epilepsy, 133–134
Queueing model
  distribution of latent period, queueing model, 316–319
  elaborated, and rate of infection of MS, 319–321

•

Radiation effects on CNS development, proposed mechanisms for, 251–253
residence, place of, and stroke, 101
Retroviruses, 109
Risk-taking behavior of elementary school children, 332
Rubella (German measles), 13

•

Salk vaccine for polio, 3
Sampling methodology and neuroepidemiology, 321–323
School, elementary, risk factors for injuries at, 331–333
  macroenvironment as risk factor, 333
  nonbehavioral risk factors, 331
  psychosocial, 331–332
  risk-taking behavior, 332
  socioeconomic factors, 332–333
School-related characteristics variables, 342
School-related injuries, epidemiology, 330–331
  causes, 330
  incidence, 330
  severity, 331
  types of injuries and body parts affected, 330–331
Seasonal variation of NTD births, 216–217

Sex, distribution of NTDs by, 220
Shaking palsy. *See* Parkinson's disease
Shanghi Survey of Alzheimer Disease and Dementia (SSADD), 54–55
Simple queueing model, distribution of latent period, 316–319
Simple Markov model, and natural history of MS, 310–312
Smoking and CVD
  analytical studies, 166
    introduction, 166
    prospective studies, 170–175
    retrospective case-control studies, 168–170
    retrospective studies, 166–168
  causation, 175–176
  conclusion, 177
  stroke, as manifestation of CVO, 165–166
Social activities, and stroke, 99–101
Social phobia, following stroke, 103–104
Sociocultural aspects of alien hand, 187–191
  as folk illness, 189
  prehistory, 187–189
  signs versus syndromes, 189–190
  social construction, 191
Socioeconomic factors and risk taking of school-age children, 332–333
Socioeconomic status (SES) of NTD births, 218
Soil, lead poisoning in, 268
Spina bifida, 213, 216
  anencephaly and spina bifida by outcome type in San Diego County and California, 225
  by outcome type in San Diego County and California, 227
  by sex in San Diego County and California, 229
Stroke, 6–7
  as manifestation of CVD, 165–166
  and National Institute of Neurological and Communicative Disorders and Stroke (NINCDS), 6

thrombotic stroke, 7
transient ischemic attack (TIA), 6
Stroke banks, utility of in epidemiology
    of cerebrovascular disease
    applications, 303
        clinical trials, 304
        diagnostic intervention, 303–304
        prognosis, 304–305
        stroke etiologies, 302–303
    description of, 289–297
    potential applications of, 290
    requirements for reliability in,
        289
    stroke data banks, 287–289
    stroke therapies, 288
    summary, 305
    University of California, San Diego
        stroke data bank, 297–302
    methods, 297–298
    results, 298–302
        data from other stroke data
            banks, 299–302
        data from UCSD data bank,
            298–299
    strengths and weaknesses, 298
Stroke-related disability, epidemiology
Australia, cerebrovascular disease
    study in, 93–94
    cerebral vascular diseases, 90
    conclusions, 105–106
    methodological issues, 92–93
    Perth community stroke study,
        94–105
    aims and methods, 94–97
        ascertainment of cases, 95
        assessment instruments, 96–97
        follow-up schedule, 95–96
    discussion, 101–105
    results, 97–101
        emotional disorders, 98–99
        physical disability, 97–99
        residence, 101
        social activities, 99–101
    stroke, etiology, 91–92
    studies, 89–90

Student's personal characteristics
    variables, 340–342
Swine flu and Guillaine-Barre
    syndrome, 13–14

•

T65DR dosimetry, studies of head
    circumference among atomic
    bomb survivors, with radiation
    exposure based on, 245–247
Thrombotic stroke, 7
Transient ischemic attack (TIA), 6, 90
Transmission
    of HTLV-1, 115–116
    of MS and models thereof, 41–47
        Faroe Islands parishes and
            populations, 44–45
        primary MS affection (PMSA), 43
Tropical ataxic neuropathy (TAN), 110
Tropical neuropathies, 109–111
Tropical spastic paraparesis (TSP),
    109–110

•

United States, frequency of NTD births
    in, 214
University of California, San Diego
    stroke data bank, 297–302
    methods, 297–298
    results, 298–302
        data from other stroke data banks,
            299–302
        data from USCD data bank,
            298–299
    strengths and weaknesses, 298
Unusual sources of lead poisoning,
    270–271

•

Verbal Fluency Test, 58–59
Viruses, other human T cell, 121–122

•

Water, as source of low-dose lead
    poisoning, 269
Wernicke-Korsakoff syndrome (WKS)
    and related disorders due to
    alcoholism
    descriptive studies, review, 151–157
    public health intervention, 161–162
    research topics
        current research topics, 157–159
            continuity hypothesis, 157–158
            relationship of WKS to other
                alcoholic disorders,
                158–159
        future, 160–161

Wernicke's encephalopathy (WE),
    149–150
    women, effects of alcohol in, 159–160
Wernicke's encephalopathy (WE),
    149–150
Western Pacific ALS, update on
    epidemiology
    data from Guam and Mariana
        Islands, 75–80
    environmental considerations, 81–84
    patterns of distribution and etiologic
        implications, 80–81
WKS. *See* Werner-Korsakoff syndrome
Women, effects of alcohol in, 150–
    160

ISBN 0-12-504220-5

90038

9 780125 042208